W9-BBV-941

THE
FACTS ABOUT DRUG USE

Coping with Drugs and Alcohol in Your Family, at Work, in Your Community

Barry Stimmel, M.D.,
and the Editors of
Consumer Reports Books

Consumer Reports Books
A Division of Consumers Union
Yonkers, New York

Copyright © 1991 by Barry Stimmel
Published by Consumers Union of United States, Inc.,
Yonkers, New York 10703
All rights reserved, including the right of reproduction
in whole or in part in any form.

Library of Congress Cataloging-in-Publication Data
Stimmel, Barry, 1939–
The facts about drug use : coping with drugs and alcohol in your family, at
work, in your community / Barry Stimmel and the editors of Consumer
Reports Books.
p.m.
Includes bibliographical references and index.
ISBN: 0-89043-235-X
1. Psychotropic drugs. 2. Drug abuse. I. Title.
[DNLM: 1. Social Support. 2. Substance Abuse—psychology. WM
270 S858f]
RM315.S8918 1991
362.29—dc20
DNLM/DLC   90-15170
for Library of Congress   CIP

Special permissions appear on page iv.

Design by Tammy O'Bradovich

First printing, April 1991
Manufactured in the United States of America

To Barbara

The excerpt on page 3 is reprinted from *Phantastica: Narcotic and Stimulating Drugs—Their Use and Abuse* by L. Lewin, translated by P. A. Wirth. London: Kegan, Paul, Trench, Trubner, 1931. Reissued by Routledge and Kegan, London, 1964.

The quote on page 59 is reprinted from *Alcoholism: The Facts* by D. W. Goodwin. Toronto: Oxford University Press, 1981. Reprinted by permission of Oxford University Press.

The quote from Sigmund Freud on page 189 is reprinted from *The Cocaine Papers by Sigmund Freud*, edited by R. Byck. New York: Stonehill Press, 1974.

Contents

Preface

Drug use permeates all levels of our society, from the poor to those with the resources to disguise their problem or surreptitiously seek treatment. Whether it's alcohol or nicotine or prescription or over-the-counter medications, or illicit drugs, the effects of addiction on the individual are great; the cumulative effects on society are staggering. Annual U.S. expenditures for treatment and prevention in 1991 have been calculated at more than $2.9 billion, not including losses because of crime and lower productivity, plus the costs of law enforcement. In 1988 the U.S. Alcohol, Drug Abuse, and Mental Health Administration estimated the total annual costs for illicit drug use and alcoholism at $144 billion. These estimates are probably low.

Eliminating use of all such substances from our culture is impossible. It isn't even desirable, because many are medically valuable. But there are considerable differences in the psychological and physical effects of various mood-altering drugs, as well as in the effects someone using a particular substance might have on other people.

A multitude of books have been published on drug use, mostly for health professionals. The pharmacologic effects, medical complications, and behaviors resulting from the use of mood-altering drugs can be complex, but it's still realistic and advisable for everyone to know about them. Knowledge of the adverse effects of such drugs, why they're used excessively, how to identify persons at risk, available resources for users, and the problems an addict encounters trying to become drug-free helps us form an appropriate response to a drug problem and decide what position on drug use society should take.

The Facts About Drug Use was conceived to accomplish those objectives. To enable those with little or no background in science or health care to understand the often complex issues of drug use, the information is presented clearly, concisely, and without jargon.

Considerable research and professional experience provide the underpinnings of the book, but no annotated references are included. Instead, selected references are listed in a separate section at the end. Publications by individuals mentioned in the text are listed in this section. To allow a more comprehensive overview of the material, a few citations refer to secondary rather than primary sources. For those interested in a more thorough or technical view, several general works used in writing the book are listed at the beginning of the references.

The first sections present a nonjudgmental view of the effects of all licit and illicit mind-altering substances. This approach is sure to offend the "abolitionists," who believe all use of such substances is harmful, and the "libertarians," who view benignly any drug use by informed adults.

I believe that any substance taken primarily to produce a profound mood-altering effect—other than for defined medical reasons—is inappropriate or risky, but not criminal. Acts associated with or resulting from such use *may* be criminal, and those who commit such acts should be held accountable.

Some may disagree. But I hope that chapter-by-chapter the book will create a better understanding of the effects of mood-altering substances and the reasons many continue to use them despite the consequences. Unless we understand the nature of dependency and addiction, and the external forces (including poverty and homelessness) that promote such behavior, we will never even approach a solution to one of our greatest problems.

Acknowledgments

The preparation of a book such as this requires the help of many. I am grateful to the editorial staff of Consumer Reports Books, as well as additional others, for the editorial and secretarial assistance I received. Leslie Barovick was particularly helpful in the completion of the initial manuscript. David Rose, M.D., carefully reviewed the chapter on AIDS and drug use. The extensive bibliography was checked and verified through the efforts of Jeanine McAdam, Harriet Meiss, Lynn Kasner Morgan, Margie Prasek, and Jean Sullivant. Mary Kennedy, as always, was available to take up the slack and offer quality assistance. Finally, to my sons Alexander and Matthew for putting up with the encroachment on what little free time there exists in life and to my wife, Barbara, who, in addition, critically assessed several key chapters, I am especially thankful.

The editors of Consumer Reports Books give special thanks to Joseph R. Botta for his sagacious commentary and thorough review of this book. And a special thanks to Thomas Blum for the help he provided in developing the text of this book.

PART I

BASIC CONCEPTS

Chapter 1

Who Uses Drugs

From the first beginning of our knowledge of man, we find him consuming substances of no nutritive value, but taken for the sole purpose of producing for a certain time a feeling of contentment, ease, and comfort. Such a power was found in alcoholic beverages and in some vegetable substances, the same that are used for the purpose at the present day.

—Lewin in *Phantastica:*
Narcotic and Stimulating Drugs

One of the features that most distinguishes humans from other species is our ability to adapt to and alter environments to promote our survival. But we often fail to recognize that we have been altering our *internal* milieu since prehistoric times—experimenting with a wide variety of plants and substances to improve our psychological and physical well-being. At times, the resulting experiences were so profound that the mood-altering substances became integrated into a culture's religious practices or way of life.

The history of the poppy, for example, begins in antiquity. Its seeds and pods have been found in the area of the Stone Age Lake Dwellers. The poppy was cultivated between 4000 and 3000 B.C. by the Sumerians in Mesopotamia (present-day Iraq) to provide opium, known as gil, and meaning "happiness and joy." Similarly, *Cannabis sativa* (marijuana) has been known almost since the beginning of recorded history. Practically every human malady has been treated with one form or another of this plant. Caffeine, cocaine, nicotine,

3

and alcohol have all been used for centuries, sometimes playing integral roles in different cultures. More recently, advances in technology have been applied to synthesizing mood-altering substances. New and highly potent synthetic products are available, along with those "primitive" substances that probably will be around forever.

Our concern over drugs often focuses on the mood-altering substances that are outlawed by society. Yet to understand why millions of people choose to break the law to consume these drugs, the use and effects of *all* mood-altering substances taken for nonmedical purposes must be considered. These include drugs obtained in supermarkets and liquor stores, those prescribed by physicians, and "street drugs."

We must also consider the accuracy of statistics about drug use. Determining legitimate medical use of mood-altering drugs is difficult because reporting may violate confidentiality between physician and patient. Illegal drug users aren't apt to identify themselves; users of alcohol aren't necessarily alcoholics. As a result, most data are gathered from a cross section of the population and applied to the general population. Some surveys review data from people entering treatment programs, or from pharmaceutical databanks that keep track of prescribed medications. In addition, a considerable number of epidemiological surveys have been conducted by investigators interested in the use patterns of specific drugs or drug use among specific populations. But these surveys may vary greatly in their definitions of current use and lifetime use. Moreover, in any cross-sectional survey, groups at high risk for drug use (high school dropouts, the homeless, the unemployed) may not be included.

Most of the data in the book are from relatively few sources (see Appendix A) and must be viewed as estimates rather than absolute figures.

DRUGS AND THE YOUNG

In 1988 the annual Drug Use, Drinking, and Smoking Survey reported continuing declines in the use of marijuana, stimulants, and sedatives among high school seniors, college students, and young adults. These findings were confirmed by the 1988 National Household Survey on Drug Abuse, tracking substance use among 12- to 17-year-olds. This is significant, because other researchers have shown that people rarely start using drugs—except for cocaine—once they reach their mid-twenties. Periods of highest use decline sharply after adolescence.

Nevertheless, the survey noted that almost 80 percent of young adults have tried an illicit drug by their mid-twenties, with 60 percent having tried a drug other than marijuana. Use of alcohol has slightly diminished, but cigarette use changed little from 1981. Of high school seniors, 57 percent were current drinkers. Approximately 5 percent of them were drinking daily, and 32 percent had five or more drinks in a row at least once in the previous two weeks. Approximately 29 percent of high school seniors are current smokers, with 18 percent smoking daily. After high school, 25 percent of 19- to 28-year-olds smoke daily, with 20 percent consuming at least one-half pack a day.

The number of high school seniors reporting cocaine use in the preceding 12 months decreased from 13 percent in 1986 to 5 percent in 1990. The decrease among college students was from 17 percent to 6 percent. For the second time, use of crack by high school seniors decreased, from 4 percent in 1986 to 2 percent in 1990. But that's no cause for complacency. The number of schools reporting that their students have access to crack jumped from 50 percent in 1986 to 76 percent in 1988. So while use may have stabilized, more students are being exposed to the drug. However, wide variations in the use of cocaine and crack are seen in different geographic areas.

Use of "legal" drugs by teenagers often goes unreported. According to the Drug Use, Drinking, and Smoking Survey, over-the-counter (nonprescription) medications, such as diet pills, have already been used by 22 percent of students, with "stay-awake" pills used at some time by 37 percent. As for "medically supervised" psychoactive drugs, nearly one in five high school seniors in the class of 1985 reported having used one or more prescribed opiate drugs, such as codeine, 8 percent had prescriptions for amphetamines, 5 percent for barbiturates, and 12 percent for minor tranquilizers.

ADULTS AND DRUG USE

Although the National Household Survey showed a decrease in illicit drug use among all age groups, races, and both sexes from 1985 to 1988, the number of current users was still estimated at 14.5 million, with an estimated 7.25 million having used an illicit drug in their lifetime. Only 41 percent of adults between the ages of 18 and 25, and 36 percent of adults between 26 and 34, reported no history of illicit drug use. The figure for adults age 35 and up was 77 percent. Some might argue that the survey doesn't provide a typical picture of illicit drug use, but a 1989 *New York Times*–CBS News poll reported almost identical findings, with use of various illegal drugs varying from 38 to 50 percent among 18- to 44-year-olds.

Tobacco consumption remains alarmingly high. Of young adults in the 1988 National Household Survey, 30 to 35 percent were current smokers. The lifetime prevalence of cigarette use did not change significantly between 1985 and 1988 as compared to a significant decrease in lifetime use of ''any illicit drugs.'' Similarly, while the past month prevalence rates for any illicit drug decreased significantly between 1985 and 1988, the prevalence of cigarette use remained about the same.

Pinning down use of mood-altering substances in older adults is difficult. Some researchers estimate that the number of alcoholics age 60 and above is slowly rising. And health professionals are more and more recognizing late-onset alcoholism, a problem that may grow as the number of older people increases.

Inappropriate (nonmedical) use of psychotherapeutic drugs that can be prescribed by physicians is also of concern. The 1988 National Household Survey on Drug Abuse found 12 percent or 23.5 million of the U.S. household population to have used these drugs nonmedically, with 3.4 million using them within the past month of the survey. Adults between the ages of 26 and 34 had the highest lifetime prevalence rate of 22 percent.

ETHNICITY AND DRUG USE

A long-standing societal perception is that drug use has always been major among poor African-Americans and Hispanics. Epidemics of heroin use in lower-income areas have been documented. And so have high rates of poverty and broken homes, which unquestionably play substantial roles in promoting drug use.

More than likely, our perceptions about drug use are probably related more to socioeconomic levels and the conditions under which drugs are taken than to racial and ethnic differences. After all, individuals with similar drug dependencies—but with greater economic resources—can hide their drug use more effectively.

Careful studies show that overall use of mood-altering drugs among minorities is similar to that of the general population. But certain differences may exist with respect to specific drugs. Alcohol use, for example, is of great concern among the Native American population. Use of inhalants among Native Americans is also frequent, with up to 30 percent trying these substances, compared with 10 percent of the general population. Marijuana use is widespread as well; 75 percent of those beyond the sixth grade have tried the drug at least once, compared with 30 percent of the general population.

More research is needed to define differences in susceptibility to drug use among various populations. The National Institute on Drug Abuse states that most studies of minority drug use have been poorly designed and hence haven't been able to capture all the required data. But it's more than fair to say that neither race nor ethnicity protects someone from using mood-altering substances or condemns someone to use them.

DRUGS AND THE WORKPLACE

Approximately 65 percent of young adults entering the work force have probably used illegal drugs, and 10 to 23 percent of all U.S. workers may continue to use dangerous drugs while working. In a 1989 nationwide survey of employers, 80 percent identified alcohol and other drugs as significant problems in their organizations.

A survey by the National Institute on Drug Abuse found that 10 to 20 percent of all job applicants to private corporations were actively using drugs. Eight percent of the men admitted getting high on marijuana while working, and 2 percent did so on cocaine.

Such use is incompatible with personal safety and in certain jobs can endanger others. Alcohol plays a well-documented and publicized role in accidents, homicides, and suicides. In 1987, 38 percent of all fatally injured drivers were legally intoxicated. Almost 50 percent of all traffic fatalities are alcohol-related. Intoxication is a factor in approximately one-third of all homicides and deaths from boating and aviation accidents. Nearly half of those in prison were intoxicated when they committed their crimes.

Becoming more evident in recent years is the role of other substances, notably marijuana and cocaine, in plane crashes, train wrecks, and of course, automobile accidents. Considerable debate has been engendered on how to eliminate such drug users from certain jobs (Chapter 5).

DRUG USE AMONG THE AFFLUENT

The relationship between drug use and socioeconomic status is elusive. Data on drug use are frequently gathered from large federally funded programs, and these programs typically serve people from the lower or middle economic groups. People with sufficient financial resources avoid entering such programs. Instead, they seek treatment from the psychiatric departments of voluntary hospitals or private treatment facilities, often located in secluded areas.

From available information, however, it's clear that the rich are as susceptible as the poor to effects of drug dependency. Indeed, a number of studies have suggested that excessive drinking is more prevalent among the affluent. In a study of more than 630 members of Alcoholics Anonymous, 35 percent were in managerial and professional positions.

In one well-conducted 1984 study of New York State householders, consistently high usage rates of illicit substances turned up among those with annual incomes of $50,000 or more. The upper-income group tended to favor marijuana, sedatives, tranquilizers, and cocaine. In the six months prior to the survey, 25 percent of those surveyed used one of those substances, compared with 17 percent of the general population. The favorite combination of substances was marijuana and alcohol, used by 14 percent of the group as opposed to 10 percent of the general population.

In another survey, of 70 cocaine users with average annual incomes of $83,000, half admitted addiction. And despite their high incomes, more than one-third were dealing the drug to support the cost of their habit—at times exceeding $3,000 a week.

Use of alcohol and mood-altering drugs by members of the health, legal, and education professions is not new but has recently become a genuine cause for concern. As noted by Blum and Associates, psychiatrists (along with other mental health professionals) and lawyers were among the first to use hallucinogens for nontherapeutic reasons. They were often introduced to these drugs—particularly LSD—by friends who were using them as part of legitimate research projects. These observations demonstrate that inappropriate use of mood-altering drugs can occur despite professional status or awareness of their adverse effects.

Chapter 2

Classifying
Mood-Altering Drugs

Mood-altering drugs can be classified by their availability or perceived harm to the public, effects perceived by the user, action on the brain, actual mood-altering effects, and legitimate medical use.

AVAILABILITY OR PERCEIVED PUBLIC HARM

This classification separates substances into three categories—those that can be bought in stores, those that require a physician's prescription, and those that are considered illicit. This classification is valuable in determining the risk that society assigns to particular drugs but really doesn't help in understanding their effects. And despite their assigned risk, some illicit substances have only relatively minor effects—unless they're consumed frequently or in large quantities, or are contaminated.

THE USER'S PERCEPTION

Drugs are often classified by users with street jargon such as uppers, downers, mind messer-uppers, and spacers. Such categories are also not an entirely clear means of classification. Some drugs fall into several categories, depending on the person describing their effects, and substances that produce markedly different physiological effects are sometimes grouped together. What's more, a drug's effects vary with the user, the setting in which it's used, frequency of use, quantity, and how it is administered.

PRIMARY ACTION ON BRAIN RECEPTORS OR NEUROTRANSMITTERS

The action of mood-altering drugs on the brain is the basis for an essential classification for physicians and researchers. But it is less helpful to the public than classification by the actual effects experienced when taking drugs.

PRIMARY MOOD-ALTERING EFFECT

Actual mood-altering effects is the classification that health professionals generally accept. But controversy can arise over placement of a drug in a particular group because that can mask critical similarities among groups. For example: Narcotics are central nervous system (CNS) depressants, as are drugs in the alcohol-barbiturate-sedative group. Combining them can result in severe breathing problems, even death.

Nevertheless, this classification is useful. All drugs in a group have similar effects and can usually be interchanged easily—except for such minor stimulants as nicotine and caffeine with the much more potent amphetamines and cocaine.

LEGITIMATE MEDICAL USE

Appropriate medical indication is one of two criteria for classifying drugs under the federal Controlled Substances Act of 1970. The other is potential for inappropriate use.

The characteristics of each drug group (Table 2.1) are discussed in detail in subsequent chapters, but several points should be mentioned here.

Interchangeability Within a Group. Interchangeability is important when considering treatment. For example, any drug in the CNS group mimics the effects of alcohol. So substituting a minor tranquilizer, say, diazepam (Valium) or chlordiazepoxide (Librium), allows an alcohol-dependent person to avoid withdrawal symptoms.

But dependency on the tranquilizer continues in the same way as

---

TABLE 2.1
Mood-Altering Drugs by Primary Effect

Group	*Examples*
Central nervous system depressants (CNS)	Alcohol; chloral hydrate; barbiturates; benzodiazepines (Ativan, Dalmane, Valium, Librium, Xanax, Serax, Halcion, etc.); hypnotic sedatives (Parest, Quaalude, Doriden); and other tranquilizers (Equanil, Miltown, Noludar, Placidyl, Valmid)
Narcotics (opiates)	Opium, codeine, heroin, morphine, Demerol, Pethidine, Dilaudid, methadone, Percocet, Percodan, Darvon, Tussionex, Fentanyl, Lomotil, Numorphan, agonist-antagonists (Talwin, Stadol, Buprenex, Temgesic, Nubain)
Stimulants	Amphetamines, caffeine, cocaine, nicotine, Preludin, Ritalin, diet pills, khat
Hallucinogens (psychedelics)	Amphetamine variants (2, 5 DMA, PMA, STP, MOA, DOM, MMDA, TMA, DOB); LSD, mescaline, peyote, phencyclidine and analogues, psilocybin, psicocyn and miscellaneous compounds (DMT, DET)

TABLE 2.1 (continued)
Mood-Altering Drugs by Primary Effect

Group	Examples
Cannabinoids	Marijuana, hashish, THC
Inhalants and volatile solvents	Nitrous oxide, various paints and paint thinners, glues
Antidepressants	
Tricyclic antidepressants	Amitriptyline (Elavil, Endep, Amitril, Emitrip) and related drugs
Monoamine oxidase (MAO) inhibitors	Isocarboxazid (Marplan), phenelzine (Nardil), tranylcypromine (Parnate)
Tetracyclic antidepressants	Maprotiline (Ludiomil)
Miscellaneous antidepressants	Trazodone (Desyrel), fluoxetine (Prozac)

dependency on alcohol, and the ability to use inappropriately the substitute drug to obtain a similar mood-altering effect will also continue. Little is gained, therefore, by substitution alone. Yet gradually reducing the dosage of the tranquilizer or barbiturate can detoxify someone with alcohol dependency.

Dependency on any drug in a group can be maintained by any other drug in that group (Chapter 3). Depending on potency, more or less of the second drug may be needed. A heroin-dependent person may be maintained on methadone, meperidine (Demerol), or proproxyphene (Darvon) without going into narcotic withdrawal. But much higher doses of meperidine or proproxyphene are needed to obtain the same effect as methadone.

Detoxification from a drug can be accomplished with any drug in a similar group, but not with drugs from another group. Thus narcotic withdrawal can't be treated adequately by alcohol or another CNS depressant.

All narcotics are interchangeable and can be substituted for one other if the doses are equivalent. Nevertheless, problems can arise. Some narcotics have both narcotic (agonist) and antinarcotic (antagonist) properties. When such a drug is given to someone dependent on a purely narcotic agent, immediate withdrawal is possible. Drugs with dual properties displace the pure narcotic from receptors in the brain, as do antagonist-only drugs. Substituting pentazocine (Talwin) for pain relief in a person who has been on meperidine (Demerol) for several days, causes withdrawal—nausea, vomiting, and extreme discomfort (Chapter 9).

But drugs classified as hallucinogens *always* cause hallucinations, even when relatively small amounts are used. Hallucinogens include some amphetamine derivatives capable of causing hallucinations on extremely low doses. A number of drugs not classed as hallucinogens can cause hallucinations in excessive amounts. Toxic doses of stimulants, narcotic antagonists, and even drugs not usually used inappropriately—steroids and drugs used to treat ulcers, for example—can produce hallucinations.

Cannabis (marijuana) and its synthetic analogue, THC, are considered a separate group. Although image distortions and hallucinations can occur at high doses, they are rare with common usage. Hashish, although more potent, has similar effects.

The potency of stimulants varies greatly. Nicotine and caffeine are obviously much less stimulating than amphetamines or cocaine. Khat, derived from leaves of the cathaedulis plant, is pharmaceutically distinct from other stimulants, but its actions are similar to those of amphetamines and cocaine—two extremely potent stimulants whose toxic effects are often indistinguishable.

A common misconception is that use of antidepressants does not lead to dependency. Recent evidence suggests that inappropriate use of certain antidepressants with a predominant sedative effect, say amitriptyline (Amitril, Elavil, Emitrip, Endep, Enovil), may be considerable in those with a history of inappropriate use of mood-altering drugs.

It should be emphasized that any drug in any group can be used inappropriately, but use alone does not imply automatic dependency. Drugs within a group can vary greatly in ability to produce habituation, dependency, and addiction. Even those with the greatest dependency-producing potential can, in theory, be used intermittently for long periods without producing dependency (Chapter 3). More important, even when these drugs are consumed intermittently, their pleasurable effects often encourage greater use (positive reinforcement), and that can lead to dependency. The process is most common with the more potent central nervous system depressants, narcotics, and stimulants.

Too often, people begin taking drugs thinking they can easily control their drug use. Yet animal testing shows that habitual *self-administration* of narcotics, barbiturates, alcohol, and stimulants can develop quickly (Chapter 3). With some drugs, such as narcotics, use occurs at a steady rate once dependency has been established, mainly to prevent unpleasant withdrawal. With others, notably cocaine and amphetamines, the reinforcing effects are particularly great. Sometimes laboratory animals press levers up to 4,000 times to self-administer a single injection of cocaine. When given free access, the animals increasingly choose the substance over food and water, if necessary, until they die. In short, mood-altering drugs are neither equal in their effects nor equal in their potential to produce dependency.

Controlled Substances Act. The Controlled Substances Act of 1970 created five schedules for drugs (Table 2.2).

Schedule I drugs have the highest potential for inappropriate use and have no commonly accepted medical use in the United States. These drugs cannot be prescribed and are available only for research after special application to federal agencies.

Schedule II drugs have a currently acceptable medical use, along with a high potential for inappropriate use and for causing heavy psychological and physiological dependency. To prescribe Schedule II drugs, physicians must be registered with the federal Drug Enforcement Administration (DEA) and must comply with certain requirements.

Schedule III, IV, and V drugs have currently acceptable medical uses; their potential for inappropriate use and dependency is lower in each succeeding schedule. Schedule V drugs may, under certain well-defined conditions, be dispensed without a prescription if that practice doesn't conflict with other federal, state, or local laws.

TABLE 2.2
Schedules for Federally Controlled Substances*

Schedule	*Common Examples*
I	Heroin, marijuana, LSD, DMT, DET, peyote, psilocybin, mescaline, hashish, dihydromorphinone, methaqualone, nicocodeine, PCP, marijuana
II	*Narcotics:* opium (Pantopon), morphine, codeine, hydromorphone (Dilaudid), methadone (Dolphine), meperidine (Demerol, pethadol), oxyymorphone (Numorphan), oxycodone (Percocet), Fentanyl, sublimaze *Stimulants:* cocaine, amphetamine group, phenmetrazine (Preludin), methylphenidate (Ritalin) *Cannabinoids:* dronabinol (Marinol), nabilone (Cesamet) *Barbiturates:* amobarbital, Pentobarbital, Seconal, etorphine hydrochloride
III	Paregoric, glutethimide (Doriden), methyprylon (Noludar), nalorphine, various weight-reducing pills
IV	Pentazocine (Talwin), propoxyphene (Darvon), phenobarbital, chloral hydrate ethchlorvynol (Placidyl), meprobamate (Miltown, Neuramate, Equanil, Sedabamate), benzodiazepines (Valium, Librium, etc.)
V	Drugs containing moderate quantities of narcotics, usually in antidiarrheal agents and cough suppressants, includes diphenoxylate preparations (Lofene, Logen, Lomotil, Lonox, Lo-Trol, Low Quel, Nor-mil, Lomanate)

*Selected substances—schedule of a particular drug may change with time.

Many Schedule I and II drugs can produce a high degree of physical dependency and considerable withdrawal symptoms. But as noted earlier, *any* drug with mood-altering properties can be used inappropriately and produce intense "highs," depending on how much and how often it's used. So someone who needs to get high when the preferred drug is unavailable will take any available drug—in large quantities, if necessary—to obtain the desired effect.

Perhaps the most striking example was an episode of paregoric use in Detroit in the early 1950s. At that time paregoric, commonly used to treat diarrhea, was sold over the counter. Addicts unable to get heroin bought paregoric, boiled it with the antihistamine tripelennamine, and injected it intravenously. Users called it Blue Velvet; its high was almost identical to heroin's.

More than two decades later, a similar use was perpetuated with the narcotic agonist-antagonist pentazocine (Talwin). Another substitute, propoxyphene (Darvon), was initially promoted as a nonnarcotic painkiller. But it's a derivative of methadone, and when taken in large doses can produce narcotic dependency and withdrawal symptoms. Drug users quickly spotted Darvon's mood-altering effects, but the public became aware of its potential for inappropriate use only recently.

The Controlled Substances Act has been a mixed blessing. It has helped highlight drugs that create dependence and withdrawal symptoms, but ironically has lulled the public and the medical profession into incorrectly believing that Schedule III, IV, and V drugs can be used with little concern about dependency. Periodically drugs are reclassified based on reports of increased inappropriate use or decreased effectiveness. The Drug Enforcement Administration within the Department of Justice is responsible for assuring compliance.

Drug scheduling fosters other ironies. Drugs that some professionals deem worthwhile are considered by others to have no medical value.

- Heroin, a Schedule I drug, is available in England as a potent pain reliever. But most doctors in the United States oppose making it available even for terminal patients in excruciating pain.

- Marijuana, medically useful in well-defined situations, is listed in Schedule I, while its principal psychoactive component, dronabinol (Marinol), and its synthetic counterpart, nabilone (Cesamet), are available as Schedule II drugs to ease nausea and vomiting following chemotherapy.
- Peyote, a Schedule I drug, is not available for medical purposes. But until recently it had been "approved" for use by various Native American groups in religious ceremonies. This freedom was revoked by a U.S. Supreme Court decision in 1990, allowing federal and state laws to exclude exemptions for use of illicit drugs for religious purposes.

As stated previously, any drug that alters moods can be used inappropriately. That's not to say these drugs should be prohibited when there are medical reasons for their use. Risk of disabling dependency is low when a drug is taken for medical reasons for a defined period. Someone incapacitated by pain can be helped by the temporary use of narcotics. But using any substance for the primary purpose of getting high carries the potential for habituation and—depending on the drug—addiction.

DESIGNER DRUGS

In the 1980s a new group of substances was synthesized. These new drugs have effects similar to those of existing drugs but differ slightly in chemical structure (see Table 2.3). They've been termed designer drugs because their chemical structure is developed specifically to avoid accusations of illegal manufacture. Many designer drugs can produce potent highs with such small quantities that they're virtually undetectable in blood or urine tests. And the change in chemical structure often results in unanticipated—sometimes fatal—toxic effect.

The three major groups of designer drugs are fentanyl (Sublimaze) analogues, meperidine (Demerol) analogues, and amphetamine analogues. Drugs in the first two groups are used instead of heroin; those in the third group in place of hallucinogens. By the late 1980s,

TABLE 2.3
Designer Drugs

Street Name	Clinical Name	Class
China White	Fentanyl derivatives	Narcotic
Ecstasy, XTC, Adam, MDM, MDMA	3–4 methylenedioxy methamphetamine	Hallucinogen
Eve, Love Drug, MDEA	3–4 methylene dioxyamphetamine	Hallucinogen
Ice	Methamphetamine derivatives produced in smokable form	Stimulant
MPPP	Meperidine derivative: N-methyl-4 phenyl-4 propionoxy piperidine	Narcotic
MPTP	Meperidine derivative: N-methyl-4 phenyl-1, 2, 3, 6 tetrahydropyridine	Narcotic
Marijuana	Synhexyl	Marijuana
PMA	Paramethoxyamphetamine	Hallucinogen

methamphetamine derivatives in smokable form began appearing with increasing frequency as a substitute for cocaine.

These drugs are extremely potent. One fentanyl analogue, for example, is 3,000 times more potent than the same amount of morphine; a meperidine analogue is 25 times more potent than meperidine itself.

For producers and dealers, the advantages of designer drugs are great. Since routine toxicology can't detect and identify these substances, they enjoy licit status for a while until laws can be passed making their production, sale, or purchase illegal. They're also fairly easy to manufacture—and with legally obtained chemicals. (This eliminates the necessity of becoming involved with criminal organizations to buy opium or the morphine base, cocaine, or marijuana.) And designer drugs are easy to market because they produce highs that are often indistinguishable from those of naturally derived products.

The biggest advantage, however, is the enormous profit. By 1986, the annual market for these substances ran to an estimated $1 billion.

Designer drugs carry significant risks. Overdosing is common; users often do not realize that the new drug may be 1,000 times more potent than the drug they usually take. Side effects of a meperidine analogue (MPPP) include drastic loss of muscle control (similar to symptoms of Parkinson's disease, which can lead to permanent neurologic damage). Serious complications from the amphetamine analogues, Eve and Ecstasy, vary from extreme restlessness and agitation to convulsions.

The National Narcotics Act of 1984, part of the Comprehensive Crime Control Act, an early effort to put legal restraints on designer drugs, wasn't particularly effective. As a result, the more stringent Anti-Drug Abuse Act of 1986 contains the Controlled Substance Analogue Act, which requires that any analogue of a Schedule I substance be included as a controlled substance in Schedule I.

PERFORMANCE-ENHANCING DRUGS

Athletes often use drugs to improve their performance. They take stimulants to give them more energy, narcotics to relieve pain, and anabolic steroids, cortisone, and growth hormone to increase muscular strength. Drugs in the third category don't produce mood changes, but their excessive use can affect behavior (Chapter 19).

Chapter 3

Habituation, Dependency, and Addiction

Although mood-altering substances have been used since antiquity, clear definitions of and terminology for their effects weren't developed until the early 1980s. And some terms have still not been accepted fully by the drug-treatment community. One reason is the emotional response generated in various individuals by such terms as "dependency," "addiction," and "addict."

Recognizing the need for clear and uniform terminology, the American Medical Association established a special task force in 1983 to survey 99 experts in various professions. That first attempt produced a common—though not perfect—vocabulary. The effort also provided a core of understanding for developing a consensus about patterns of use of mood-altering drugs. To help clarify the AMA's terminology, some additional definitions have been provided by the author.

DEFINING TERMS

Patterns of mood-altering drug use form an eight-stage continuum: nonuse, appropriate use, misuse, experimental use, abuse, habituation, psychological and/or physical dependency, and addiction.

1. *Nonuse* denotes just that—not using a substance at all.
2. *Appropriate use* means using a substance for sound reasons in an accepted and approved manner. But "appropriate" is a relative term.

    Minor tranquilizers are appropriate treatment for extreme

anxiety that is otherwise uncontrollable: Medical consensus also holds that mood-altering drugs are appropriate in a variety of situations, such as stimulants for hyperactivity syndrome in children, opiate (narcotic) analgesics for unremitting pain that doesn't respond to nonnarcotic analgesics, cocaine as a topical anesthetic, tranquilizers for severe anxiety, antidepressants for severe depression, and sleeping medications for incapacitating insomnia.

Other uses for mood-altering drugs are accepted—though not unanimously—by the medical community. They include stimulants to lessen the need for morphine in cases of acute postoperative pain, antidepressants for chronic pain, marijuana for controlling nausea following chemotherapy, antidepressants for cocaine users, and methadone for heroin users.

3. *Misuse* is taking a drug for its prescribed purpose but not in the way it is supposed to be taken. Two examples are taking sleeping medication more frequently than prescribed in order to sleep longer, and using more analgesics than indicated for headache in the hope of getting faster and better relief.

4. *Experimental use* may be unintentional misuse. But more commonly it's a conscious effort to see what effect the drug will have. Experimental use implies trying a drug only once or twice.

5. *Abuse* is taking a drug for *other* than its intended purpose and/or in a way other than that prescribed. It's also use of any illicit drug that can result in physical, psychological, economic, legal, or social harm, either to oneself or to others. Abuse begins as experimental use, progresses to casual use, and then moves along the continuum to more serious patterns of use. Drugs can be classified by their potential for dependency.

6. *Habituation* is the result of continued casual use and can be characterized as the need to take a drug at given times to avoid the anxiety associated with not taking it. At this stage, the intervals between uses are long enough to prevent dependency. Habituation doesn't usually progress to dependency or addiction but is frequently observed in weekend drinkers, in smokers

who need a cigarette on awakening, and even in the many people who need a morning cup of coffee to ''get started.''

7. *Psychological and/or physical dependency* usually follow habituation to a substance with high potential for dependency (see Table 3.1). Typically, dependency is characterized by three responses:

- the need to take a drug to experience its pleasurable effects
- the appearance of behavioral changes—psychological and/or physiological—when the drug is abruptly discontinued
- the need continually to increase the dose and/or frequency of use to sustain its initial effects

Psychological dependency is an emotional state of craving a drug either for its positive effects or to avoid the negative effects caused by its absence. All mood-altering drugs can create psychological dependency.

Psychological dependency often motivates drug-seeking behavior. A common misconception is that drugs with low degrees of physical dependency are less likely to be used inappropriately. Cocaine, for example, is thought to produce little physical dependency, but no drug is more psychologically reinforcing. Trying to differentiate the ''addictive potential'' of drugs by their degree of physical dependency is of little value.

Physical dependency is reached when the body has adapted to a drug and cannot function normally without it. Unpleasant symptoms—withdrawal—appear when the drug is suddenly discontinued. Physical dependency is associated with many medications and is usually—but not always—characterized by increasing tolerance to one or more effects of the drug. In fact, dependency is acceptable if the drug is for a specific medical condition and is necessary to maintain normal functioning. For example, individuals with epilepsy are dependent on barbiturates prescribed to prevent seizures. Discontinue the medication and they suffer withdrawal. On barbiturates or similar drugs, however, they function without having their lives disrupted by seizures. Similarly, people with chronic or incapacitating cancer pain are able to resume normal, productive lives with use of narcotic (opiate) analgesics. Their dependency on these drugs may be quite pronounced, and they may need increasingly higher doses to function normally, but they rarely take the drugs for their euphoric effect. Problems begin when a person becomes dependent on the euphoria or high produced by the drug and takes it solely for that purpose.

8. *Addiction*, characterized by the compulsive use of a substance resulting in physical or psychological dependency, is usually accompanied by increased tolerance. The person is unable to restrict drug use. As addiction develops, individuals lose control over intake and invest their energies in obtaining the drug. Today, the drug with the greatest addictive potential is cocaine or crack.

"Addiction," unlike "dependency," is always used in the negative sense. Within this powerful negative context, many people lose the ability to see the addict as a person or to think clearly about appropriate approaches to addiction.

Putting addiction in perspective requires a look at features associated with dependency.

TOLERANCE

One definition of "tolerance" is the physiological adaptation to the effects of a drug. In other words, the user needs larger and larger quantities to obtain the same effect and can consume those greater doses without untoward side effects. Tolerance to any drug in a particular class is usually accompanied by cross-tolerance—that is, tolerance to *other* drugs in that class. Tolerance to barbiturates, for example, would be accompanied by cross-tolerance to the benzodiazepines or alcohol. Tolerance may develop at different rates to the various effects of a specific drug. A person may become tolerant to the sedative and euphoric effects of barbiturates relatively quickly, but tolerance to the lethal level rises much more slowly. The result can be an overdose when the person tries to get high with those drugs.

TABLE 3.1
Dependency Potential of Commonly Used Drugs

Scale: 0–5, with 5 indicating most severe degree of dependency

Drug	Psychological	Physical	Withdrawal
Alcohol	4	4	4
Other CNS depressants	2–4	2–4	2–4
Narcotics	3–4	3–4	3–4
Stimulants			
Caffeine	1	0–1	0–1
Tobacco	3–4	3	0–2
Amphetamines	4	2	1–2
Cocaine	5	2	1–2
Marijuana	2–3	1	2
Hallucinogens	2	0	0
PCP	2	1	1
Inhalants and volatile solvents	2	0–1	0

Different groups of drugs produce dependency at different rates (Table 3.1) and intensities, depending on their potency, quantity taken, and the individual's sensitivities. For example, both narcotics (opiates) and central nervous system (CNS) depressants—such as alcohol—can lead to a high degree of dependency and tolerance, and withdrawal follows if they are suddenly discontinued. But withdrawal from alcohol is much more severe than withdrawal from narcotics, and if untreated may cause death.

Cocaine generates very rapid psychological dependency. Its markedly positive (euphoric) and short-lived effect fosters development of dependency because the user immediately wants to repeat the experience. Dependency on alcohol develops over a much longer period, and with responsible use may never develop. Nevertheless, the degree of physical dependency on alcohol is much greater than on cocaine. And so is the severity of withdrawal.

WITHDRAWAL

Withdrawal is what happens after a drug-dependent person abruptly stops taking the drug. The resulting physiologic changes vary according to the kind of drug it is or the degree of dependency on it. Withdrawal can always be suppressed by the drug that caused the dependency or by another drug in the same group when cross-tolerance exists.

Detoxification. The process by which the daily dose of a dependency-producing substance is slowly diminished is called detoxification. This gradual decrease lowers the level of tolerance while preventing withdrawal symptoms. Detoxification can be carried out using the actual dependency-producing drug or a drug with cross-tolerance. Examples include diazepam (Valium) for alcohol and methadone for heroin.

EFFECTS OF DRUGS ON THE BRAIN

In general, most behavior is modified by chemical substances called neurotransmitters, neuromodulators, and neuromediators acting on the brain and other parts of the nervous system.

Neurotransmitters, contained in nerve cells (neurons), may be released to transmit information to another cell. Although production and destruction of neurotransmitters may vary with the specific substance, simply put, neurotransmitters are usually synthesized in the neuron by a variety of enzymes acting on basic precursor substances. Once synthesized, neurotransmitters are stored in vesicles in the nerve ending and released after an electrical impulse passes through the nerve or by the action of a specific substance given to the body (Figure 1.) Once released into the space between nerve cells (synapse), a neurotransmitter moves across the synapse and attaches itself to a receptor site located on a postsynaptic neuron. Specific receptors exist for each neurotransmitter, with the fit described as a "lock-key" interaction. This combination initiates a chain of bio-chemical events that ultimately results in either excitation or inhibition.

The neurotransmitter may then be: (a) broken down by enzymes at the receptor site; (b) released into and metabolized at the area of the synapse; or (c) returned to the originating neuron to be broken down by enzymes located in the cell. Mood-altering drugs can therefore affect the neurotransmitter-receptor reaction in a variety of ways (Figure 2). They may interfere with the enzymes required to synthesize the drug in the neuron or, once the drug is synthesized, may prevent it from being stored in the vesicle, resulting in its being broken down in the nerve cell prior to being released into the synapse. Drugs may cause a release of neurotransmitters from the vesicles into the synaptic space. A given drug may occupy the receptor site, preventing neurotransmitter-receptor binding and resulting in an increased concentration of the transmitter in the synaptic space. When this occurs, the drug may mimic the effect of the neurotransmitter or may be "neutral," that is, not cause any interaction. Uptake of the neurotransmitter may be inhibited or breakdown of the transmitter may be prevented through the drug's action in blocking the enzymes responsible for the degradation. Although receptor sites for specific mood-altering drugs as opiates, benzodiazepines, and most recently marijuana have been identified, almost all mood-altering drugs in a variety of ways affect neurotransmitter-receptor interaction. These are discussed more fully later.

Neurotransmitters related to mood-altering drug action include the endogenous endorphins and enkephalins (opiates), dopamine (cocaine), gamma aminobutyrate (alcohol, benzodiazepines), norepinephrine (opiates, stimulants, LSD), epinephrine, and 5-hydroxytryptamine or serotonin (alcohol). Neuromodulators aren't secreted by the nerve cells, but they influence their activity or excitability. Neuromediators may act in conjunction with neurotransmitters to produce a final effect.

Many neurotransmitters act by combining with other parts of the cells. This combination is the basis for an actual effect. Such mood-altering drugs as opiates and benzodiazepines combine with specific receptors to exert their effects.

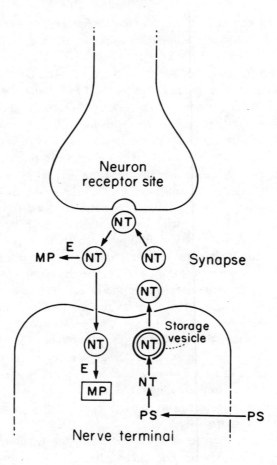

Figure 1 Functioning of neurotransmitter at receptor sites
PS = precursor substance; NT = neurotransmitter; E = enzyme;
MP = metabolic product: the substance formed when NT is broken down

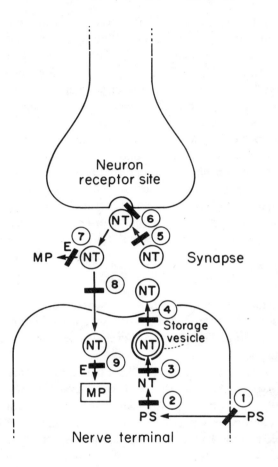

Figure 2 Sites of possible interference of mood-altering drugs with neurotransmitter-receptor interactions

PS = precursor substance; NT = neurotransmitter; E = enzyme; MP = metabolic product as breakdown of NT

(1) inhibition of uptake precursor substance; (2) inhibition of synthesis of (NT); (3) prevention of storage of NT in vesicle; (4) prevention of release of NT from vesicles in nerve terminal into synapse; (5) prevention of NT-receptor binding; (6) actual binding of drug with receptor; (7) prevention of breakdown of NT either in synapse or after return to cell (9); (8) prevention of uptake of NT at neuron

Drugs that mimic or enhance the effect of the body's own neurotransmitters are termed agonists. Drugs that prevent the neurotransmitter or a like substance (drugs) from combining with a receptor
are termed antagonists. Drugs may also act independently of receptor
activity. Some may combine with smaller molecules in the cells.
Others, such as those used in cancer chemotherapy, may be incorporated into the genetic material of cells.

Also located in the brain are anatomical areas called pleasure or
reward centers. When subjected to stimulation of these centers during
laboratory experiments, animals continue the pleasurable effects by
pressing a lever to receive direct electrical stimulation or a mood-
altering drug, say, cocaine. How specific mood-altering drugs act on
the reward centers and receptors is discussed in Chapter 4, as well
as in chapters on the use of specific drugs.

DEPENDENCY

Development of Dependency.   A grasp of how dependency develops is the key to understanding why it's so hard to stop using a
particular drug. The course of heroin use best illustrates the process
(Figure 3).

When someone injects heroin for the first time, the amount of the
drug reaching the brain slowly rises. The rate of rise depends on the
strength of heroin, speed and amount of its consumption, and the
body's ability to metabolize it. Initial use may result in an uncomfortable feeling that reaches a peak and then slowly diminishes. But
with subsequent use, the effect is pleasurable and promotes continued
use.

Tolerance buildup is avoided if the user spaces the heroin injections so that the brain isn't consistently exposed to concentrations of
the drug. The pleasurable effects are achieved, but the person won't
become dependent. Users who take heroin that way are known as
"chippers." They inject once or twice a week without becoming
physically dependent. Similarly, using alcohol in that manner—a
pattern termed "binge drinking"—does not lead to physical dependency (see Figure 3, graph A).

Trouble comes when the user takes more of the drug while levels of previous doses are still in the brain tissues stimulating the pleasure centers. That's when a tolerance threshold (TT) begins to develop. The user gets a high when the threshold is crossed (see Figure 3, graph B). Dropping the drug level below the threshold results in withdrawal symptoms.

Taking the drug at constant doses at regular intervals raises the threshold so that a high is no longer experienced (see Figure 3, graph C). Rather than stop the drug, lose the highs, and face withdrawal, the user injects more heroin and/or shortens the time interval between injections (see Figure 3, graph D). That pushes the drug level above the threshold and allows a high to be produced.

This simplified description points up some important facts about drug use:

- Tolerance to the high from most drugs continues to rise with constant administration, thus necessitating greater and greater intake to achieve a high.
- When the amount taken is much higher than the tolerance threshold, the result is overdose and possibly death.
- When the tolerance threshold is slowly increased, the user can be maintained on very high levels of the drug—levels that could kill a nontolerant person.
- Tolerance to specific effects of a drug may not occur at the same rate.
- When tolerance to the high is reached faster than tolerance to the lethal dose, escalating drug use may cause death.
- When the tolerance threshold is gradually lowered by giving smaller and smaller doses of the drug (detoxification), withdrawal will follow with relatively little discomfort.

Treating Dependency: Learning from Animals. A common assumption is that dependency and addiction are moral weaknesses; that the alcohol, narcotic, or cocaine addict can use will power and "just say no." It simply isn't that easy, as studies of laboratory animals clearly show.

Animals can be taught to self-administer drugs, including stimulants (cocaine and amphetamines), narcotics (morphine and heroin), and minor tranquilizers. But they're selective. They won't, for ex-

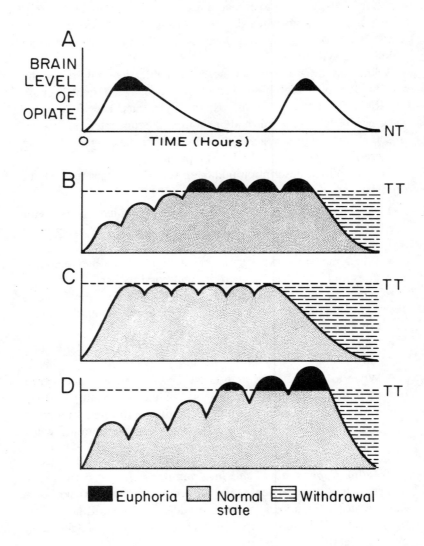

Figure 3

ample, self-administer hallucinogens or marijuana. And they'll consume alcohol-containing solutions only when forced. Once dependent on alcohol, however, they'll take it regularly. (Mice can be bred to choose alcohol.)

More significant, the animals quickly become dependent on cocaine and narcotics, and their self-injections increase markedly under stress. Dependent animals will choose drugs over food and water.

One conditioned response in animals is similar to human behavior. Put a drug-dependent animal through withdrawal while a light flashes in its cage. Months later, that drug-free animal will go through the withdrawal process when the cage light flashes. Similarly conditioned is the heroin addict—drug-free while hospitalized or incarcerated—who feels the need to shoot up as soon as he or she is back in his or her drug-taking environment.

Stress and environment are important considerations in treating addiction and are discussed in Chapter 4 and Chapter 5. Any approach to treatment, however, must recognize the difficulty of stopping any addiction—cigarettes, alcohol, heroin, or even food. After treatment, the proportion of people who return to their addictions is about the same for all those substances.

Chapter 4

Why People Use Drugs

The topic for a panel at a national meeting of experts on drug use was "Why do people take drugs?" The panelists—a psychologist, psychiatrist, general physician, sociologist, and a drug user—were allotted 10 minutes each. All the professionals ran overtime, of course. Finally, the moderator asked the user to describe why he takes drugs.

"They give me great pleasure" was all he said.

Despite the vast amounts of time, effort, and money spent trying to discover why people use drugs, no uniformly accepted theory can consistently predict drug dependency. The "feel good" response is only a partial answer to a complex question; drug use often continues long after the pleasure has gone. But that answer must be taken seriously. In addition, some biologic determinants and psychological factors are associated with, and may be powerful reinforcers of, alcohol and drug dependency.

BIOLOGIC DETERMINANTS

Scientists and clinicians have been searching for many years for a genetic disposition to chemical dependency. Hereditary patterns have long been recognized in the development of alcoholism (see Chapter 6) but not clearly demonstrated in relation to other drug dependencies. The identification of brain receptors and neurotransmitters has led many researchers to propose that the use of mood-altering drugs could be a response to a genetic defect causing an abnormal balance between the neurotransmitters and receptor sites. Taking a mood-altering substance might correct this imbalance but at the same time compel the individual to continue to take the drug in order to feel well.

One of the first hypotheses on the biochemical basis of addiction to drugs other than alcohol dealt with heroin dependency. The idea of giving the drug methadone to heroin users was developed by Drs. Vincent Dole and Marie Nyswander, who believed that once heroin use was regularized, certain biochemical changes occurred in the body, resulting in a need or craving to take heroin or opiates in order to function normally. But whereas heroin is a short-acting drug and therefore produced "highs" because of rapidly changing levels in the brain, methadone is a long-acting opiate that can satisfy this craving over a greater time period. Although this hypothesis has never been proven, the effectiveness of methadone in the treatment of heroin dependency has been amply demonstrated.

Neurotransmitters.   The identification of opiate receptors in the brain and the presence of endorphins and enkephalins soon led to the hypothesis that those deficient in neurotransmitters or opiate receptors would be predisposed to anxiety and anger. To curb these feelings, they may take heroin. The feeling of well-being produced by the drug then reinforces its continued use. There has been no convincing evidence, however, that heroin addicts have deficiencies in either endorphins or opiate receptors.

The effects of stimulants on the brain have been shown to be related to the ability of these drugs to block the uptake of the neurotransmitter dopamine at the receptor site (Chapter 3). It has been hypothesized that depression is related to decreased levels of dopamine. Those who are depressed may be more susceptible to amphetamine and cocaine use. An alternate hypothesis is that those whose dopamine levels are too high might be sensitive to small changes, with resulting depression or anxiety. These individuals may take stimulants to increase their dopamine levels even further to maintain a feeling of well-being.

The neurotransmitters gamma amino butyrate (GABA) and serotonin have both been shown to be elevated by alcohol. It has been hypothesized, though not proven, that an indirect relationship exists between serotonin levels and the presence of aggression or violence.

Low serotonin levels are believed to occur with greater frequency in those with poor impulse control and aggressive behavior. Drinkers with low brain levels of serotonin or GABA may be particularly susceptible to develop alcoholism. Most recently, investigators have suggested that a specific gene affecting dopamine receptors exists in a much higher proportion of alcoholics as compared with others (Chapter 6). In addition, investigators at the National Institute of Mental Health have identified receptor sites for marijuana in the brain.

These hypotheses are particularly attractive because they appear to offer a quick way to eliminate a craving for a specific drug. Since it is the craving that compels continued use, its elimination would not only diminish drug use but also enable individuals to remain in treatment for longer periods (recurrent drug use is one of the most common reasons for leaving treatment). For this reason, the Alcohol and Drug Abuse and Mental Health Administration has been increasingly promoting research on the biologic effects of mood-altering substances on the brain. However, even with such relationships, whether these deficiencies predate the use of these drugs or are caused by them remains to be determined. In addition, biologic determinants do not address the known environmental and psychological factors promoting drug dependency. Indeed, an overreliance on these biologic effects may inadvertently detract attraction from providing alternatives to drug addiction, an essential part of the rehabilitative process.

PSYCHOLOGICAL FACTORS

Psychological explanations for drug dependency range from classic analytic theory to more superficial explanations of personality. But an ''addictive'' personality has never been clearly defined. Characteristics commonly seen in the drug-dependent are seen just as frequently in those without signs of alcohol or drug problems. However, some experiences can increase (or decrease) the likelihood that someone may use or become dependent on drugs.

Parent-Child Interactions. Deficient parent-child interactions show up as lack of intimacy, failure to praise the child's achievements, criticism, inability to set clear limits to behavior, lack of closeness between parents, and lack of communication. A positive family relationship usually deters drug initiation, or at least minimizes chances that drug experimentation will progress to inappropriate drug use.

Contradictory and sometimes hypocritical attitudes often exist between licit and illicit drug use. Most parents are quite aware of the dangers of illicit drug use and aren't reluctant to advise against it. But they may have a benign attitude toward alcohol. They may be heavy drinkers themselves and even provide alcohol for their children's parties. The message that "drinking as I do is all right" is one reason excessive alcohol use by parents is often associated with problem drinking among adolescents.

It's a small step from excessive alcohol use to illicit drugs such as marijuana or other substances. But that progression isn't automatic. Although most people who use heroin or cocaine tried marijuana first, the overwhelming majority of marijuana users don't progress to heroin or cocaine.

The importance of developing a strong family bond can't be overemphasized. This relationship is increasingly difficult to achieve, especially when both parents work or in single-parent families. Lack of appropriate role models in the family leads to increased reliance on peers and other adults.

Peer Relationships. Drug-related behavior in the absence of a secure family bond is strongly associated with drug experimentation among friends. Peer influence is especially strong during early adolescence, when the sense of appropriate and inappropriate behavior is established. And peer influence is particularly powerful when it comes to marijuana and cigarette smoking. Conversely, inability to form adequate peer relationships—alienation from others and such antisocial behavior as chronic anger or fighting—also places a child at risk for illicit drug use.

Expectations about school performance have also been associated with drug use. Lower commitment to education, diminished likelihood of going on to college, and poor academic performance are all risk behaviors.

Adults as Role Models.   The impact of adult role models other than family members seems to be strong, particularly in the absence of good parent-child relationships. In general, children tend to make role models of people they view as successful, usually in terms of financial success or physical prowess. When athletes endorse beer and ''smokeless'' tobacco, for example, they promote feelings of approval for the product, encourage its use, and even associate the product with success (Chapter 19).

The beverage and tobacco industries claim that these ads are targeted to informed adults, but an overwhelming majority of adolescents see the ads and try to emulate the life-styles portrayed in them.

Those who deal drugs may appear glamorous and daring. Dealers have large sums of ready money, and the excitement of ''making it'' on the street is a strong incentive for youths who have little else to occupy their time.

PHYSIOLOGY AND CONDITIONING

As explained in Chapter 3, stimulating the reward system of the brain with a drug results in a craving that requires frequent use to achieve a pleasurable response. As the reward system becomes less sensitive to the drug's effects, higher dosages, administered more frequently, are necessary to achieve pleasure.

Discontinuing the drug—abruptly stopping the stimulation of the reward system—intensifies craving for the drug and results in increased drug-seeking behavior, even if there is no dependency. With dependency, however, abrupt discontinuation results in an increased sensitivity of neurons or an outpouring of neurotransmitters, the probable culprits responsible for withdrawal symptoms. Some heroin addicts who have developed sufficient tolerance not to get high still continue to inject for fear of withdrawal.

Environmental stimuli promote continued drug use. Anticipating a high when injecting heroin often results in a high even when the substance contains only contaminants. In settings associated with drinking, study subjects tend to get high when unknowingly consuming drinks without alcohol. Associating pleasurable situations with prior drug use can also create a craving. Ex-smokers, for example, often experience the greatest desire for a cigarette when having morning coffee or when having alcohol in the late afternoon or evening. All those occasions had been moments of pleasure associated with cigarettes. Former heroin addicts returning to neighborhoods where they had previously shot up begin to experience drug cravings, even when they've been abstinent for prolonged periods.

In addition, drug-free former users who've experienced withdrawal symptoms in certain places may experience similar symptoms when they return to those environments. In an experimental setting, merely showing videotapes of someone undergoing withdrawal to former heroin users often makes them uncomfortable.

Chapter 5

Identifying and Treating Drug Dependency

Differentiating between acceptable drug use—smoking, social drinking, or even occasional marijuana use—and problem use of drugs is far from easy.

Most of those who become habituated to and dependent on drugs follow a fairly standard progression: cigarettes and/or alcohol to marijuana, then on to other mood-altering substances with greater dependency potential. Yet the majority of those who smoke or drink don't follow that path. Understanding why some people progress from socially acceptable behavior to illicit drug use is extremely important. Unfortunately, a behavior pattern that consistently leads to drug use is yet to be determined.

SIGNS AND SYMPTOMS OF DRUG USE

Early signs of drug use tend to be similar, regardless of the drug. Behavior at school or work often changes: the person has trouble paying attention; levels of efficiency fall dramatically; work or study habits change; and there is a lack of concern about physical appearance or dress. At home, the person may appear distracted, often expresses anger, and loses interest in his or her usual pursuits. Someone injecting usually wears long sleeves to hide needle marks. Unexplained absences sometimes occur, leading to defensiveness and anger when questioned. Need for money begins to surface; the person often tries to borrow from friends, relatives, co-workers, and employers.

Most important: the circle of friends may change; the new group often includes one or more people known to use drugs.

Identifying a user of mood-altering drugs is essential if help is to be offered before patterns of drug-taking behavior become established. Specific signs vary with the type of substance consumed.

Alcohol and Other Central Nervous System Depressants. There are a number of signs of excessive use of alcohol:

- obvious impairment in individual relationships and social functioning, plus need for ''social drinking'' early in the day
- decreased productivity in school or at work
- increasing absenteeism
- loss of control over amount consumed
- possible ''binge'' drinking sprees

Symptoms of the physiological effects of alcohol may include increasing anxiety and tension, inability to sleep, chronic heartburn, rapid heart rate.

Other central nervous system depressants such as the benzodiazepines (Valium, Librium), glutethimide (Doriden), and methaqualone (Quaalude) produce the following symptoms: occasional drowsiness, slurred speech, inability to concentrate, and altered perceptions. When the drug is not readily available, those symptoms may alternate with periods of increased anxiety, sweating, and agitation. Judgment is often impaired, as are motor skills. The symptoms are quite similar to those of alcohol intoxication.

Stimulants. Stimulant dependency is most often associated with weight loss (despite a voracious appetite at times), difficulty sleeping and concentrating, hyperactivity, and impulsivity. Stimulant-dependent people have difficulty maintaining a conversation. Pupils may be dilated, and vision may be blurred. When use stops abruptly, extreme fatigue may set in with long periods of sleep. With extreme use, paranoia and even hallucinations can occur.

Those who snort cocaine also have nasal irritations, alternately manifested by a running nose and nasal stuffiness. Weight loss may be pronounced at times, associated with loss of interest in food. The pupils are often dilated; coughs and colds may be present. Crack, when used in high doses, frequently intensifies all those signs and symptoms, sometimes leading to sudden death.

Narcotics. Narcotic use is readily identifiable when the individual is high, or immediately after an injection when he or she is sleepy or drowsy. But once the high has subsided, it's very hard to tell if someone is using narcotics. The user may establish behavior patterns that indicate a frequent need to take drugs and become anxious and irritable anticipating the next dose. The user's eyes are watery, and the pupils are often constricted, even between injections. Signs of injections—track marks or drug paraphernalia—are obvious clues, but they are often hidden. Detection is difficult when narcotics are taken orally.

Marijuana. Intermittent use of drugs in the cannabis group is also hard to detect. Frequent use produces a dreamy state with no desire for productive activity, the antimotivational syndrome. The smoker may have a distorted sense of time and distance, and feel considerable anxiety. Appetite is often increased. Physical signs include red eyes, dry mouth, rapid heartbeat, and facial pallor.

Hallucinogens. Hallucinogen use is relatively easy to identify when the user is observed soon after the drug is taken. A hallucinogen high may produce euphoria, anxiety, panic, and odd behavior. Even hours later, the user may experience visual hallucinations and lose the sense of self. Persons on a hallucinogen may have trouble expressing thoughts or describing events. Phencyclidine (PCP) can cause extreme hyperactivity, mood disturbance, and sometimes impulsive or violent behavior and "pressured" speech. Such behavior may last for hours.

Inhalants. Breathing volatile substances is most likely to be done by children and adolescents, and by adults who have specific access to such substances in the workplace. Signs of inhalant use can include sneezing, coughing, nosebleeds, and difficulty concentrating.

URINE TESTING

Urine tests to detect drug use have been available since the late 1970s (see Appendix B). The issue of widespread testing didn't become a major public concern until 1986, when President Ronald Reagan issued an executive order requiring all federal agencies to achieve a "drug-free workplace." Congress subsequently required implementation of that order to include testing all job applicants, plus employees suspected of drug use. The mandatory requirements specify testing for marijuana, cocaine, opiates, amphetamines, and phencyclidine.

More recently, the Department of Transportation has required the testing of private employees involved with mass transit. This group comprises employees of businesses that do work for the Federal Aviation Administration, Federal Highway Administration, Federal Railroad Administration, U.S. Coast Guard, Urban Mass Transit Administration, and the Special Research and Special Program Administration (including workers operating pipelines and those who produce and store liquid natural gas). All told, more than 4 million employees will be affected.

In a decision that will accelerate the move toward mandatory testing of new employees outside federal agencies and the military, the U.S. Supreme Court in March 1989 upheld the constitutionality of drug testing over challenges by employees of the U.S. Customs Service and the Federal Railroad Administration. However, as far as local municipalities are concerned, in June 1990 a federal judge declared the mandatory urine testing of all New York City Transit employees unconstitutional, deciding that mandatory testing was appropriate only for "safety sensitive positions." And, in November 1990, a U.S. Court of Appeals in the District of Columbia struck down regulations allowing the Department of Agriculture to test employees suspected of off-duty drug use if such use did not impair performance. This issue is thus still far from resolved.

According to a 1984 survey by the Employees Management Association, only 3 percent of the surveyed companies conducted urine tests of job applicants or new employees. By 1988, the numbers had risen to 30 percent, with 21 percent also testing current employees.

Moreover, half of the larger Fortune 500 companies engaged in urine testing in 1988, compared with only 18 percent in 1985. Fueled in no small way by the Office of Management and Budget's 1989 directive to firms with federal contracts to screen all employees, many smaller companies can be expected to begin testing programs. In 1989, the Bureau of Labor Statistics estimated that 20 percent of Americans work in businesses with drug-testing policies.

Concern about drugs in the workplace is understandable. In 1985 drug use cost U.S. industries more than $36 billion in lost productivity, medical expenses, thefts, and damages. The National Institute on Drug Abuse estimates that one in every five employees between the ages of 18 and 25, and one in every eight employees between 26 and 34, uses drugs at work.

VALUE OF IDENTIFYING THE DRUG USER

Use of illegal substances by people in sensitive positions, or in jobs critical to the safety of others, cannot be condoned. In fact, these people should not use *any* mood-altering drug, and that includes alcohol, probably responsible for most of the breaches of security and accidents at work. The existence of a drug-testing program states clearly that such use will not be condoned, and may serve as a deterrent to some employees. But when a person tests positive for, say, alcohol, but there's no evidence of impaired job performance, is further action warranted?

That's not an academic question. Some years ago several transit system employees in a large city were summarily dismissed when methadone was found in their urine. Their dismissal was upheld by the U.S. Supreme Court, based on the ability of the transit system authority to hire and fire whomever it pleases.

The former president's executive order makes clear that illegal drug use by itself is incompatible with federal employment. But again, if use is sporadic, recreational, and not accompanied by impairment, should the person be at risk of losing his or her job? The order establishes Employees Assistance Programs and states that no employee can be discharged or disciplined if he or she voluntarily seeks counseling or treatment. Thus identification may facilitate treatment. But it is unclear whether counseling is needed or effective for sporadic use of such drugs as alcohol or marijuana if such substances are not used on the job or when the person must report to work.

REFERRAL FOR TREATMENT

An impressive array of programs exists for the treatment of alcoholism and drug dependency. They're supported to varying degrees by public funds, third-party carriers, and private fees. Interest in providing more insurance coverage is growing; more than 36 states now require that some degree of "substance-abuse" coverage be offered.

On October 30, 1987, approximately 600,000 people were being treated in 6,866 alcohol and drug programs nationwide. Those are the most recent statistics from the National Drug and Alcoholism Treatment Survey (NDATUS), a joint effort by the National Institute on Drug Abuse, the National Institute on Alcohol Abuse and Alcoholism, the Veterans Administration, and the Federal Prison System. Other NDATUS findings for that date:

- Of the treatment programs, 14 percent were private for-profit facilities, 65 percent private nonprofit; 17 percent were run by states, 2 percent by the federal government. The majority of patients—60 percent—were in private nonprofit facilities.
- Of all patients, 57 percent had a primary alcohol problem; 43 percent were mainly drug dependent. Of the drug-dependent, 42 percent had been using drugs intravenously.
- In the previous 12 months, the programs treated approximately 2.2 million people—63 percent primarily for alcohol, 37 percent primarily for drugs.
- Approximately 15 percent of each group were treated primarily as inpatients, the rest as outpatients.

The National Institute on Drug Abuse estimated that there were 4 million drug users in the United States in 1988. Further estimates are that 25 percent could stop using drugs with the support of friends, family, and clergy; that 25 percent are unwilling or unable to stop;

but that the rest—2 million people—would benefit from well-designed treatment programs.

Whether enough programs are available to provide such care has been debated, as has the estimate of 4 million serious drug users. Those who urge rapid expansion of treatment programs cite long waiting lists (especially for intravenous users) to get into maintenance programs. Critics claim that many place their names on multiple waiting lists and don't bother to remove their names once they're accepted for treatment.

According to the NDATUS data base, overall utilization of treatment slots was 81 percent, with private for-profit programs having the lowest rates (64 percent) and public-funded state programs the highest (90 percent). Seven states had a utilization rate over 90 percent, with New Hampshire, Utah, and Louisiana reaching 100 percent, and West Virginia reporting 107 percent.

So while a considerable number of people are in treatment, treatment on request is far from guaranteed. What's more, the relatively low utilization rates for private for-profit facilities suggest that many who want help have neither the personal resources nor the necessary insurance coverage to afford treatment.

AVAILABLE TREATMENT MODALITIES

The types of treatment opportunities are varied and frequently cut across specific types of drug dependency. Often a facility or modality will use more than one therapeutic alternative. Below are brief descriptions of the various treatment programs and modalities, presented in alphabetical order. Additional information is given in chapters that describe specific treatment for a particular drug.

Acupuncture.   Acupunture has been used for several years—primarily for narcotic addiction but also for other addictions (Chapter 11). Proponents claim good success rates in decreasing withdrawal symptoms, promoting general relaxation, and enhancing the ability to remain drug-free. But those claims have not been evaluated objectively. A National Acupuncture Detoxification Association was formed in 1985 to evaluate and support acupuncture in treating drug dependency. As of this writing, only a few well-designed studies have been conducted.

Behavioral Therapies. Behavioral therapy is based on the belief that dependence on mood-altering drugs is learned behavior, maintained and reinforced by conditioning caused by the drugs independent of other psychosocial conditions. It teaches the user to understand the relationship between the thought process that initiated use and the actual initiation. Therapy is directed toward developing behaviors that are incompatible with drug use and avoiding situations associated with a high risk of recidivism.

Behavior therapies range from contingency contracting (an agreement between patient and therapist that results in rewards and/or punishment) to aversive conditioning to extinction of conditioned behavior.

Aversive conditioning diminishes use or the desire to use drugs through the administration of unpleasant stimuli, for example, disulfiram (Antabuse) for alcoholism (Chapter 6). In "extinction" behavior therapy, the addict takes a prescription drug to block the pleasure and other positive reinforcement associated with drug use; the narcotic antagonist naltrexone (Trexan) has been used in this way with heroin addiction. Relaxation techniques, biofeedback, and desensitization procedures are other forms of conditioning that are also employed. Unlike the classic psychotherapeutic approach, conditioning is usually a time-limited process.

Comprehensive Outpatient Treatment. Outpatient programs offer a variety of services from drop-in centers to free clinics and formal counseling. They provide educational, medical, psychological, and rehabilitative services related to substance use, and may meet other medical needs of the community. Such programs account for half of the people in treatment, and they allow easy access for those unwilling or unable to make a greater time commitment. In that respect, they can serve as the second step after detoxification.

Counseling and Employee Assistance Programs. Counseling is conducted by trained counselors, social workers, and psychologists,

as well as by those without formal degrees whose experience and
training equip them for the job. In itself, counseling is the most basic
form of therapy. It deals with the practical problems of both client
and family members, providing support and appropriate referrals.

In the workplace, counseling is offered through Employee Assistance Programs (EAPs). They serve as resources for those identified as having an alcohol or drug problem. A good EAP provides
education to employees and their families about alcohol and drug
use, and develops among management a better general knowledge
of drug dependency and how to spot it before it becomes a major
problem.

EAPs were slow in getting started because of the costs involved.
But they've been increasing at a growing rate since the Office for
Work Place Initiatives was instituted by the National Institute on
Drug Abuse. Acknowledgment by many states that health-care insurance should be made available for drug dependency treatment has
also facilitated their development.

Even though there are an estimated 10,000 EAPs across the United
States, and despite evidence that they're effective for both employer
and employee, only 30 percent of the work force has access to these
programs.

Detoxification.   The first step in starting drug therapy in cases
involving a high degree of physical dependency is detoxification. It
allows gradual withdrawal with minimal discomfort. Both inpatient
and outpatient detoxification units can provide immediate relief from
heroin use. But detoxification is not rehabilitation. It merely sets the
stage for entering a therapeutic relationship.

Detoxification is often accomplished by decreasing the dose of the
drug on which the patient is dependent, but more commonly by
substituting another cross-tolerant drug. Thus diazepam (Valium) or
phenobarbital is used to detoxify from central nervous system depressants, and methadone from heroin. At times, a drug such as
clonidine (Catapres) may be administered for quicker withdrawal
from heroin without withdrawal symptoms (Chapter 11). Clonidine
is also recommended to relieve nicotine withdrawal symptoms
(Chapter 14). Cocaine withdrawal can be accomplished without med-

ication, but symptoms are often severe enough to require treatment. In such cases, the antidepressant desipramine (Norpramin) has been found to be effective (Chapter 13).

Detoxification has a number of benefits beyond serving as the first step in drug therapy:

- It protects the dependent user from the hazards of seeking illicit drugs.
- It protects society from the user's antisocial behavior to get money for drugs.
- It encourages the user to consider a longer and more productive therapeutic relationship in a suitable facility.
- It allows existing medical problems to be identified and appropriately addressed.
- It offers users the opportunity to get their lives in order once the cycle of drug dependency has been broken.

Family Therapy.   This therapy helps foster development of a healthy interrelationship among family members as a prime motivating factor in getting off drugs.

Pharmacologic Therapies.   After detoxification, a number of pharmacologic methods exist to help a person stay off drugs.

Antabuse therapies.   Disulfiram (Antabuse) is one of the oldest forms of "modern" pharmacotherapy (Chapter 6). It causes an unpleasant and sometimes frightening reaction when combined with alcohol, thus preventing the alcohol user from drinking. For this therapy to be effective, however, the alcoholic must be sufficiently motivated to take Antabuse every day, and sufficiently frightened by the intensity of the reaction to refrain from drinking.

Maintenance therapies.   These therapies are provided for those who can't stop using narcotics despite repeated attempts at detoxification or other therapies. Any narcotic drug can be used in maintenance, but the only approved drug is methadone (Chapter 11).

Narcotic (opiate) antagonists.   The rationale for administering a narcotic antagonist is to prevent the addict from experiencing the pleasurable effects of a narcotic. That lowers the addict's incentive to continue exposing himself or herself to risks. It's a form of behavioral therapy involving a process called "extinction." The FDA approved drug is naltrexone (Trexan) (Chapter 10). Like Antabuse, the drug must be taken regularly to be effective.

Miscellaneous drug therapies.   Other drugs, known as psychotropic agents, are used when an underlying psychologic disturbance exists regardless of drug dependency. A variety of drugs have been suggested to eliminate the craving for cocaine: amantadine (Symmetrel), bromocryptine (Parlodel), various antidepressants, buprenorphine, an opioid antagonist (Chapter 10), and flupenthixol, an antidepressant agent. Effectiveness of all these agents remains to be determined.

Psychotherapy.   Provided by psychologists, social workers, rehabilitation counselors, and/or psychiatrists, psychotherapy may be part of a comprehensive outpatient program or just a one-to-one relationship with a therapist. It can vary in intensity, depending on the client's needs and the particular training and belief of the therapist. By allowing the client to understand his or her behavior, a rationale for change is developed. Initially thought to be ineffective because of the severe personality disturbances accompanying addiction, psychotherapy alone, or in combination with other modalities, is now known to be helpful.

Self-Help Groups.   Well-organized self-help groups have had a major impact on helping alcoholics and others with chemical dependencies to maintain productive, drug-free lives. The oldest and best known, Alcoholics Anonymous (AA), has chapters in every major city in the United States, as well as in many other countries (Chapter 6). It was developed and is run by "nonprofessionals." The only qualification for admission is self-recognition of a dependency problem and a desire to be helped.

Residential Therapeutic Communities.   Changing the personal characteristics that led the drug user into taking drugs is the target of residential therapeutic communities (Chapter 11). Since Synanon was founded in the 1950s, a large number of such programs have been developed. As described by George DeLeon, therapeutic communities can be distinguished from other forms of treatment in two main ways:

1. Almost all their primary therapists and staff have themselves completed a recovery process. As successful role models, they offer continuous support as they instill appropriate behavior backed by their own rehabilitation experience.
2. Addiction or drug use is viewed more as a symptom than as a problem. Detoxification, therefore, becomes a preliminary step toward entering the therapeutic process, rather than the goal. The ultimate objective is being able to cope with stress without needing any pharmacologic support.

As a result of that philosophy, many therapeutic communities—unlike other treatment facilities—are amenable to admitting people with multiple drug problems, including alcohol. The therapeutic experience may require living in the community for up to two years and passing through successive stages of increasing responsibility, ending in the reentry phase: maintaining contact with the community while living outside it and being engaged in productive activity. Commitment to the process must be total, so there is a large dropout rate.

CIVIL COMMITMENT

Civil commitment entails forcing drug users into therapy regardless of their desire for help. It is not a new idea. By 1938, facilities to treat and rehabilitate narcotic offenders had been established at Lexington, Kentucky, and Fort Worth, Texas. Ostensibly under the auspices of the U.S. Public Health Service, the facilities were in fact supervised by the Federal Bureau of Narcotics and the Justice Department. The result was closer to a prison than a rehabilitation center.

In 1944, the Public Health Service Act led to a program for management of narcotic dependency at these centers. Since then, thousands of persons have entered the hospitals at Lexington and Fort Worth. But while these facilities have produced a great deal of clinical research on the complications and effects of narcotics, their effect on rehabilitation has been minimal, with relapse rates as high as 90 percent.

A number of states have experimented with varying forms of civil commitment. Under California's 1962 Metcalf Voker Law, arrested narcotics addicts could request civil commitment in lieu of prosecution. Charges would be dropped if they successfully completed this program and then practiced abstinence and good behavior over the next three years. The California civil commitment program then established comparable guidelines, allowing a person to request commitment in a state rehabilitation center from several months to years.

In 1966 the Narcotic Addict Rehabilitation Act (NARA) empowered the federal government, rather than the state, to commit narcotic users not previously charged with any criminal offense. But those committed under this act had a high recidivism rate, with up to 45 percent using an opiate almost as soon as they left the program. To date, the general experience with civil commitment has been unsatisfactory.

Nevertheless, advocates of civil commitment programs say they can be successful only when rehabilitation facilities are effective *and* when those who leave treatment prematurely are forced to return to the legal system for sentencing. As concern over escalating drug use has risen, so has consideration of civil commitment. So far, 19 states have civil commitment laws. They vary from those that let parents commit children suspected of drug use to those that commit individuals convicted of violating state drug laws. New York State, for example, had considered large drug treatment compounds, or "campuses," on federal lands for rehabilitating addicts after civil commitment, as well as for those seeking voluntary treatment. A variety of treatment strategies may be implemented on these "campuses" along with stringent sanctions against those who have been committed but leave before completing therapy.

EVALUATION OF TREATMENT

Despite the wide variety of facilities, evaluation of their effectiveness has not been satisfactory. Published studies are usually subject to serious criticism.

Failure to develop well-designed studies isn't surprising. It's difficult to find treatment and nontreatment groups adequately matched for age, sex, socioeconomic levels, and reasons for seeking treatment. Incentive to enter treatment is often related to the need for keeping a job, staying out of jail, or maintaining a family.

Success is usually measured in terms of the number of patients who complete the program and remain abstinent rather than by the number who drop out. Success also may be measured in terms of continuing abstinence from the drug that caused dependency rather than abstinence from alcohol and all other mood-altering drugs. Follow-up studies tend to be relatively short and depend on questionnaires completed by former clients, which may not be reliable. Underlying psychological disturbances can also skew the outcome. Some approaches to treatment may not be socially acceptable and therefore can't get funding for studies. Such approaches include controlled drinking and acupuncture. Correspondingly, the intense feelings of some professionals toward specific techniques can prevent opposing findings from being heard. Studies have revealed no differences in success rates of inpatient versus outpatient treatment of alcoholism, but they have shown a much more favorable cost-benefit analysis for outpatient treatment. Yet inpatient therapy remains more commonly accepted.

Several large-scale, nationwide evaluations of drug treatment have been made. The first, the Drug Abuse Reporting Program (DARP), under the auspices of the Institute for Behavioral Research of Texas Christian University, followed more than 44,000 clients in 52 programs from 1969 through 1974. The study compared methadone maintenance programs, therapeutic communities, outpatient programs, and detoxification clinics. Leaving out detoxification clinics, there were no differences in effectiveness among the other three modalities.

The Treatment Outcome Prospective Study (TOPS) followed 11,000 drug-dependent people in 41 programs in 10 cities who entered treatment from 1979 through 1981. They were followed from one month after starting treatment and at three-month intervals during treatment. Representatives from each group were interviewed three months after leaving treatment, and then at one-, two-, and three- to five-year intervals.

The TOPS study found that treatment was effective for up to five years after a single treatment episode, regardless of treatment program used. The time spent in treatment, regardless of treatment program, was the single most important contributing factor.

Compared with those who stayed in therapeutic communities less than three months, those who stayed more than one year were significantly less likely to report regular use of drugs and were three times more likely to be employed full-time. Similar results were observed for those in outpatient treatment for at least six months or on methadone maintenance continuously for at least two to three years. Those on methadone for at least one year were less likely to use heroin than those on the drug for less time; those on methadone for two to three years were four times less likely to use heroin and three times less likely to commit crimes.

The cost-benefit analysis of drug treatment as opposed to jailing addicts and treating their medical complications was decidedly positive. Both methadone and residential programs showed a tax-dollar savings ratio of 4:1.

Unfortunately, but not surprisingly, the TOPS found considerable limitations in the ability of treatment programs to appreciably change the lives of those in therapy by reintegrating them into society and providing full-time employment.

Social use of marijuana and alcohol changed minimally. Depression improved considerably during treatment, but deteriorated somewhat immediately after treatment, then leveled off in subsequent years. That's to be expected, unless the reasons that people turn to drugs are viewed as equally important as the actual drug use. Abstinence can be maintained for long periods only by a few.

Despite controversy over the "best method" for a specific addict or addiction, there's little doubt that treatment is better than no treatment. And it's reasonable to assume that people tend to choose the type of therapy that's most comfortable for them, thus maximizing their own success rates. Matching patients to treatment alternatives through careful evaluation of individuals is most likely to produce the greatest success.

AFTER TREATMENT

The depression that can follow completion of treatment for drug dependency has been described by Dr. Forrest Tenant as Post Drug-Impairment Syndrome (PDIS): on returning to the community at large, the individual feels fragile in the face of the everyday stresses of life and has difficulty relating to friends and concentrating on ordinary problems. The urge to resume drug use begins to resurface.

Intensity of the syndrome varies and doesn't always cause problems. But certain steps can help minimize its effects and thus maximize chances for successful abstinence. Counseling during the last phases of treatment, and afterward, is of prime importance. So is community involvement in job placement. A job provides a purpose in life and lessens the amount of aimless free time that breeds a craving for drugs.

A strong social environment, especially a stable family unit, is also essential. The lack of such an environment is particularly significant for the homeless. Many are amenable to entering treatment facilities, but they quickly go back to drug use when they're released.

Coercing a person into treatment and abstinence with "or-else" threats of jail or job loss is effective only to the extent that the person has something to lose by not complying. Treatment is often successful among such top-dollar professionals as airline pilots and physicians. Their attractive and highly paid work serves as strong motivation to get off and stay off drugs.

PART II

MOOD-ALTERING DRUGS

Chapter 6

Alcohol

If, when you say whisky, you mean the devil's brew, the poison scourge, the bloody monster that defiles innocence, yea, literally takes the bread from the mouths of little children; if you mean the evil drink that topples the Christian man and woman from the pinnacles of righteous, gracious living into the bottomless pit of degradation and despair, shame and helplessness and hopelessness, then certainly I am against it with all of my power.

But, if when you say whisky, you mean the oil of conversation, the philosophic wine, the stuff that is consumed when good fellows get together, that puts a song in their hearts and laughter on their lips and the warm glow of contentment in their eyes; if you mean Christmas cheer; if you mean the stimulating drink that puts the spring in the old gentleman's step on a frosty morning; if you mean the drink that enables a man to magnify his joy and his happiness, and to forget, if only for a little while, life's great tragedies and heartbreaks and sorrows; if you mean that drink, the sale of which pours into our treasuries untold millions of dollars, which are used to provide tender care for our little crippled children, our blind, our deaf, our dumb, our pitiful aged and infirm, to build highways, hospitals and schools, then certainly I am in favor of it.*

—a state senator addressing Mississippi legislature, 1958

* From D.W. Goodwin, *Alcoholism: The Facts* (Toronto: Oxford University Press, 1981).

Alcohol remains the one mood-altering substance viewed with considerable ambivalence by the American public. It's been around since the founding of the country, when its use was widespread and considered almost a necessity at every social gathering. The erratic or rowdy behavior associated with excessive drinking during the eighteenth century was blamed more on a person's companions than on the drinking itself. Average Americans then consumed greater quantities of alcohol than they do today.

Concern over the adverse effects of alcohol developed during the nineteenth century and grew into the temperance and prohibitionist movement, culminating in 1919 with ratification of the Eighteenth Amendment (prohibiting the production, sale, and transportation of alcohol for use in beverages) and passage of the Volstead Act to enforce it. Prohibition lasted until 1933, when the Twenty-first Amendment repealed the Eighteenth.

Since then, drinking has become an accepted part of our way of life. But there is still controversy. Advocates claim that *moderate* social drinking facilitates communication, allows a person to relax after a hard day, assists those unable to sleep, and diminishes chances of heart attack. Critics say that drinking increases antisocial behavior that puts the user and public at risk, causes severe illness and death, places unborn children at risk, and facilitates the use of illicit drugs. Without question, *excessive* consumption of and dependency on alcohol is associated with a wide array of adverse psychological, physical, and societal effects.

PATTERNS OF USE

In 1985 approximately 10 percent of adult Americans (18 million) were using alcohol excessively, including some 7.5 million who had undergone a serious crisis such as loss of job, divorce, or a medical problem as a result of drinking.

Four to five times more people use alcohol than use any other mood-altering drug; three to four times more use alcohol excessively or are dependent on it than any other mood-altering drug. Roughly one-third of Americans are nondrinkers, one-third light drinkers, and one-third light to moderate drinkers.

In 1987, the most recent year for which reliable figures are available, the average per capita consumption of pure alcohol (in all beverages) by Americans was 2.54 gallons. Take the one-out-of-three nondrinkers out of the calculation, and per capita consumption jumps to almost four gallons. That's equivalent to 56 gallons of beer, 20 gallons of wine, or six gallons of distilled spirits. Not to be overlooked is that almost half the alcohol was consumed by only 10 percent of the population. These figures are lower than those reported in the previous three decades. Nonetheless, that year over 1.4 million people in this country were treated for excessive alcohol consumption or dependency. And, as documented in the 1988 National Household Survey on Drug Abuse, approximately 106 million of the U.S. household population age 12 and over had consumed alcohol within the month preceding the survey.

COSTS OF DRINKING

Alcohol is responsible for a multitude of medical problems—up to 40 percent of general medical hospital admissions, and perhaps 20 percent of the nation's total expenditure for medical care.

Estimates of alcohol-related deaths range from 50,000 to 200,000 per year. These include accidents, homicides, and suicide—where alcohol is implicated in about half the cases. One study shows a significant relationship between number of drinks per occasion and incidence of fatal injury: those who had five or more drinks were more than twice as likely to die from injuries as those who drank less.

Excessive drinking doesn't affect only the drinker. Approximately 40,000 newborns each year are at risk of fetal alcohol syndrome (Chapter 18), one of the three leading causes of birth defects. Up to 15 million school-age children live with at least one alcoholic parent. Altogether, about 28 million (one out of every eight) Americans are children of alcoholics. Many experience a wide variety of emotional problems that often last well into adulthood.

Alcohol use also puts children in general at risk. A survey by the National Council on Alcoholism indicated that almost 30 percent of fourth graders were encouraged by peers to try alcoholic beverages.

Three of every 10 teenagers (4.6 million) have experienced problems with alcohol. A New York State survey found that 11 percent of students in grades seven through 12 were "hooked" on alcohol: the average age at which they began drinking was 13.

Money lost because of alcohol use, put at $117 billion in 1987, may reach approximately $150 billion per year by 1995. Half of those arrested on criminal charges are believed to have been drinking while committing the crime. Traffic accidents are the leading cause of death in young adults. Of the 47,093 traffic fatalities in 1988, alcohol was implicated in approximately 40 percent. Roughly half the daytime fatalities on weekends involve drunk driving. The numbers climb to about 60 percent on weekend nights. Alcohol and other drugs are believed responsible for more than a half million nonfatal injuries a year; two out of five Americans will be involved in an alcohol-related accident in their lifetimes, and nearly half of all fatally injured drivers will have significant levels of alcohol in their blood. Total cost to society for these accidents is approximately $74 billion a year.

COMMON ALCOHOLIC BEVERAGES

The three basic types of alcoholic beverages are wines, beer, and distilled spirits. Fermented fruit juices and their distillation produce brandies; addition of sugar or other flavorings produce liqueurs or cordials. Wines, dessert wines, wine coolers, and sherry or port can be produced by varying the quantity of alcohol or sugar. This results in a total of seven groups of beverages (Table 6.1): beers and ales, distilled spirits, liqueurs (brandies, cordials, port, sherry), table wines, dessert wines, wine coolers, and hard cider. The volume of alcohol in those beverages varies, so consumption must be compared in terms of absolute alcohol. For example, one ounce of absolute alcohol is considered equal to two cans of beer, or two glasses of wine, or two 1.5-ounce drinks of distilled spirits. The term "proof," used to describe potency, refers to twice the alcohol content by volume. Thus a drink that is 80 proof is 40 percent alcohol.

The concept of equivalency is important because of the common

TABLE 6.1
Alcohol in Common Beverages
Based on serving sizes of 12 ounces for beer,
4 ounces for table wine and hard cider, 3 ounces for dessert wine,
8 ounces of a wine cooler, and 1.5 ounces for liqueurs and
distilled spirits

Beverage	Percent by Volume	Proof	Amount per Serving oz	gms
Beers and ales	3–6	6–12	0.36–0.72	10–20
Distilled spirits	25–50	50–100	0.52–0.75	7–21
Hard ciders	8–15	16–30	0.32–0.60	9–17
Liqueurs	20–55	40–110	0.30–0.90	6–15
Wines				
Dessert wines	15–20	30–40	0.45–0.6	14–17
Table wines	8–14	16–28	0.32–0.56	9–17
Wine coolers	1.5–3	3–6	0.12–0.24	3–7

misconception that a glass of wine or beer has less alcohol than a mixed drink or a "shot." In fact, all have roughly the same quantity of alcohol. A person who drinks two double shots a day is consuming a considerable quantity of alcohol, but no more than someone drinking four beers or four glasses of wine.

Popularity of particular alcoholic beverages changes. In 1988 beer accounted for 51 percent of the alcohol consumed, wine 14 percent, and distilled spirits 35 percent. Wine coolers, the newest type of beverage, were increasingly consumed through most of the 1980s until their popularity began to lessen. Currently, nonalcoholic or dealcoholized wines and beers are becoming popular. It is important to realize that some of these drinks may not be completely alcohol free but contain less than 0.5 percent alcohol. Those sensitive to

TABLE 6.2
Components of Alcoholic Beverages

Aldehydes	Fusel oils	Sugars
Amino acids	Ketones	Sulfites
Esters	Minerals	Tannins
Ethanol	Other alcohols	Vitamins
Fungal products		

alcohol should make certain the beverage is labeled alcohol free rather than nonalcoholic.

OVER-THE-COUNTER (OTC) MEDICATIONS

A large number of over-the-counter (OTC) medications—antihistamines, cough syrups, mouthwash, asthma medications, and other drugs—contain alcohol in varying amounts, up to 60 percent in some. The alcohol content of these drugs is usually of little concern because they're taken in relatively small quantities. But not always. Someone with asthma or chronic bronchitis who takes three tablespoons of a theophylline elixir four to five times a day is consuming up to 1.5 ounces of pure alcohol. That's roughly equivalent to 10 ounces of table wine, 2.4 ounces of distilled spirits, or 30 ounces of beer. In such instances, especially in the presence of other underlying medical problems, the alcohol could produce adverse effects.

HOW ALCOHOL IS HANDLED BY THE BODY

Alcohol's effects on the brain depend on quantity consumed, rates of absorption, distribution, which in turn is affected by weight, elimination, and the sensitivity of particular tissues to alcohol or its metabolites.

Absorption of Alcohol. Alcohol is readily absorbed into the bloodstream from the stomach and intestinal tract (about 25 percent of alcohol from the stomach; the rest from the small intestine). The rate of absorption, however, varies greatly among people, as well as in the same person, depending on a number of factors. They include the pattern of drinking, rate of consumption, tolerance to alcohol (based on previous exposure), food in the stomach, and type of beverage. Food in the stomach can decrease the blood alcohol level by about 30 percent; an empty stomach results in a markedly increased absorption.

Distribution of Alcohol. Once absorbed, alcohol is quickly distributed throughout the body, with the concentration in the brain about the same as in the bloodstream. However, for a given quantity of alcohol, blood alcohol concentrations are less in a heavier person than in a thin one, and the effects are felt more acutely earlier on.

Metabolism of Alcohol. Almost all alcohol is completely metabolized (broken down) in the liver. New research has demonstrated that alcohol begins to be metabolized first in the stomach, not in the liver as previously believed. This first breakdown results from the action of alcohol dehydrogenase, an enzyme. When the enzyme's action is diminished—as happens when drinking on an empty stomach and in chronic alcoholics—the body's tissues receive greater amounts of alcohol.

The investigators also showed that women tend to have less alcohol dehydrogenase in their stomach linings and therefore absorb more alcohol than men. Thus women tend to become more intoxicated than men and are more vulnerable to the damaging effects of alcohol on the liver, and to the potentially detrimental effects on the fetus of even small quantities of alcohol.

Alcohol is mainly oxidized by enzymes in the liver, forming acetaldehyde. Two enzyme systems are involved in the metabolism of alcohol to acetaldehyde: the microsomal enzyme oxidizing system (MEOS) and alcohol dehydrogenase. The MEOS also breaks down several other drugs, such as acetaminophen (Tylenol) and many barbiturates and tranquilizers. The effect of alcohol on the MEOS can result in alcohol-drug interactions that either increase or diminish the effects of the other drugs.

Alcohol dehydrogenase accounts for most of the metabolic process at low blood alcohol levels. As the levels increase, the MEOS becomes more active, an important phenomenon because of the effect that the system has on metabolism of other drugs.

When isoniazid (INH), a drug used to treat tuberculosis, is metabolized by the MEOS, a metabolite toxic to the liver is produced. For that reason, adverse effects of INH are common in alcoholics.

The commonly used painkiller acetaminophen is acted upon in a similar manner. Since Tylenol and other similar drugs are taken in large doses by alcoholics to relieve headaches, the potential for liver damage exists. It is important to note that once activated, the MEOS may remain active for some time, even in the absence of alcohol. So toxic effects can result when acetaminophen is taken for withdrawal symptoms.

Although long-term administration of alcohol activates the MEOS, acute drinking of a large quantity of alcohol has the opposite effect. Thus the metabolism of other drugs usually deactivated by the MEOS is inhibited. That affects tranquilizers, barbiturates, and methadone, the blood and brain levels of which are enhanced with consumption of large amounts of alcohol. So when someone who has been drinking large quantities of alcohol takes one of those drugs to get to sleep, the potential for overdose is real.

Acetaldehyde is extremely toxic. When it accumulates in the bloodstream, it can cause flushing, headaches, and rapid heartbeat. This reaction is the basis of the disulfiram (Antabuse) reaction.

A diet consisting mainly of alcohol lacks vitamins and minerals. Relying on alcohol as the main source of calories (even when caloric intake is adequate) leads to deficiencies and breakdown of the body's protein stores, resulting in a number of medical complications. Even when a healthy diet is eaten, chronic alcohol use can prevent the body from effectively using the nutrients, impairing absorption as well as metabolism of vitamins, proteins, carbohydrates, and minerals.

Approximately 2 percent of alcohol is excreted unchanged through the kidneys and the lungs. Excretion through the breath reflects the alcohol concentration in the blood, the basis of the Breathalyzer test for intoxication.

INTOXICATION

Alcohol is popularly perceived as a stimulant. It isn't. It's a depressant. As consumption progresses, the areas in the brain that normally inhibit behavior are depressed, leaving unopposed those brain centers that facilitate behavior. Virtually everyone has witnessed the strong antisocial behavior that sometimes results when large quantities of alcohol are drunk. But as the amount consumed goes up, general central nervous system depression sets in. So at low doses alcohol appears to be a stimulant, until its actual depressant effects become visible as the dose increases.

How fast an individual becomes intoxicated depends on many factors—body weight, food in the stomach, alcohol metabolism rate in both stomach and liver, tolerance to specific alcohol, beverage strength, other mood-altering drugs in the system, and even the environment.

The most common way to correlate impairment with alcohol consumption is through alcohol content in the body. Alcohol is easily measured in the blood and urine, but blood alcohol level is the standard measurement for impairment and intoxication. Breathalyzer tests are frequently administered by police. They're both quick and fairly accurate in pinpointing blood alcohol concentrations.

Blood alcohol levels (BAL) are expressed as milligrams per deciliter (mg/dL), grams per deciliter (g/dL), or more commonly as percent by volume. In most states intoxication is defined as a blood alcohol concentration of 100 mg/dL (0.10 g/dL), or 0.10 percent.

Performance can be affected at much lower levels. In various studies, 14 to 68 percent of tested subjects were diagnosed as intoxicated with blood levels of 0.05 to 0.10 percent. On an individual basis, impairment may be detected at levels as low as 0.02 percent (Table 6.3). Clearly, using a 0.10 percent BAL to define the threshold for driving while intoxicated is not very helpful—a shortcoming recognized by the surgeon general, who recommended decreasing the level to a 0.08 percent BAL by 1990, and to 0.04 percent by the year 2000. And for those under 21 years of age, no BAL would be acceptable.

TABLE 6.3
Effect of Blood Alcohol Levels on Performance

Level	Volume (%)	Impairment	Number of Drinks Consumed*
20–30	0.02–0.03	Increased reaction time, altered mood, diminished critical thinking, diminished fine motor control	1
50–99	0.05–0.09	Possible impairment resulting in accident	2 to 3
100	0.10	Evidence of driving while intoxicated	3 to 4
150	0.15	Grossly intoxicated	4 to 5
400	0.40	Average concentrations in fatal cases; death usually the result of depression of brain's respiratory center	

* Numbers given are estimates based on a person weighing 150 pounds. Effect varies depending on body weight and other factors that affect absorption.

Food in the stomach greatly affects BAL. A BAL of 0.10 percent can be reached quickly after two glasses of wine (or equivalent) on an empty stomach; after three glasses if drunk an hour or two after a meal. Four ounces of whisky on an empty stomach result in a BAL of 0.67 to 0.92 percent; the same amount after a meal would result in a BAL of about 0.3 to 0.5 percent.

EFFECTS OF ENVIRONMENT

What an individual expects from a drink, and the setting in which it's consumed, are also important determinants of intoxication. People who don't know they're drinking alcohol become intoxicated at a slow rate. People who think they're drinking beverages containing alcohol (but which don't) show remarkable mood changes. A person can become high drinking in a social setting more quickly than when drinking alone. Compared with people who don't anticipate positive mood changes from alcohol, those who expect pleasurable effects tend to be more likely to become heavy drinkers, to drink when confronted with stress, and are less able to handle stress when they're abstinent.

Alcohol is metabolized in an adult at a rate of approximately one-fourth to one-third of an ounce (7 to 10 grams) per hour—about equal to two-thirds to one ounce of distilled spirits, or 8 to 12 ounces of beer. Limiting consumption to the rate of metabolism can keep a person's BAL under 0.10 percent. Genetic variations cause some people to metabolize alcohol much more slowly than others. These people rarely get drunk because even one glass of wine can produce headache, flushing, or dizziness.

As tolerance develops, larger quantities of alcohol must be drunk to produce intoxication. Tolerance results from either a more rapid metabolism rate or a function of alcohol on the central nervous system. With tolerance, some people can appear to perform at acceptable levels with a BAL higher than 0.20 percent. But tolerance doesn't always rise to lethal levels of blood alcohol, so respiratory depression and death can follow soon after rapidly drinking large quantities of alcohol. Drinking large amounts in a relatively short time can also cause an alcoholic blackout, an acute loss of memory surrounding the immediate drinking episode without impairment of long-term memory.

INTERACTION WITH OTHER DRUGS

As a central nervous system depressant, alcohol exhibits cross-tolerance and cross-dependence with all other CNS depressant drugs (Chapter 3). As discussed earlier, chronic drinking increases activity of the MEOS in the liver that breaks down CNS drugs, making higher dosages necessary to provide the same effect. But when alcohol is taken acutely, or the BAL rises swiftly, the MEOS is inhibited, and the person is then susceptible to the combined depressant effects of alcohol and the other CNS depressant. Overdose is a frequent complication, so taking sleeping pills after a night of heavy drinking can be hazardous.

Alcohol can also interact with other drugs, including oral anticoagulants, anticonvulsants, antidepressants, and painkillers. When interacting with drugs for diabetes, a marked lowering of blood sugar (hypoglycemia) can result. The same effect is likely with insulin, because alcohol can decrease the rate at which insulin is broken down in the body.

The use of aspirin and alcohol may increase the chances of gastrointestinal bleeding, especially in persons with a history of peptic ulcers. Medications taken by people with peptic ulcers or hyperacidity, called histamine H_2 receptor blockers (Tagamet, Rantidine), may also effect alcohol metabolism by decreasing the activity of the enzyme alcohol dehydrogenase in the stomach. As discussed in the section on Antabuse, a drug used to prevent drinking, a number of drugs have Antabuse-like activity and, in susceptible individuals, can cause adverse reactions when a person taking these medicines drinks.

DEPENDENCY AND WITHDRAWAL

Chronic and excessive alcohol consumption leads to dependency and then leads to severe withdrawal symptoms when drinking stops. Untreated, the withdrawal reaction progresses through four stages,

TABLE 6.4
Alcohol Withdrawal Symptoms Requiring Treatment

Rapid heart rate, shortness of breath, chills, fever of 100.5° F
Chest pain
Nausea with recurrent vomiting
Abdominal pain
Hallucinations
Seizures

based on severity of symptoms. Withdrawal can be prevented by treating the person with appropriate medications—or even with alcohol. Indeed, detoxification from alcohol should never allow symptoms to progress further than the stage at which medical help is first sought (Table 6.4).

Stage One usually sets in from six to 12 hours after the last drink. Anxiety, restlessness, increased heart rate, sweating, difficulty sleeping, and increased blood pressure are common. At this point, if dependency is not extreme, the discomforts may be minor and treatable without medication, but with reassurance.

Stage Two begins after 12 hours, often peaking at 24 to 36 hours. It combines Stage One symptoms with visual and auditory hallucinations, notable because of relatively clear intervals. When not hallucinating, the person is well oriented and aware of having hallucinated. Medical treatment should *always* be given.

Stage Three begins from 12 to 48 hours after the last drink. Seizures may occur. In susceptible individuals, these may come as early as seven hours after the last drink.

Stage Four begins up to 72 to 96 hours after consumption. This is when delirium and tremors (delirium tremens, or DTs) appear, characterized by increasing confusion, disorientation, agitation, and paranoid hallucinations. Without treatment, the DTs can persist for several days and result in death up to 50 percent of the time, especially when there's an underlying medical problem. Recovery usually takes five to seven days.

DTs should never be allowed to develop because withdrawal

symptoms can be treated so effectively in their earliest stages. The rare cases that show up today are the result of not recognizing—during the early stages of withdrawal—that the person is dependent on alcohol. The individual begins to experience withdrawal, but denies his or her alcohol-dependent problem, tries to hide it from family and friends, feels capable of "going it alone," or is too embarrassed to seek medical help.

That's why family and friends of a chronic drinker should be alert to withdrawal symptoms. When that person stops drinking and starts to develop a rapid heart rate, shortness of breath, chills, low-grade fever, or nausea with recurrent vomiting and/or abdominal pain, immediate medical attention is necessary.

ADVERSE EFFECTS

When used excessively, alcohol is a toxic drug responsible for both acute and chronic complications (Table 6.5). Such problems involve a variety of systems and organs in the body.

Gastrointestinal Tract and Liver.   Even mild social drinking can cause impairment of motor function and gastrointestinal upset felt as heartburn. Increased short-term use, even a single episode, can cause inflammation of the stomach (gastritis) with abdominal pain and bleeding, peptic ulcers, and inflammation of the pancreas. When an episode of heavy drinking is superimposed on chronic complications, such as enlarged esophageal veins (portal hypertension) and liver disease, severe bleeding and liver failure can occur.

Not uncommon are such accompanying problems as decreased absorption of nutrients, diminished intestinal activity, fatty liver, cirrhosis with liver failure, and pancreatic cysts and inflammation (pancreatitis). Most of those complications are seen in people who've been drinking large amounts of alcohol for long periods, but recent evidence suggests that such damage can show up in susceptible people after much less drinking. Chronic liver disease and cirrhosis is a frequent cause of death in alcoholics.

TABLE 6.5
Complications of Heavy Alcohol Use

Acute Use	*Chronic Use*

Gastrointestinal tract and liver
  Gastritis and peptic ulcer,*
  dilated and bleeding
  esophageal veins, pancreatic
  inflammation (pancreatitis),
  liver failure
	Gastrointestinal tract and liver
	  Gastritis, dilated esophageal
	  veins (portal hypertension),
	  peptic ulcer, malabsorption,
	  diminished esophageal
	  motility, fatty liver, cirrhosis
	  with liver failure, pancreatic
	  cysts and inflammation
	  (pancreatitis)

Heart
  Irregularities of rhythm,
  elevated blood pressure
	Heart
	  Enlargement (cardiomyopathy),
	  high blood pressure, stroke

Metabolic abnormalities	Nutritional General malnutrition, anemia
Decreased temperature	Infections Lungs and urinary tract

Allergic reactions
  Flushing, urticaria, headache
	Cancer
	  Mouth, larynx, esophagus,
	  pancreas, liver, stomach,
	  colon, breast

Neurologic effects
  Intoxication, blackouts,
  withdrawal
	Neuropsychiatric effects
	  Wernicke's Syndrome,
	  Korsakoff's psychosis,
	  cerebellar degeneration,
	  polyneuropathy, optic
	  neuropathy, myopathy,
	  dementia, central pontine
	  degeneration, Marchiafava-
	  Bignami disease

* Usually when taken with a gastric irritant such as aspirin

Cardiovascular System. Chronic alcohol consumption can lead to enlargement of the heart (cardiomyopathy). Although this condition is seen only in 1 to 2 percent of excessive drinkers, it can cause heart failure and death. Even nonchronic alcohol use has been associated with rises in blood pressure, and an increased incidence of stroke shows up among those who drink more than 300 grams (about 10.5 ounces) a week. It is estimated that 5 to 24 percent of hypertensive patients may have elevated blood pressure because of alcohol consumption—in this instance, three drinks per day.

A number of studies, however, have suggested that minimal to moderate drinking can have a "protective effect" against coronary artery disease, as opposed to no such effect from either abstinence or heavy drinking. One reason may be that alcohol increases the blood levels of one type of high density lipoprotein (HDL). HDLs are believed to be a protective factor in preventing heart attacks. But some say that the type of HDL that's increased by alcohol has no connection with the protective factor and that any significant decreases in heart attacks occur only among those who already have heart disease. The latter hypothesis draws strong support from a British study of 7,700 men, which found that increased mortality among nondrinkers was the result of their changing from drinkers with cardiovascular disease to nondrinkers after evidence of heart disease.

Except for that study, reduced risk of heart attack among light drinkers has remained a fairly consistent finding. A reduced risk of severe narrowing (stenosis) or obstruction of the coronary arteries with moderate alcohol consumption has also been noted. However, the association of heavy drinking with increased death rates from coronary heart disease (and other causes) has been noted in all studies.

Even in healthy people, acute consumption of alcohol causes an increased heart rate, and a slight—but definite—decrease in muscular contractions of the heart. Relevance of that effect to a specific disease process has not been determined. Irregular heart rhythms have also been reported, particularly in regular drinkers. This phenomenon is known as the "holiday heart syndrome" because it was first described following drinking during the Christmas-New Year holiday season.

Neuropsychiatric Effects. A wide variety of neuropsychiatric complications have also been noted, ultimately leading to dementia and inability to function with excessive alcohol intake. Researchers have demonstrated that even two drinks can temporarily alter brain function and affect memory. Chronic neurologic effects of excessive alcoholism are well known (Table 6.5).

Wernicke's encephalopathy, primarily due to thiamine deficiency, consists of disordered cerebral function, including memory impairment, confabulation, organic psychosis, paralysis of eye muscles, and difficulty walking. Treatment with thiamine can reverse many of those symptoms, but residual effects may remain, including Korsakoff's psychosis, a memory disorder associated with apathy.

A more severe and much less common syndrome, Marchiafava-Bignami disease, is characterized by inability to walk, dementia, and muscle spasticity. Difficulty walking and speech disturbances associated with long-term drinking are because of degeneration of the cerebellum.

Destruction of another part of the brain, the pons, leads to paraplegia and inability to speak or swallow (central pontine myelinolysis).

Cognitive deficits can be demonstrated in chronic alcoholics following detoxification. Approximately 50 to 70 percent of people with a long-term alcohol dependency show impairment in cognitive function, including problem solving, memory, and perception. Although this may be related to the presence of coexisting disease, notably cirrhosis with low levels of encephalopathy, such findings have been observed in individuals without any evidence of severe liver disease. In such cases CAT scans of the brain have revealed structural abnormalities. Some of these deficits have diminished when the person stopped drinking. Extensive studies on this aspect of alcoholism have recently begun and in the future will be the subject of much research.

Other Effects on the Body. Almost every system can be affected by long-term excessive drinking. Next to nicotine, alcohol is associated with the most serious and widespread complications of any mood-altering drug.

Especially in combination with smoking, alcohol has been associated with increased risk of cancer of the head and neck, esophagus, pancreas, stomach, colon, rectum, liver, and even the breast.

Endocrinologic effects of alcohol have been described for almost every hormonal system in animal studies. The relevance of some of these observations to humans remains to be determined. But it has been frequently observed that chronic alcohol intake can alter hormonal function relating to human sexuality.

Men can show decreased levels of testosterone, a female pattern of hair distribution, and breast enlargement. Impotence isn't uncommon. As Shakespeare put it, "It [drink] provokes the desire, but it takes away the performance."

In women, menstrual abnormalities and infertility are the most common effects. Alcohol causes fetal alcohol syndrome, a condition seen in 0.1 to 0.3 percent of live births, with the most serious effects resulting from the daily consumption of four or more glasses of an alcoholic beverage during pregnancy. But much smaller amounts also can have deleterious effects (see Chapter 18).

The nutritional disturbances that go with heavy drinking include less attention to a balanced diet, substitution of alcohol calories for those usually obtained from carbohydrates, protein, and fat in other foods, diminished absorption of other nutrients, loss of appetite, vomiting, and deficiencies of fiber, protein, calcium, iron, folate, zinc, and vitamins A, B_1 (thiamine), B_6 (pyridoxine), and C.

Disorders of peripheral nerves (peripheral neuropathy) and muscles (myopathy) are fairly common. Symptoms and signs include numbness, tingling or burning in the extremities, and muscle cramps, tenderness, and weakness. Chronic alcoholism affects the immune system, predisposing the drinker to common and uncommon infections.

DIAGNOSIS

Inordinate drinking is bad for your health; occasional or responsible drinking has minimal, if any, proven adverse effects. But the

TABLE 6.6
Signs and Symptoms of Alcoholism
Modified from National Council on Alcoholism guidelines

Definite	*Probable*
Physical dependency on alcohol, with tremors, hallucinations, seizures on abstinence	No control of consumption
	Surreptitious and/or morning drinking
Mental changes directly related to alcohol	Repeated, conscious attempts at abstinence
Major effects on brain	Medical excuses from work for a variety of reasons
Alcohol-associated complications	Shifting from one type of alcoholic beverage to another
Drinking despite strong medical or social contraindications	Loss of interest in activities not associated with drinking
Blatant, indiscriminate use of alcohol	Rages and suicidal thoughts with drinking
Consuming one-fifth gallon of whiskey or alcohol-equivalent in beer or wine daily for more than one day	Drinking to relieve insomnia, anger, fatigue, depression
Alcoholic blackouts	
BAL over 0.15% without gross evidence of intoxication, or 0.30% at any time	

dividing lines between responsible use, excessive use, and alcoholism are fuzzy, even to experts in the field.

Some believe heavy drinking means having more than one ounce of pure alcohol (two drinks) a day. Others focus on the amount consumed per occasion (five drinks or more), and frequency of consumption, with heavy drinkers defined as those who take five or more drinks at one time more than once a week.

The National Council on Alcoholism has developed a list of signs and symptoms for diagnosing alcoholism, divided into *definitive* and *probable* groups (Table 6.6). Most important, however, is early recognition of inappropriate alcohol use by family, friends, teachers, or employers.

Both the American Psychiatric Association (APA) and the World Health Organization (WHO) have been working to establish a more quantitative definition of inappropriate use of alcohol, separate from alcohol dependency. The new WHO guidelines and the APA guidelines have moved closer together to allow for unified diagnostic criteria. A consensus of these guidelines now defines inappropriate use of alcohol as a harmful, maladaptive state characterized by at least one of the following:

- continued use despite knowledge of alcohol causing actual psychological or physical harm to the user
- recurrent use in situations in which alcohol is physically hazarddous.

According to the guidelines, the pattern of inappropriate use must exist for at least one month or recur repeatedly over a longer period for a diagnosis to be confirmed.

By comparison, the guidelines consider alcohol dependency to exist in the presence of at least three or more of the following:

- compulsion to drink
- loss of control in managing alcohol use
- alcohol taken to relieve or avoid withdrawal symptoms
- presence of a physiologic alcohol withdrawal state
- evidence of tolerance, with markedly increased amounts of alcohol needed to achieve intoxication or the desired effect
- progressive neglect of social, occupational, or recreational activities

---

TABLE 6.7
Early Signs of Drinking Problems

Anxiety relieved by drinking
Frequent job and/or residence changes
Gulping drinks
Choosing jobs that facilitate drinking
Frequent traffic violations and/or accidents
Social disorganization in family
Complaints by spouse over drinking
Denial
Depression alleviated by drinking

- continued use despite knowledge of adverse consequences
- frequent intoxication or withdrawal when expected to fulfill major social obligations or when alcohol use is known to be hazardous
- prolonged periods spent drinking or recovering from the effect of drinking

Dependency is established when these symptoms exist for at least one month or recur repeatedly during the prior 12 months.

Many questionnaires have been developed to identify problem drinkers early, as have certain laboratory tests. In conjunction, they provide a fair degree of predictability. Unfortunately, these techniques are valuable only in a medical setting. Their widespread use among the general population is still impractical.

Some of the early signs of alcoholism, however, are not difficult to spot (Table 6.7). They include periods of depression alleviated by taking a drink, needing several quick drinks in order to relax (accompanied by increased anxiety if alcohol isn't available), marked increase over previous drinking, drinking at inappropriate times, and undue denial or anger when questioned about drinking behavior. Frequent change of jobs, absences for nonspecific medical reasons, accidents at work or when driving, or coming to work with alcohol on one's breath should all serve as warning signs.

REASONS FOR EXCESSIVE DRINKING

The greatest controversy in trying to determine the reasons for alcoholism centers on the roles of nature and nurture, or genetics versus environment. Many studies have shown that alcoholism is three to five times more common among children whose parents were alcoholic, regardless of whether they were reared with biologic or adoptive parents. Other studies have shown a predominance of alcoholism among adopted children whose biologic parents were alcoholics. One of the largest studies included 862 men and 913 women adopted between 1930 and 1949. The incidence of alcohol dependency among the adoptive parents showed no association with increased risk of alcohol dependency among the children. Excessive alcohol consumption among the biologic parents, however, was linked to an increased risk for alcoholism among the children. Two distinct patterns came to light (Table 6.8)

Type I appeared when at least one biologic parent consumed large quantities of alcohol *and* the situation in the adoptive home was similar. Both men and women were three times more likely to develop alcoholism than those in a control group. This high-risk group is termed "milieu-limited," meaning that a drinking-conducive environment had to have existed. Excessive drinking in this group usually developed after age 25, with the person experiencing frequent guilt over his or her drinking. These people can seldom abstain from drinking, but they are less likely to be antisocial when they drink.

Type II (male-limited) were men whose biologic fathers abused alcohol. Their risk of alcoholism existed regardless of environment—from 17 to 18 percent had problems later on in life, compared with fewer than 2 percent of those who didn't fit that pattern. Women who matched that pattern appeared to develop increased anxiety in later life, but not actual alcoholism. The men began drinking before age 25 and were frequently able to abstain for periods of time. But they consistently engaged in aggressive behavior, were often arrested while drinking, and rarely experienced guilt over their drinking episodes.

However, more recent studies have been unable to confirm the existence of a Type II pattern of primary alcoholism. It is now be-

TABLE 6.8
Genetic Patterns of Alcoholism

Characteristics	Milieu-Limited (Type I)	Male-Limited (Type II)
Age of onset	After 25	Before 25
Ability to abstain	Infrequent	Frequent
Aggressive behavior and arrests when drinking	Infrequent	Frequent
Loss of control	Frequent	Infrequent
Guilt over drinking	Frequent	Infrequent

lieved by many in the alcohol field that those thought to have Type II alcoholism have a primary personality disorder with a secondary drinking problem. This inability to validate what had been previously considered a characteristic of primary alcoholism illustrates the difficulties inherent in separating genetic from environmental influences.

Ability to metabolize alcohol. Support for the genetic theory is given by the fact that different ethnic groups metabolize alcohol at different rates—because of variations in enzyme activity. Asians and Native Americans metabolize alcohol at a much slower rate than other groups. That leads to an increased concentration of acetaldehyde in the body, resulting in a strong adverse reaction to only small amounts of alcohol. It could be assumed, therefore, that such cultures would have a lower incidence of alcohol use. But this is not so.

The adverse biochemical reaction is unarguable, but improper use of alcohol among Native Americans is high; indeed, it is one of their leading causes of death. And while excessive drinking is relatively rare among Asians, the 1980s have seen an increase, especially in those cultures that are developing highly competitive industrial societies. Note that even though the rate at which alcohol is metabolized may be genetically determined, there's still little evidence that this metabolism is related to excessive drinking.

Other genetic factors.   Other genetic factors have been identified in laboratory studies. But their relationship to an inevitable genetic predisposition to alcoholism remains to be determined. Recently, a gene thought to be responsible for placing one at risk for alcoholism was identified in the brain of deceased alcoholics. The dopamine D2 receptor was identified in 77 percent of the brains of dead alcoholics as compared with 28 percent of nonalcoholics. If confirmed by further studies, this would be a major discovery, but the number of people studied was small and the relevance of this finding still needs to be established.

Neurophysiology.   Studies have also found differences between children of alcoholics and other children in tests of general intelligence, memory, attention, and organizational abilities. These studies involved relatively small samples, so it's hard to ascertain whether genetic influences or environment played a role in the findings.

Environment.   The evidence is convincing that a genetic risk for excessive drinking exists in some people. Yet it's clear that such patterns don't follow simple Mendelian distribution, which would make alcoholism in a parent the basis for predicting with certainty the proportion of children who will become alcoholic.

Studies of the drinking habits of twins would appear to be a good way to build a case for genetic determinants of alcoholism. But one must be aware of confounding variables such as social interaction between twins, even when living with separate adoptive parents, as well as the environment in which twins may live when reaching adulthood, especially the stability of their own family unit. Investigators who have reviewed these factors have found that identical twins tended to have more social contact with each other during adulthood than fraternal twins. This frequent social contact seemed to affect their drinking patterns. However, it did not fully explain the strongly similar drinking habits; there must still be a significant genetic contribution. This finding existed only for men, not women. With respect to women twins, marital status appears to play a role, with genetic factors accounting for 60 to 75 percent of the variance in drinking habits in twins who are not married, but only for 31 to 59 percent of the variance in those who are married.

In a study of genetic and social determinants in adolescent alcohol use, family influence was found to be quite important, accounting for 51 percent of the variance in men and 58 percent in women. More than 80 percent of children in the male-limited susceptibility group do not go on to abuse alcohol. Nor do the majority of alcoholics fit either pattern. Less than one half of children of alcoholics develop drinking problems, and an even smaller proportion become dependent on alcohol.

So environment is important in fostering improper use of alcohol. This includes the family, use of alcohol by peers, role models, and society's view of alcohol consumption—favorable if consumed in reasonable amounts in social settings.

A DISEASE OR A DISORDER?

Almost everyone involved in treating alcoholism considers it a disease, largely because that's supposedly the official stand of the American Medical Association, the American Psychological Association, the American Psychiatric Association, the American Society of Addiction Medicine, and the World Health Organization. But a closer look shows that the consensus among a few of these groups holds excessive alcohol use to be a recognized "disorder" rather than a stated disease.

In the strictest sense, excessive alcohol consumption fits the commonly acknowledged definition of "disease": a change of normal body function as demonstrated by specific signs and symptoms whose causes are known or unknown. And excessive alcohol, of course, is recognized as causing a host of changes in the body. But there's no question that alcoholism also fits the definition of "disorder": a derangement or abnormality of function caused by a specific agent.

So why the disagreement? Opponents of the alcoholism-is-a-disease school say that that judgment tells alcoholics they're victims, helpless to control their drinking, and doomed to continuing alcoholism if they should take even one drink. That relieves the alcoholic of personal responsibility to control his or her behavior.

Critics of the disease model say that because alcoholics can control their drinking for varying periods, because most people with genetic predisposition to alcoholism don't become alcoholics, and because large numbers of alcoholics don't even have the predisposition, clearly alcoholism is not a disease. These observations, however, are really independent of the disease model.

As for mandatory insurance coverage for treatment, it hardly matters whether alcoholism is a disease or a disorder. Impaired function, whether the result of a character disorder, generalized anxiety, or alcohol, should be covered in the same way as organ system damage because of high cholesterol (coronary artery disease), nicotine consumption (lung cancer), or liver disease (alcohol).

Both sides are talking at, rather than to, each other. Recognizing that excessive drinking can cause a definable syndrome neither negates the disease concept nor relieves an individual of responsibility for his or her behavior. Simply acknowledging that fact would allow more energies to flow into prevention programs and assessment of treatment alternatives.

PREVENTION

Many prevention efforts can help to diminish excessive drinking behavior. They include general education campaigns for those most likely to identify potential problems, particularly teachers, health-care professionals, and employers; and intervention techniques aimed at such high-risk groups as children of alcoholic parents.

Raising the economic and social costs of drinking can also be effective. Such efforts include increasing the cost of alcoholic beverages, raising the legal drinking age, establishing severe penalties for driving while intoxicated, and establishing shared liability between drinker and server when an accident occurs.

While several studies of advertising alcoholic beverages have documented a positive effect in increasing alcohol consumption, others revealed no consistent relationship. However, advertising, especially that on television, may be more pernicious in encouraging children and adolescents to drink. Although alcohol accounts for only 6 percent of total beverage use in the United States, it is the third most common drug used on television and the most frequently televised beverage. Those portrayed drinking in print and on television are often role models for children as well as adults.

TREATMENT

Each of the many approaches for treatment of alcoholism has its advocates and detractors. Unfortunately, not one has been objectively evaluated. On an anecdotal basis, however, compelling evidence of effectiveness has been offered by advocates of various treatments. The authors of an extensive review of treatment-outcome studies concluded that the approaches that appeared to be most effective had one common characteristic: they were rarely used consistently in treatment programs.

Competition among treatment facilities for funding and for patients has often prevented rational dialogues among professionals who advocate different approaches and has also stymied attempts at objective studies to document effectiveness. The best solution would be to have a comprehensive array of services from which anyone needing therapy could select the most appropriate. Individualized therapy results in the best outcome.

Available therapeutic options used alone or in combination include inpatient detoxification and subsequent rehabilitation, outpatient detoxification and rehabilitation, such self-help groups as Alcoholics Anonymous and Al-Anon, such drug therapies as disulfiram (Antabuse) and lithium, short- and long-term behavioral therapy, and controlled drinking.

Detoxification and Short-Term Rehabilitation. An inpatient setting for detoxification isn't always necessary, but it becomes so when a person simply can't stop drinking or has a severe underlying medical problem such as heart disease or uncontrolled high blood pressure, which can make ambulatory detoxification risky. In addition, detoxification may be more effective in such a setting if the patient does not have an adequate support system.

A complete medical assessment and relevant laboratory tests are performed before inpatient detoxification. Diet is adjusted, including vitamin supplements when appropriate, and a suitable therapy to follow withdrawal is chosen. Detoxification by itself rarely eliminates the drinking problem; it must be considered just a first step in the entire rehabilitative process.

Detoxification is usually accomplished with a drug in the benzodiazepine group (Librium, Valium, Serax, or Ativan) in doses high enough to keep the person comfortable during the first few days. The drug is then decreased about 25 percent a day, subject to considerable variation. When dependency is low and withdrawal symptoms minimal, medication may not be needed. That's preferable because developing dependency on other depressants is always a concern in those who are alcohol-dependent.

Drugs called Beta-blockers (Inderal, Tenormin) have been assessed for control of withdrawal symptoms. Early withdrawal from alcohol and several other mood-altering drugs is associated with increased activity of the sympathetic (adrenergic) nervous system; the B-blockers prevent activity by the neurotransmitters in that system (Chapter 3). In outpatient use, for example, the B-blocker atenolol (Tenormin) has lowered the intensity and shortened the duration of withdrawal symptoms, and lessened the craving for alcohol. Clonidine, which has been used to treat hypertension and also to prevent symptoms of heroin withdrawal, has also been shown to be helpful in alcohol withdrawal.

Withdrawal symptoms may persist for a number of weeks after detoxification has been accomplished. This protracted withdrawal is most often manifested by anxiety, insomnia, and, at times, a craving for alcohol. During this time support is essential.

Inpatient Versus Outpatient Treatment After Detoxification. Whether to treat alcoholics as inpatients or outpatients is a long-standing controversy among health professionals. Sometimes, the patient makes an independent decision. But that decision is usually based on how the options were presented—or not presented at all.

Inpatient treatment, with detoxification plus four to eight weeks on a rehabilitation unit, is the established method of dealing with alcoholics. It became the best method decades ago, largely because it was the only practical approach.

But as far back as 1965, both the American Psychiatric Association and the National Association of Mental Health recognized the value of outpatient treatment, stating that outpatient clinics should be the backbone of services. By no means does that constitute a call to eliminate inpatient treatment, clearly necessary for some alcoholics. Rather, it reflects evidence that—for the majority of alcoholics, who won't develop severe withdrawal symptoms—well-run outpatient programs have the same success rates at one-eighth to one-tenth the cost of inpatient programs, which nevertheless continue to dominate initial treatment of alcoholics.

Alcoholics Anonymous and Al-Anon. Alcoholics Anonymous (AA), founded in 1935 by two former alcoholics, remains a self-supporting, self-help organization with over 73,000 groups worldwide. Its only requirement is for a participant to want to stop drinking. AA's Al-Anon, a separate but parallel program, is for family or friends whose primary concerns are to keep AA members sober and help others achieve sobriety.

AA has no affiliation with any organization or institution, takes no political stand on any issue, and doesn't allow members to identify themselves for any political purpose.

The basic premise of participation is acceptance of an alternate way of life without drinking and acknowledgment that alcoholism is an incurable, progressive disease that can be managed only through abstinence. The nondenominational, yet religious, nature of this group is apparent in its 12-step program. Full participation requires considerable soul-searching and total commitment—not easy tasks.

AA was initially thought best able to help healthy, stable, middle-class, severe alcoholics. But its membership probably mirrors the general population of drinkers. AA meetings are held in the United States and many other countries. Directories are available from any local AA chapter. Some people can be helped through periods of acute stress by attending only a few meetings; others can't adjust to the process and find it of little value. But the many who continue to participate are intensely committed to the program and profoundly believe in its effectiveness.

AA's abstinence approach leaves many chapters with an unkindly view of dependency on other mood-altering drugs, even when prescribed by a physician. Thus former heroin users with alcohol problems who are on methadone maintenance may have trouble joining AA or may be pressured to detoxify from methadone. And since many alcoholics may have underlying psychologic disorders that require psychotropic medication, discouraging the use of such drugs can prevent an individual from staying abstinent.

Evaluations of AA's effectiveness have produced varying results. Among the reasons for this are the voluntary, informal nature of the organization and the difficulties in obtaining membership lists. Its success is connected to the long-standing commitment of members who serve as sponsors of new members. Yet the dropout rate can be high. In one study of people who attended an AA meeting one month after being discharged from a detoxification unit, only 11 percent were still participating a year later. In other studies, 68 percent dropped out before the tenth meeting. But of those who attended regularly, an estimated 26 to 50 percent remain abstinent after one year.

This success rate matches those of other treatments. AA is most effective in conjunction with other therapies, such as individual or group therapy, or Antabuse. Such a combination may well increase the possibility of success.

Disulfiram Therapy.   Disulfiram (Antabuse) has been used since the 1940s. Antabuse inhibits the breakdown of alcohol in the body, which causes high levels of acetaldehyde. Elevated blood levels of acetaldehyde result in nausea, vomiting, sweating, restlessness, flushing, chest pain, headaches, increased heart rate, palpitations, generalized weakness, and changes in blood pressure that can cause loss of consciousness or severe, irregular heart rhythms.

Disulfiram becomes partially effective within an hour of administration and its effect lasts four to seven days. Even small amounts of alcohol will produce the bad reactions in five to 15 minutes, and they can last from 30 minutes to several hours.

Just the fear of a disulfiram reaction is enough to motivate most

TABLE 6.9
Drugs That Interact with Disulfiram

Generic Name	Brand Name
Barbiturates	Ambarbital, Phenobarbital, Seconal
Benzodiazepines	Ativan, Librium, Serax, Xanax
Caffeine	Coffee, tea
Metronidazole	Flagyl
Phenytoin	Dilantin
Rifampin	Rifadin, Rimactane
Theophylline	Aerolate, Bronkodyl, Elixophyllin, Theon
Tricyclic antidepressants	Elavil, Tofranil, and other tricyclic antidepressants
Warfarin	Coumadin

people to refrain from alcohol. The dose used in many disulfiram programs is actually too low to cause a severe reaction. Many people on disulfiram, told what they can expect, have never challenged its effect.

Side effects to disulfiram include allergic skin reactions, drowsiness, fatigue, occasional impotence, and a metallic aftertaste. More severe, but unusual, are loss of coordination, behavioral disturbances, seizures, bleeding into the brain, liver dysfunction, and damage to the optic nerve.

Disulfiram can also intensify the effects of other medications (Table 6.9). Many of these drugs are widely prescribed, so a careful medical history should be taken before starting disulfiram therapy. Some drugs act similarly to disulfiram and produce a mild disulfiram-alcohol type reaction when alcohol is consumed (Table 6.10). A disulfiram reaction can occur when *any* beverage containing alcohol is drunk, including those not usually thought of as containing alcohol.

TABLE 6.10
Drugs That Cause Antabuse-Alcohol Reactions
Reaction varies depending on dose, individual sensitivity, and quantity of alcohol consumed

Generic or Group Names	Brand Name
Amitriptyline	Elavil and others
Calcium Carbimide	Temposil
Cephalosporins	Cefaclor, Keflex, Duricef
Chloramphenicol	Chloromycetin
Chlorpropamide	Diabinese
Griseofulvin	Grisactin, Grifulvin, Gris-PEG, Fulvicin
Metronidazole	Flagyl, Metryl, Protostat, Staric
MAO inhibitors	Pargyline, Nardil, Parnate
Nitrofurantoin	Furadantin, Nitrofan, Macrodantin
Phenylbutazone	Azolid, Butagen, Butazolidin
Procarbazine	Matulane
Quinacrine	Atabrine
Sulfonylureas	Orinase, Dymelor, Tolbutamide, Tolazamide, Ronase, Tolinase, Chlorpropamide, Diabinese, Glucotrol, Dibeta, Micronase

Disulfiram must not be given when there's an acute infectious disease, asthma or respiratory insufficiency, cardiac disease, epilepsy, psychosis, liver or renal disease, or pregnancy. A history of prior adverse reactions to disulfiram itself, or an allergy to rubber, are also absolute contraindications.

To be most effective, disulfiram must be taken daily (usually a

250- to 500-milligram dose), thus requiring motivation for continued use. Disulfiram capsules have been developed to be implanted in the body, but this form of treatment is still experimental and can't be put into general use. Besides, the drive to drink is sometimes so great that some continue to drink even while on the drug.

New studies have generated less enthusiasm for disulfiram as the sole, long-term therapy for alcoholism. Little or no evidence exists to indicate that disulfiram—unaccompanied by another therapy—has any marked beneficial effect in helping to sustain abstinence. It's now considered most effective for short-term use to prevent drinking while the individual starts outpatient therapy.

Lithium Carbonate. Lithium, a drug used for manic depression, has been under evaluation as a treatment for alcoholism, typically in conjunction with other therapies. But its use is still experimental.

Drugs That Affect Neurotransmitter Activity. The discovery of the role that neurotransmitters and receptors may have in promoting drug use, including alcohol (Chapter 3, Chapter 4), has led to the development of drugs that may affect those receptors and neurotransmitters particularly sensitive to alcohol. Much of this work remains experimental; however, some of the findings may well prove to have future application. The narcotic (opiate) antagonists naloxone and naltrexone have been shown to diminish alcohol consumption in laboratory animals as well as to reduce alcohol-induced respiratory depression. Bromocriptine (Chapter 13), a dopamine agonist, has been suggested to reduce both alcohol craving and consumption. Drugs reducing uptake of serotonin by nerve cells also diminish alcohol consumption. These drugs include fluvoxamine, fluoxtine, citalopram, and the nonbenzodiazepine antianxiety drug Buspirone.

Counseling and Psychotherapy. Counseling, family therapy, marital therapy, and forms of recognized individual psychotherapy have been used for a long time, alone or together with other therapies. Psychotherapy may be exceptionally helpful for those drinkers with underlying psychological disturbances. Family therapy, to identify the settings that promote drinking and help family members relate appropriately to the problem, is also valuable.

Employee Assistance Programs (EAPs). Recognition of the effects of excessive drinking in terms of days lost, inadequate job performance, and high health-care costs has led to development of programs that help identify and refer employees with drinking problems. Most large companies have such programs, staffed by trained personnel. When an employee voluntarily seeks help from an EAP, and follows EAP staff recommendations, the situation is kept confidential from the employer. But if the employee is referred by a supervisor and doesn't follow the recommendations, a pink slip may result. Evidence to date suggests that EAPs provide valuable resources for early identification of problem drinkers and subsequent referral to long-term therapy.

Behavioral Therapy. Studies of short-term therapy based on negative conditioning (aversive therapy) designed to control drinking behaviors have produced mixed results. Aversion therapy, based on producing physical or emotional discomfort when in a setting that promotes drinking, remains controversial. But several studies have supported the effectiveness of some of these approaches.

Controlled Drinking. Probably no treatment has aroused more controversy than training the alcoholic to control his or her drinking. Proponents of the abstinence approach believe that the term "controlled drinking" is itself a fallacy because it's impossible to moderate an alcoholic's drinking patterns. "One drink, one drunk" and "One drink is too much, and two are not enough" embody the prevailing philosophy of the alcohol-treatment community in the United States.

The fear that deemphasizing recovering alcoholics' ability to abstain might cause them to revert to alcoholism may be warranted. But several studies suggest that some alcoholics can moderate their drinking behaviors, either as part of a controlled-drinking program or by returning to drink at greatly reduced levels. Formal programs of controlled drinking exist in other countries but not in the United States, where approaches other than abstinence have not met with either public or professional acceptance.

In many instances, chronic drinkers have been able, over time, to moderate their drinking. But in equal—if not greater—numbers of instances, drinkers have lapsed into excessive alcohol consumption, believing they have failed. As treatment methods and evaluation techniques become more refined, well-designed, objective studies of controlled drinking may be undertaken.

Chapter 7

Central Nervous System Depressants

The central nervous system (CNS) depressants comprise a variety of chemically unrelated compounds, all capable of altering mood. Their effects are generally similar to that of alcohol, and withdrawal symptoms are often indistinguishable from those of chronic alcoholism.

The first drug in this group to be synthesized was chloral hydrate, in 1832. Several years later, barbituric acid, parent drug of the barbiturates, was developed. The first drug, barbital (Veronal), was introduced into clinical practice in 1903, with phenobarbital following close behind. The ability of these drugs to produce sedation, relieve insomnia, and decrease seizure activity resulted in their ready acceptance by the medical profession.

Their adverse effects weren't widely recognized until the late 1940s, when health professionals realized that such drugs could cause highs and dependency. Yet their popularity continued. More than 2,500 barbiturates were synthesized; 50 available for medical use. In 1976 an estimated 18 million prescriptions were written for barbiturates, enough to allow each adult in the United States 24 doses of 100-milligram pills. Barbiturate usage has since declined considerably with development of newer agents. In 1950 meprobamate (Equanil, Miltown) came on the market as an effective tranquilizer. It was promoted as having lower potential for dependency and fewer prominent side effects than the barbiturates. But it quickly became apparent that chronic use could induce meprobamate dependency.

Chlordiazepoxide (Librium), first of the benzodiazepines, appeared in 1961. Since then, more than 3,000 benzodiazepines have been synthesized, with more than 25 in clinical use. The ability of benzodiazepines to relieve anxiety, relax muscles, prevent seizure activity, and treat sleep disturbances resulted in remarkable acceptance by both the medical profession and the public.

In 1967 prescriptions for psychotropic drugs added up to 17 percent (170 million) of the 1 billion written, with Librium and Valium accounting for one-third (or 56 million) of that number. More than 70 million prescriptions were written in 1972 for those two drugs combined, and an estimated 7 percent of all adults between the ages of 18 and 25 were taking some kind of tranquilizing drugs.

Concern over inappropriate prescriptions for these drugs led the FDA in 1975 to classify diazepam as a Schedule IV drug, permitting no more than five refills within a six-month period, and recommending reevaluation of need after four months of continuous use. But that measure did little to stop use. Four years later, the percentage of 18- to 25-year-olds who ever used tranquilizers had risen to 15 percent.

Flurazepam (Dalmane), introduced in 1970 for treatment of sleep disorders, was responsible for 7 million prescriptions by 1976. In 1978 more than 68 million prescriptions were written for the benzodiazepines (half for Valium) despite increasing concern over adverse effects reported even with "appropriate" use. That statistic was accompanied by another: diazepam ranked second only to alcohol in combination with other drugs in drug dependency related episodes treated in emergency rooms nationwide.

In 1985 prescriptions for benzodiazepines reached 61 million, with more than 8 million written in New York State alone. Of the top 50 drugs prescribed in 1987, five were benzodiazepines (Xanax, Halcion, Valium, Ativan, and Tranxene). Xanax ranked fourth highest of any type of drug.

Nonmedical use of these drugs appears to be on the decline. In 1981 the National Household Survey on Drug Abuse reported that approximately 25 percent of the population had taken one of these drugs daily within the past four months. The 1988 survey reported 1 percent or approximately one million members of the household population to have used sedatives or tranquilizers nonmedically within the past month. All CNS depressants have similar side effects, but they vary considerably in potential for overdose and intensity of the withdrawal syndrome.

PATTERNS OF USE

Depressant drugs are prescribed for a number of reasons. Perhaps the most common reason for appropriate use is their ability to relieve stress and facilitate sleep. Until recently, the ease of getting a prescription introduced many people to their beneficial effects. The positive mood-altering effects of the depressants often led to continued use, first for anxiety, then to feel comfortable, and ultimately in a few individuals to get high.

A paradoxical stimulant effect is seen as tolerance develops in people taking depressants on a regular basis. A heightened high can be reached when additional doses are taken irregularly, thereby reinforcing continued use. A depressant is often taken to counteract the actions of other drugs that are being simultaneously used, cocaine or amphetamines, for example. That's common in those using relatively large amounts of stimulants at frequent intervals in order to counteract the stimulant's effect (Chapters 12, 13).

Use of one CNS depressant to intensify a high from another also occurs. Excessive drinkers, fearful of having alcohol on their breath during working hours, may switch to a depressant drug to avoid detection. It offers a high and affects behavior in almost the same way as alcohol. Drinking a great deal of alcohol sometimes results in increased awareness several hours later, along with difficulty sleeping. This often leads to taking a depressant to facilitate sleep. When alcohol is unavailable, those who use illicit narcotics and those on methadone maintenance programs may also take depressants to enhance or produce a mood-altering effect.

Combining CNS depressants and alcohol or narcotics accentuates the respiratory effects of these drugs. That's why depressants are frequently identified in overdose cases. Diazepam (Valium) is perhaps the most commonly improperly used prescription drug seen in emergency room admissions and is the legal drug most commonly found in deaths resulting from unnatural causes, such as multiple drug overdose and accidents. Although the benzodiazepines have a relatively low overdose potential when taken alone, the consequences can be deadly when they're taken in combination with alcohol or other CNS depressants.

These drugs can best be described by dividing them into three groups: barbiturates; nonbarbiturate hypnotics and sedatives; and benzodiazepines, the group most often prescribed and most frequently used inappropriately.

BARBITURATES

The barbiturates can be classified by duration of their action: ultrashort, short, intermediate, and long-acting (Table 7.1). Those with ultrashort duration of action include hexobarbital (Evipal), methohexital (Brevital), thiamylal (Surital), and thiopental (Pentothal), and are administered by injection to produce rapid anesthesia. They are rarely used inappropriately. But short- and intermediate-acting barbiturates are frequently used to get high.

Absorption from the gastrointestinal tract varies when barbiturates are taken orally. Ultimately, they're widely distributed in the body and metabolized in the liver. They produce a generalized depression, with the mood-altering effects ranging from mild sedation and euphoria to coma. The latter is caused by marked depression of the brain's respiratory center as a result of overdose.

The effects of barbiturates and related hypnotics and sedatives on the heart and blood vessels is relatively minor. So are their actions on other organ systems, except for the liver. As is the case with alcohol, they can interfere with other drugs metabolized in the liver and increase or decrease the effects of the other drugs.

Tolerance, Dependency, and Withdrawal. Tolerance for barbiturates develops easily. They have a relatively narrow tolerance-toxicity ratio. That is, someone tolerant to a given dose of barbiturates may show little mood-altering effect, but even a slight increase above the tolerance threshold can result in intoxication and overdose.

TABLE 7.1
Common Nonmedically Used Barbiturates

Brand Name	Generic Name	Street Name
Long-acting		
Luminal, Phenobarbital, Barbita, Solfoton	Phenobarbital	Barbs, Beans, Biscuits, Blockbusters, Bullets, Downers, Downs, Dolls, Fool Pills, Goofballs, Green Dragons, Greenies, Mexican Reds, Pajao, Pink Ladies, Purple Hearts, Rojo, Sleeping Pills, Stumblers
Gemonil	Metharbital	
Mebaral	Mephobarbital	
Intermediate-acting		
Amytal	Amobarbital	Bluebirds, Blue Devils, Blue Heaven, Blues
Alurate	Aprobarbital	
Butisol	Butabarbital	
Lotusate	Talbutal	
Short-acting		
Nembutal	Pentobarbital	Nebbies, Nimbies, Yellow Jackets, Yellows
Seconal	Secobarbital	Red Birds, Red Devils, Reds, Seccies

TABLE 7.1 (continued)
Common Nonmedically Used Barbiturates

Brand Name	Generic Name	Street Name
Combinations		
Tuinal	Amobarbital, secobarbital	Christmas Trees, Rainbows, Tooies, Toolies, Trees, Tuiys
Tri-barbs, SBP	Phenobarbital, butabarbital, secobarbital	

Considerable cross-tolerance exists among all hypnotic and nonbarbiturate sedatives and alcohol. Withdrawal from any of these drugs can be relieved immediately by administering any other drug in the group.

Abruptly stopping high doses of barbiturates and related drugs leads to the characteristic severe withdrawal syndrome indistinguishable from that seen with alcohol. Depending on the barbiturate or hypnotic, symptoms appear within 10 to 24 hours with the short-acting drugs, or within two to three days with longer-acting drugs. Restlessness and anxiety appear first, accompanied by cramps, nausea, and vomiting. Next come tremors of hands and feet, followed by seizures and ultimately hallucinations, delirium, disorientation, increases in blood pressure, and—if untreated—collapse of the respiratory and cardiovascular systems. Hallucinations can reappear for several months after withdrawal has been completed.

NONBARBITURATE HYPNOTICS AND SEDATIVES

A number of nonbarbiturate hypnotic and sedative drugs with potential for excessive use are listed in Table 7.2. Several of the more common ones are discussed below.

Glutethimide (Doriden). Doriden was promoted as a nonaddictive alternative to barbiturates when it was introduced in 1954.

TABLE 7.2
Nonbarbiturate Hypnotics and Sedative Drugs

Brand Name	Group*	Generic Name	Street Name
Doriden	NBH	Glutethimide	Hits***
Equanil, Meprospan, Miltown, Nevramate	C	Meprobamate	
Noctec	CH	Chloral hydrate	Green Frogs, Knockout Drops, Peter
Noludar	NBH	Methyprylon	
Optimil**	NBH	Methaqualone	
Parest**	NBH	Methaqualone	
Paraldehyde, Paral	O	Paraldehyde	
Placidyl	NBH	Ethchlorvynol	Plastivil
Quaalude**	NBH	Methaqualone	Ludes, Mean Greens, Quads, Quas
Sopor**, Somnafac**	NBH	Methaqualone	Soapers, Soaps
Valmid	C	Ethinamate	

*C = Carbamate; CH = Chloral hydrate; NBH = Nonbarbiturate hypnotic
**No longer legally manufactured.
***Combined with codeine

But its potential for inappropriate use was quickly recognized. Although its CNS depressant effect is similar to that of the barbiturates, it is particularly long-lasting, with a half-life—the time it takes to eliminate half of a substance—in the blood of up to 100 hours. Severe withdrawal symptoms and prolonged aftereffects can show up in people who are dependent on even moderate doses.

One of the newer street drugs, ''Hits'' (500 milligrams of glutethimide and 60 milligrams of codeine), is particularly dangerous because it depresses the central nervous system's respiratory center.

Chloral Hydrate.   This medication was one of the earliest hypnotic-sedative drugs used to treat alcohol withdrawal, anxiety, and insomnia before the synthesis of the benzodiazepines. With the alternative of benzodiazepines available today, chloral hydrate is not often prescribed. Historically, it was used as a knockout potion (a Mickey Finn). Taking alcohol and chloral hydrate results in decreased breakdown of the alcohol (by the chloral hydrate) and enhancement of chloral hydrate activity (by the alcohol).

Methaqualone.   Formerly manufactured under the brand names Quaalude, Sopor, Parest, Optimil, and Somnafac, this drug was withdrawn from legal use in the United States and classified as a Schedule I drug. Nevertheless, methaqualone continues to be sold illegally. Like other nonbarbiturate hypnotic and sedative drugs, methaqualone was at first considered nonaddictive. But it was quickly discovered to produce heightened feelings of pleasure and became known as the ''love drug.''

Its increasing inappropriate use led the Food and Drug Administration in 1973 to make it a Schedule I drug. Its use continued to grow; not even the diversion of some legal supplies to the street was enough to meet the demand. In 1979 approximately 100 tons of methaqualone were smuggled into the United States from Colombia.

By 1981, it was considered the most common drug used inappropriately after marijuana and was often associated with automobile accidents because it causes drowsiness and lack of judgment. Since then, it has become a relatively minor drug used inappropriately,

TABLE 7.3
Benzodiazepines

Brand Name	Onset Time*	Duration**	Generic Name
Ativan	I	IA	Lorazepam
Azene	R	LA	Clorazepate
Centrax	S	LA	Prazepam
Clonopin	I	LA	Clonazepam
Dalmane***	I–R	LA	Flurazepam
Doral***	I	LA	Quazepam
Halcion***	I–R	SA	Triazolam
Librium	I	IA	Chlordiazepoxide
Paxipam	S–I	IA	Halazepam
Restoril***	I	IA	Temazepam
Serax	S–I	IA	Oxazepam
Tranxene	R	LA	Clorazepate
Valium	R	LA	Diazepam
Valrelease	S	LA	Diazepam
Versed	I	SA	Midazolam
Verstran	S	LA	Prazepam
Xanax	I–R	IA	Alprazolam

*R = Rapid; I = Intermediate; S = Slow
**LA = Long-acting; IA = Intermediate-acting; SA = Short-acting
***Sleeping medications

largely because of the widespread availability of the benzodiazepines.

BENZODIAZEPINES

For the most part, benzodiazepines have replaced barbiturates and other nonbarbiturate hypnotics and sedatives in medical practice. A variety of benzodiazepines are available (Table 7.3), but it's hard to consistently find differences among them, except with those used for sleep disturbances. That causes considerable confusion for both physicians and patients in choosing the best drug with the least potential for dependency.

The benzodiazepines are thought to affect a particular neurotransmitter, gamma aminobutyrate (GABA), by triggering its calming effect. Benzodiazepine receptors have been identified in the outer part of the brain, and in its limbic system (associated, in part, with emotion and motivation).

Benzodiazepines are absorbed at varying rates, with onset of action ranging from 15 to 30 minutes, depending on the drug. (Valium acts quickest; Verstran slowest.) Levels of benzodiazepines accumulate quickly in the brain and blood, then decrease as the drug is distributed to other organs and metabolized until a "steady" state is reached. That's the point at which the amount taken is equal to the amount that's been broken down and eliminated.

Considerable mood-altering effects can be experienced during this initial period of changing brain levels. Early side effects include drowsiness, impaired thinking, diminished memory, reduced motor coordination, and slurred speech (Table 7.4). The effects differ depending on individual susceptibility, but they tend to go away after several days of consistent use.

Unlike the barbiturates and other nonbarbiturate hypnotics and sedatives (such as Doriden), benzodiazepines alone rarely produce fatal overdose. But when benzodiazepines are taken with other CNS depressants, including alcohol, fatal overdose is a real possibility.

Tolerance, Dependency, and Withdrawal. Even under medical supervision, persistent use of benzodiazepines can result in depen-

---

TABLE 7.4
Side Effects of Benzodiazepines
Drowsiness
Reduced level of consciousness
Impaired intellectual function
Impaired memory
Reduced motor coordination
Slurred speech

---

dency and withdrawal. Incidence of withdrawal has been difficult to document because the withdrawal symptoms are much like those for which these drugs are prescribed (Table 7.5). They include nausea, loss of appetite, anxiety with associated depression, depersonalization, abnormal perception or sensation. Seizures or psychotic behavior rarely may occur with barbiturate withdrawal.

The severity of withdrawal can be linked to dosage, duration of

---

TABLE 7.5
Benzodiazepine Withdrawal Symptoms

Anxiety*	Muscle aches*	Nausea
Dizziness*	Tremor*	Loss of appetite
Irritability	Sweating*	Depression
Insomnia*	Difficulty in concentration*	Depersonalization
Fatigue*	Increased sensory perception	Abnormal perception or sensation of movement
Headache*	Seizures**	Psychotic behavior**

*Common in anxiety states for which benzodiazepines are prescribed
**Rare

treatment, and to the particular drug. Ativan and Halcion have shorter half-lives and their metabolites have no activity, so they produce earlier withdrawal symptoms that can be harder to treat. Taking short-acting benzodiazepines regularly to get to sleep may, paradoxically, result in early-morning awakening. Those symptoms may be mild signs of withdrawal.

One extensive review of benzodiazepine withdrawal cases reported that withdrawal occurred 40 to 50 percent of the time with short-term use, and 40 to 100 percent of the time with use longer than one year. But when the symptoms for which these drugs were prescribed were considered, withdrawal after short-term use was no more than 5 percent of the time, and after long-term use no more than 50 percent of the time.

Eliminating such symptoms as anxiety, irritability, insomnia, muscle aches, and tremors can be misleading because they're typically seen with withdrawal from most CNS depressant drugs, including alcohol. In fact, these withdrawal symptoms have been reported to appear in patients who used medically indicated doses daily for as few as six weeks.

Potential for Inappropriate Use.   Without question, benzodiazepines are extremely valuable psychotherapeutic agents. They've been used successfully to treat a variety of disorders, including generalized and specific anxiety, panic attacks, sleep disorders, muscular and seizure disorders, and withdrawal symptoms from alcohol and other CNS depressants. They're also used to relax patients before they receive general anesthesia.

However, these drugs may not always be the best course of action, even when legally prescribed. A study of 119 patients on prescribed benzodiazepines found that one-third suffered from major depression and should have been taking antidepressants instead. Another 25 percent had panic disorders that were not relieved by the drug.

A subsequent study by the Food and Drug Administration revealed that some patients had been taking the drugs for years without medical supervision, despite their increased vulnerability to severe dependency and withdrawal after the first six months of use.

TABLE 7.6
Concerns over Regular Use of Benzodiazepine

Produces dependency and withdrawal

Easily used inappropriately

Among most common drugs identified in emergency room admissions

Commonly used in suicide attempts

Most commonly found legal drug in deaths due to unnatural causes

At least 25% of patients exceed prescribed dose, use it for other than prescribed reasons, or get it from nonmedical sources

Impairs motor skills, especially when driving

Exposes certain populations to increased risk

Withdrawal in newborns whose mothers had therapeutic levels in third trimester

Greater susceptibility to adverse reactions in the elderly, including hip fractures due to falls

Use with other CNS depressants increases depressant effects

Some benzodiazepines—diazepam, for example—are believed effective in treating certain muscular disorders, but their frequent use for lower back pain syndrome is controversial: the benefits may be attributable to decreased anxiety over the pain, rather than to actual relief of the muscle spasm. And their use in panic attacks, while effective for associated anxiety, does nothing for the underlying condition; antidepressants and other psychotropic drugs are probably a better choice. They also produce a much better outcome in treating mixed anxiety-depressive syndrome than depression alone.

As awareness of potential for inappropriate use expands (Table

7.6), prescriptions for benzodiazepines continue to decrease. The Food and Drug Administration emphasizes that appropriate studies of benzodiazepine effectiveness in treating anxiety for more than four months have not been done. New York State now requires prescriptions for benzodiazepines to be written in triplicate, just as for narcotics.

Chapter 8

Powerful Hallucinogens and Phencyclidine

Plants containing hallucinogenic substances can be grown in almost any climate, so hallucinogens have been used throughout the world from the earliest of times. In North and South America they have been used predominantly by Native Americans as part of religious observances. Peyote (mescaline), for example, continues to be used in that role today. Its religious significance has never been fully understood, but until recently its legal status has been upheld. The Native American Church of North America has been instrumental in repealing individual state laws prohibiting its use in such ceremonies. One researcher extensively reviewed peyote use by the Navajo as part of their religious practice and found no adverse reactions associated with it.

Development of lysergic acid diethylamide (LSD) by Albert Hoffman at Sandoz Laboratories in Switzerland in 1943 marked the beginning of serious interest in synthetic hallucinogenic drugs. Dr. Hoffman accidentally ingested LSD twice during its production. He found those first two experiences distinctly unpleasant, but they clearly demonstrated LSD's potent psychedelic properties.

Since then, LSD and its related compounds have been widely studied by basic researchers and psychiatrists. Enthusiasm for the beneficial effects of LSD was so great at first that some researchers encouraged friends and associates to take it for recreational purposes. Suggestions for its approved use began to flourish. They ranged from military applications (to incapacitate an enemy) to use as a palliative in cases of terminal cancer (Table 8.1). Some faculty members at

TABLE 8.1
Some Uses for LSD

Military application: brainwashing and/or disabling enemy forces
Aid in psychotherapy
Treatment of alcoholism
Treatment of opiate dependency
Palliation of cancer
Recreational use

many universities promoted LSD, leading to widespread use on college campuses during the 1960s. By the 1970s, an estimated 1 to 2 million Americans had taken LSD, and it ranked sixth in substance-involved crises at drug treatment centers. Recreational use began to decline by the end of the 1970s, but by 1982 approximately 21 percent of young people between the ages of 18 and 25 reported having tried it at some time in their lives. Estimates of use in 1989 by high school and college students are low, about 1 to 2 percent.

The response of society to use of LSD and related drugs, however, was far from enthusiastic and permissive. Concern focused on the immediate side effects and the adverse emotional reactions that occurred long after the drug had been taken. The prevailing campus theme, "Turn on, tune in, and drop out," contributed to public disapproval. LSD was classified as a Schedule I drug, similar to heroin, in the 1970s.

LSD and related compounds are relatively easy to synthesize. Illicit production and distribution began in the mid-1960s and reached such a peak that the United States had an oversupply. LSD has the unusual distinction of being the only drug illicitly synthesized in the United States and exported to Canada and Europe. Although use of LSD and some hallucinogens has greatly decreased, phencyclidine (PCP) has become more prominent.

CLASSIFICATION

Classifying a substance as a hallucinogen isn't simple. At first, the term "psychedelic" was used to describe all agents that produce visual hallucinations, usually accompanied by intensified perception or insight, and sometimes the kind of bizarre behavior and loss of contact with reality as seen in psychoses. "Psychoactive substance" describes any drug that affects the brain and subsequent behavior. Thus hallucinations can be caused by a variety of drugs, many of which share few, if any, pharmacological characteristics. Several mood-altering drugs are not primarily hallucinogens but produce hallucinations when taken in increased amounts. Still others have that effect when taken by susceptible people in small doses, or in combination with other mood-altering drugs. The hallucinogen classification in this section includes substances taken primarily to produce visual hallucinations and intensified perceptions. Although these substances themselves may differ, the psychological effects are fairly uniform: feelings of tranquillity, developing new meanings to life or watching one's life go by, and harmony with humankind and the environment—in short, mind-expanding sensations. That can be contrasted with the effects of heroin: introversion, an inward focus, and a "return-to-the-womb" environment.

Pharmacologically, it's best to classify hallucinogens according to their action on a specific neurotransmitter site (Chapter 3). But for practical purposes, classification by the subjective experiences they produce can be more helpful (Table 8.2). Thus hallucinogenic drugs can be classified as those that produce:

- effects almost identical to LSD
- effects similar but not identical to LSD
- experiences in addition to those with LSD
- completely different effects from LSD (category includes phencyclidine, PCP)

Many herbal preparations commonly used as teas contain mood-altering substances (Table 8.3). They have low potential for inappropriate use and are consumed infrequently, but purchasers may be unaware that they contain hallucinogens. Depending on the tea and quantity drunk, the effects may vary from mild dysphoria (feeling somewhat under the weather) to actual hallucinations.

LSD-like Drugs.   Hallucinogens are believed to exert their behavioral impact by modifying effects of the neurotransmitters, or messengers of the brain (Chapter 3). Depending on the drug, action on a particular neurotransmitter may be more or less pronounced.

The physiological effects of hallucinogens on the heart and blood vessels can show up within a few minutes as increased blood pressure and heart rate (sometimes accompanied by tremors), dilated pupils, elevated temperature, hyperactive reflexes, and sweating. Those signs may be accelerated when the substance is in the amphetamine (phenylisopropylamine) group (Table 8.2).

Visual hallucinations and perceptual changes appear in one to two hours. The user becomes either hypervigilant or withdrawn, perhaps changing from one condition to the other. There may be a fear of personality fragmentation, prolonged afterimages, and greatly altered time perception (feeling that the hours-long "trip" has lasted only minutes). Mood changes can range from excitability (especially with amphetamines) to tranquillity. A calming effect may appear after several hours, together with detachment and control. A clearing of mood sets in after 12 hours.

Different hallucinogens vary in how long their effects last. DMT, which has relatively short duration, is labeled the Businessman's Special. Drugs in the amphetamine group can produce effects lasting anywhere from three hours to two days. Differences also exist in potency. LSD is more than 100 times more potent than psilocibin, and 1,000 times more potent than mescaline.

Eve and Ecstasy.   Newer amphetamine derivatives continue to appear. They're part of the "designer drug" group, are often manufactured in clandestine laboratories (Chapter 2), and wax and wane in popularity. MDA combines chemical similarities of methamphetamine with properties similar to mescaline. When MDA (the Love Pill) was shown to produce damage to nerve terminals in laboratory animals, and agitation and convulsions in humans, it was replaced on the street by MDMA (Ecstasy).

MDMA was developed in 1914 as an appetite suppressant, but it was rarely used until the early 1980s when psychiatrists employed it

TABLE 8.2
Hallucinogens by Similarity to LSD Effects

Effect	Group	(NS)*	Street Name	Duration (Hours)
LSD-like				
LSD	Indolealkyamines	S	Acid, Barrels, Blotter, Blue Cap, Blue Cheer, Blue Dots, California Sunshine, Cherry Top, Camel, Candles, Cube-D, Dragon, King Tut, Man, Microdot, Mr. Natural, Orange Sunshine, Owsleys, Pape Acid, Purple Haze, 25, Wedges, White Lightning, Window Panes, Zigzag	12
Mescaline (peyote)	Phenylethyamines	A	Big Chief, Buttons, Cactus, Mesc, Mescal	4
Psilocibin	Indolealkyamines	S	Magic Mushroom, Shroom, Silly Putty	6
Morning glory seeds	Indolealkyamines	S	Glory, Mexicana	—
Similar to LSD				
DOM	Phenylisopropylamines	A	Peace, Serenity, STP, Tranquillity	Days
DMT	Indolealkyamines	S	Businessman's Special	1–2
LSD-like plus other properties				
MDA**	Phenylisopropylamines	A	Love Pill	Varies up to days

MMDA**	Phenylisopropylamines	A	
MDMA**	Phenylisopropylamines	A	Ecstasy
MDEA**	Phenylisopropylamines	A	Eve
Different from LSD Effect			
Atropine, Scopolamine	Cholinergic	C	
Muscarine	Cholinergic	C	
Physostigmine	Cholinergic	C	
Phencyclidine	Arylcyclohexylamines		Angel Dust, Crystal, Cyclone, DOA, Dust, Elephant, Goon, Itog, Killer Weed, Krystal, Loveboat, Mint, Monkey Dust, Peace Pill, PCP, Peace, Scuffle, Sherman, Supergrass, Superkool, Superpot, Surfer, T, Tac, Tran Q, Weed

*(NS) = Neurotransmitter receptor sites: A = adrenergic, C = cholinergic, S = serotonergic
**Designer drug (See Chapter 2)

Source: W. R. Martin and J. W. Sloan, "Pharmacology and Classification of LSD Hallucinogens," *Drug Addiction II: Amphetamine, Psychotogen and Marihuana Dependence,* ed. W. R. Martin. (Berlin: Springer-Verlag, 1977), 305–8.

TABLE 8.3
Hallucinogenic Plants in Herbal Teas

Plant

Popular Name	Scientific Name	Hallucinogenic Effect
Catnip	Nepeta cataria	Mild
Juniper	Juniper macropoda	Strong
Kavakava	Piper methysticum	Mild
Mandrake	Mandragora officinarum	Moderate
Nutmeg	Myristica fragrans	Moderate
Periwinkle	Cathacanthus rosens	Moderate
Thorn Apple	Datura stramonium	Strong
Yohimbe	Corynanthe yohimbe	Mild

Source: R. K. Siegel, "Herbal Intoxication: Psychoactive Effects from Herbal Cigarettes, Teas and Capsules," *Journal of the American Medical Association* 236 (1976): 473–76. Copyright © 1976 by American Medical Association.

to facilitate psychotherapy. Some don't consider it hallucinogenic, even though it has a marked psychoactive effect and hallucinations have been reported with its use. Recognition of its potential for inappropriate use and adverse effects led to its listing as a Schedule I drug in 1985. It came off Schedule I in September 1987, following a petition declaring its usefulness. But it went back on in March 1988, when the Drug Enforcement Agency ruled that MDMA had no acceptable medical use and that its safety had not been proven.

The DEA notwithstanding, those interested in promoting MDMA on the street slightly modified its structure and developed MDEA (Eve), claimed to produce effects similar to MDMA, with fewer adverse reactions.

Both Ecstasy and Eve are sold on the street in capsules or loose powders for $10 to $30 a dose. Their onset of action is less than 30 minutes, and they last four to six hours. The user feels an initial rush, followed by a feeling of increased activity (sometimes accompanied by muscle spasm) before reaching a high.

Attributing toxic reactions specifically to these drugs is difficult, but both have been associated with deaths. Whether the drugs were the sole cause of death in these cases is unknown. Use of these drugs is not widespread, but there is some cause for alarm. A late 1980s report indicated that 39 percent of students at one college had experimented with Ecstasy.

ADVERSE EFFECTS OF HALLUCINOGENS

Use of hallucinogens doesn't result in physical dependency, but there is a high degree of tolerance to the behavioral effects after several doses. Cross-tolerance exists among LSD-like drugs, but not with other hallucinogens. For that reason, a person tolerant to LSD who takes a higher dose of related hallucinogens may suffer severe toxic effects. Fatal reactions are rare and probably attributable to contaminants in the drug. Street purchases may contain strychnine, amphetamines, or PCP, among other adulterants.

Adverse psychological reactions, however, are common. They include panic reaction, suicide, post-LSD depression, flashback, and psychotic behavior.

Panic reaction—what is called a "bad trip"—is the most frequent adverse effect. Why some people almost never have a bad trip while others have one every time they take the drug is unclear. The individual's expectations undoubtedly influence the experience. So does the environment in which the drug is taken, as well as prior personality disorders. Taking a hallucinogen in too great a dose or with other mood-altering drugs can also cause a bad trip.

Suicide is a possibility during an extreme panic reaction, particularly when LSD is mixed with amphetamines. Panic reaction can be treated by placing the person in a quiet environment and providing reassurance that recovery will occur. Tranquilizers can be used but are rarely needed.

Physicians who are unfamiliar with the panic reaction caused by hallucinogens sometimes treat the condition with phenothiazines (Thorazine, Stelazine, etc.). Not only is this unnecessary, but when the panic reaction is caused by hallucinogens in the amphetamine group, it sometimes leads to intensified excitability and a drop in blood pressure. Treatment with phenothiazine is also associated with increased flashbacks.

Flashback is the phenomenon of a currently drug-free user suddenly returning to the mood-altering state of a prior "trip." It's called a "free trip" and happens to 10 to 15 percent of users. Flashbacks are more frequent among those who have combined hallucinogens with other drugs, or who are under extreme stress or anxiety. The precise cause of flashbacks is not clear. They can occur several times for up to a year following the last LSD use.

Post-LSD depression can last for months. Whether a cause-and-effect relationship exists is uncertain. Hallucinogens have also precipitated psychotic behavior; again, whether that behavior might have surfaced without use of these drugs is not known.

PHENCYCLIDINE (PCP)

Phencyclidine was first used by veterinarians in the 1950s as an anesthetic. Because it provided relief from pain (and some loss of memory) without significantly depressing the respiratory or cardiovascular systems, it was also used as an anesthetic for humans. But reports of disorientation, excitability, delirium, and even hallucinations upon awakening from anesthesia began to appear. By 1965, the adverse effects were well documented and PCP was discontinued for human use. For a time it remained available for animal use under the brand names Sernyl, Synalar, and Sernylan, but it is no longer available.

Mechanism of Action. Among the effects of PCP and related drugs are stimulation, depression, analgesia, and hallucinations. The reinforcing properties are probably the result of a combination of these effects, but none seems to dominate. Laboratory animals won't self-administer LSD or similar compounds, but they'll readily self-administer PCP, become tolerant, and undergo withdrawal when chronic use is stopped. Almost all neurotransmitters are affected by PCP, believed to bind with the sigma receptor, a type of opiate receptor (Chapter 10). Independent PCP receptors probably exist as well.

Patterns of Use. PCP wasn't popular when it first appeared on the street around 1965. It was usually taken when dealers passed it off as one of the more sought-after hallucinogens or put it in marijuana. PCP use increased from 1973 to 1979, tapered off until 1981, then rose again. Seven million people had used PCP by 1979; approximately 8.3 million by 1982. This was most apparent in metropolitan areas. In 1989 PCP was the second most frequently used drug in Washington, D.C.

PCP and its analogues are easily manufactured, making it difficult to identify and to eliminate illicit laboratories. In liquid form, PCP can be mixed with a beverage, but it is most commonly sprayed over other mood-altering substances. And as a liquid, it may contain volatile solvents that can contribute to acute reactions. PCP may be sold as cigarettes with thick brown wrappers that absorb the drug, or in small aluminum packages, from which it can be hand-rolled into cigarettes or placed in pipes.

Drugs sold as PCP are often mixed with stimulants, narcotics, or—most often—small amounts of marijuana. Of the PCP street samples that have been analyzed, up to half were contaminated with other drugs. When intentionally mixed with cocaine (Ghostbusters), it can produce marked antisocial behavior. When sold as powder (Angel Dust or Flakes), it's typically 50 to 100 percent pure. When it goes by other names, such as Rock Crystals, it's only 10 to 30 percent pure. The average dose in a PCP cigarette is about two milligrams. In one survey, up to 36 percent of first-time users didn't know they had taken PCP.

Effects of PCP can be felt within five minutes; intoxication follows within 15 to 30 minutes and lasts four to six hours. Craving after discontinuing the drug, as well as withdrawal, is possible.

Adverse Effects. As with other hallucinogens, the initial effects of PCP come from its stimulant properties (Table 8.4). These include

---

TABLE 8.4

Immediate PCP Effects

Psychologic
Combativeness
Visual hallucinations
Toxic psychosis
Disorientation

Autonomic
Rapid heart rate
Elevated blood pressure
Increased salivation
Respiratory depression

Neurologic
Coma
Convulsions

Renal
Kidney failure

---

increased blood pressure, rapid heart rate, and rapid breathing. Its other effects in the nervous system can produce flushing, wheezing, sweating, drooling, rapid eye movements, and constriction of the pupils. Users may appear clear-headed and oriented, or may have slurred speech and exhibit bizarre behavior. This can happen even with small doses. Larger doses may result in extreme mood alterations. Doses higher than 20 milligrams can cause extreme rises in body temperature, convulsions, breathing problems, coma, and cardiac rhythm disturbances—any of which may be fatal. PCP cigarettes can cause seizures, coma, and respiratory failure within one hour.

The effects of PCP have been classified into major and minor complications. The major patterns (Table 8.5) are sometimes fatal. They include coma, catatonia (total unresponsiveness), and acute brain syndrome, manifested by delirium and memory loss. Minor complications are disturbing, but usually not dangerous: lethargy, bizarre behavior, agitation, violence, and a dreamy high.

TABLE 8.5
Major PCP Complications

Coma
Less than two hours to weeks
Extremely high temperatures and blood pressures

Catatonic syndrome
Mute and staring
Muscle rigidity
Seizures, delusions, hallucinations

Toxic psychosis
Hallucinations, paranoid behavior, delusions, agitation

Acute brain syndrome
Disorientation, lack of judgment, memory loss
   without findings noted above

An acute toxic reaction is directly related to the PCP level in the blood, but a psychosis marked by impaired judgment may not be. Those with prior personality disturbances seem to be particularly susceptible to this complication.

Psychotic episodes similar to schizophrenia may continue to appear after the acute reaction and can last from four weeks to several months. This can be followed by depression, again lasting four weeks to several months, which may lead to suicide or a return to PCP.

Chronic use of PCP has been associated with memory loss, bouts of depression, recurrent psychotic episodes, and a chronic brain syndrome, called, in its most severe form, the "Alzheimer's Disease of Adolescence." This rare syndrome shows up as an inability to function and periods of forgetfulness.

PCP or related compounds have protected laboratory animals from brain damage resulting from strokes. The implications for decreasing disability from stroke and perhaps from other neurologic disorders in humans are enormous. But PCP has also shown an acute toxic effect on brain cells of laboratory animals.

Treatment.   Treatment of PCP reactions depends on the symptoms. In many cases of mild intoxication, no treatment other than reassurance is needed. For seizures, diazepam (Valium) or a similar drug can be given. Psychotic behavior is treated with such antipsychotic medications as haloperidol (Haldol). Large doses of PCP can be washed out of the stomach through a naso-gastric (nose-to-stomach) tube. A slurry of activated charcoal can also be given. And Vitamin C (ascorbic acid) increases elimination of PCP in the urine.

Depending on the severity of the effects and the patterns of use, treatment for chronic PCP use can be short-term inpatient psychiatric hospitalization or outpatient substance-abuse programs.

Chapter 9

Marijuana

Cultivation of *Cannabis sativa*, the marijuana plant, can be traced back thousands of years in both tropical and temperate climates. Its ability to alter mood, and use of its fiber in making linen, canvas, and rope, have made it a desirable crop. Mood-altering effects are obtained through eating, smoking, chewing, or drinking it. It was seen in the Americas as early as 1545, grown in Virginia around 1607 by the Jamestown settlers, and introduced into England about a decade later.

Throughout history, cannabis has been used to treat a variety of human complaints and disorders. In the United States, it was considered particularly effective for headaches, toothaches, and menstrual cramps. In fact, it was listed in the United States Pharmacopoeia until 1941. From 1913 to 1938, the Eli Lilly and Parke-Davis pharmaceutical companies maintained a farm where a highly potent strain, *Cannabis Americana*, was produced. Today, there are still some proposed medical uses for marijuana (Table 9.1), but the only use that has been generally accepted is to prevent nausea and vomiting following chemotherapy for cancer. Both dronabinol (Marinol), the principal psychoactive substances in marijuana, and nabilone (Cesamet), a synthetic cannabinoid, have been approved for that purpose.

The psychoactive effects of the plant were well known in the eighteenth and nineteenth centuries, but its use as a psychotropic agent was fairly limited in the United States until the 1920s, when the Eighteenth Amendment put an end to legal drinking. Interest in marijuana as a mood-altering substance suddenly grew. By the time

---

TABLE 9.1
Proposed Medical Uses of Marijuana

Analgesic
Anticonvulsant
Antidepressant
Antiemetic
Appetite enhancer
Bronchodilator
Preanesthetic agent
To reduce intraocular pressure in glaucoma
Sedative-hypnotic
To treat alcohol and drug dependency

Prohibition was repealed in 1933 and liquor once again became readily available, it was too late to stop the spread of the drug.

Public reaction led to efforts to restrict its accessibility. By 1937, marijuana had become illegal in 46 states. Penalties for its use were similar to those for morphine, heroin, and cocaine. The attitude toward marijuana was so negative that it was erroneously classified as a narcotic. Much of the public's thinking changed, however, as marijuana began to be perceived—especially by the young—as a relatively harmless substance whose adverse effects had been vastly exaggerated. But that thinking never permeated law enforcement agencies, which continued to consider marijuana as dangerous as other illicit substances. In the most recent turnabout, the appearance of much more potent marijuana has caused many who had been unconcerned about its use to reconsider.

PATTERNS OF USE

Despite vigorous attacks on marijuana, its use continued to increase through the general population. A 1969 Gallup poll of college students revealed that 22 percent had smoked marijuana. In December 1970 the number was 42 percent. The U.S. National Commission on Marijuana and Drug Abuse estimated in 1971 that 24 million

Americans had tried the drug. By 1979, marijuana was considered the third most common drug, after alcohol and cigarettes.

Approximately 60 percent of graduating high school students in the early 1980s had smoked marijuana at least once, and one out of eight progressed to daily use. A 1985 survey found that 5 percent of high school students (120,000 nationwide) were smoking marijuana. The same year, the National Center for Education Statistics reported that in one state, 3.5 percent of eighth graders, 9.5 percent of tenth graders, and 12.9 percent of twelfth graders smoked marijuana several times a week.

A 1990 survey (see Chapter 1) suggests that acceptance of marijuana has declined among high school students, daily use having dropped to 2.2 percent from a high of 10.71 in 1979. Nevertheless, the American Council on Education reported that 26 percent of students have used marijuana one to five times and 35 percent have used it more than five times. So marijuana is still very much with us. The 1988 National Household Survey on Drug Abuse reported approximately 66 million members of the household population to have used marijuana one or more times in their lives, with 11.6 million using it at least once in the past month.

MARIJUANA PREPARATIONS

The strength of cannabis plants is determined by the concentration of delta-9-Tetra hydro cannabinol (delta-9-THC), their major psychoactive substance. The delta-9-THC content ranges from 1.4 to 5 percent.

There are four major mood-altering products obtained from the plant (Table 9.2). Ganga comes from the dry leaves and flowering shoots. Hashish is a potent resin extracted from the top of the flowering plant; it contains 3 to 8 percent of delta-9-THC. Repeated purification of hashish yields extremely potent hashish oil, containing up to 20 percent delta-9-THC.

Marijuana is obtained from both the flowering tops and cut and dried leaves and stems. Potency varies greatly, depending on the plant (Table 9.3). A 500-milligram, U.S.-produced marijuana cigarette may contain from 0.5 to 1 percent delta-9-THC. With mari-

TABLE 9.2
Marijuana and Related Substances

Product	Origin	Street Name
Ganga	Leaf preparations	Bhang, Charas, Dugga, Goma de Mota, Kif, Machohina
Hashish	Resin from top of flowering plant	Hash, Rope, Soles, Sweet Lucy
Marijuana	Usually flowering tops, but also dried leaves and stems	Acapulco Gold, Berkley Boo, Brick, Grass, Hawaiian, Hay, Hemp, Herb, J, Jamaican, Jive, Joint, Key, Lid, Locoweed, Mary Jane, MJ, Mota, Mutah, Muggles, Pot, Reefer, Roach, Rope, Sativa, Sinsemilla, Skunk, Stick, Tea, Tocas Tea, Weed, Yerba
THC	Tetrahydrocannabinol	THC

juana imported from the West Indies, however, those numbers rise to 7 to 11 percent. In the late 1980s, law enforcement efforts lowered the amount of marijuana entering the United States. But that success has been accompanied by a more than twofold increase in domestic production, with the National Narcotics Intelligence Consumers Committee estimating it as representing 25 percent of the marijuana available in the streets. More significant, almost half the marijuana being harvested domestically is sinsemilla (from the unpollinated female plant), with a THC content of up to 14 percent. Phencyclidine (PCP), cocaine, hashish, or opium are sometimes mixed with, and sold as, straight marijuana. Of greater concern is the 1989 report by the Community Epidemiology Work Group of marijuana being laced

TABLE 9.3
Delta-9-THC Content of Street Drugs

Substance	Percent by Weight
Hashish	3–10
Hashish oil	10–30
Marijuana cigarettes	
Jamaican	0.5–4
U.S.-produced	Under 1
Sinsemilla (U.S.)	7–15

with insecticides. Identified in Phoenix and called Wac, this preparation has been associated with unusual psychiatric symptoms.

Synthetic delta-9-THC, approved by the Food and Drug Administration to combat nausea and vomiting caused by cancer chemotherapy, is occasionally diverted to the street or produced in clandestine laboratories. A potent synthetic designer drug, Synhexyl, was available through the mid-1970s and prompted considerable research.

Smoking Pot.   Marijuana can be smoked straight, mixed with tobacco, or eaten. Contrary to popular belief, marijuana smoke is carcinogenic, containing twice the amount of tar in tobacco.

When smoked, the amount of delta-9-THC that is absorbed by the lungs depends on how much is lost through burning (perhaps up to 60 percent) or through exhaled air, and how much is retained when the breath is held. From 50 to 60 percent of the THC may be delivered to the bloodstream. It's rapidly absorbed; a subjective effect is felt within minutes and continues for two to three hours.

When marijuana preparations are eaten and absorbed from the intestinal tract, first effects take 30 minutes to two hours to appear, with peak levels appearing in one to six hours. The amount of THC absorbed varies and is much less than with smoking because much is destroyed in the gastrointestinal tract and early metabolism in the liver.

Marijuana is fat soluble and enters many tissues, including the brain, heart, and liver. It's metabolized in the liver and excreted in the urine. Half of a single dose is eliminated in one day. In an infrequent user, marijuana can be detected in the blood for up to three days. In a frequent user, residual levels remain in the tissues and can be detected in urine for up to one month after the last use.

TOLERANCE, DEPENDENCY, AND WITHDRAWAL

Tolerance to the mood-altering effects of marijuana is typical; chronic users can consume, and often need, increased quantities to obtain the same feelings. Acute intoxication from marijuana is rare but has become more common with the widespread availability of the more potent varieties. It can show up as impaired learning, diminished performance, acute panic reactions, and symptoms of acute toxic psychosis. Such symptoms can include visual hallucinations, delirium, and paranoia.

Infrequent use of low doses seldom leads to withdrawal. But after discontinuing frequent high-dose use, anxiety, irritability, tremulousness, loss of appetite, and sleeping difficulties—all compatible with withdrawal—often follow.

ADVERSE EFFECTS

Adverse effects of marijuana were first described in the 1894 Indian Hemp Drug Commission Report, still considered one of the best systematic studies of the subject. In this century, a number of commission reports and books have attempted to define the effects of this drug. Some have been confirmed repeatedly; others haven't.

Effects on the Central Nervous System.   Marijuana's effects on the central nervous system vary greatly, depending on dose and the setting it's taken in. When smoked in a quiet environment, the most common positive feelings are euphoria and relaxation, accompanied by mild sedation. In a social setting, however, stimulation and increased activity are common. In such circumstances, users report keener visual and hearing abilities, and sometimes increased sexual arousal.

Taking marijuana when anxious can produce the opposite effect— an uncomfortable experience. Unlike alcohol, the high associated with a low dose of marijuana can be controlled; the person seems perfectly normal to an observer. Short-term memory can be impaired, however, and the transfer of information from intermediate to long-term memory can be slowed. Mental tasks involving complex thinking may be performed poorly.

Performance requiring coordination. Simple motor tasks may be accomplished, but complex ones, such as driving, are more difficult.

A study of teenagers who smoked the drug at least six times a month found them more than twice as likely to be involved in traffic accidents as nonsmokers. In California, one study reported detectable levels of delta-9-THC in 11 to 20 percent of drivers involved in fatal accidents. The levels were very low in most of the drivers, but blood alcohol was detected in 81 to 87 percent. Of those, 60 to 68 percent had levels high enough to cause intoxication. Those findings suggest that the combined effects of the two drugs might have precipitated the accidents.

A study of airline pilot reactions under simulated flying conditions found that 10 of 19 had substandard performances after smoking one marijuana cigarette. Impairment continued for up to 24 hours, but when tested after 24 hours, the pilots believed they were not affected by the marijuana.

Memory loss. Short-term memory loss—persisting for at least six weeks after discontinuing marijuana use—has been noted by several investigators. Their studies related the memory loss to dose and frequency of smoking. Marijuana smokers with learning disabilities or other cerebral dysfunctions might be at particular risk.

The antimotivational syndrome. The ability of marijuana to produce the "antimotivational syndrome" (Table 9.4) has been widely discussed. Chronic use is unquestionably linked to impaired function, slowed thought, and loss of coordination. But whether intermittent use in low doses results in the irreversible step toward the antimotivational syndrome is not certain.

TABLE 9.4
Antimotivational Syndrome

Loss of interest, apathy, passivity
Loss of productivity and desire to work consistently
Fatigue
Low frustration threshold
Impairment in concentration
Lack of concern with appearance
Consistent marijuana use

Laboratory animals show abnormal brain wave changes after smoking the equivalent of three marijuana cigarettes a day for three months. The changes can persist months after use is discontinued. Whether these findings are relevant to humans is yet to be determined.

Effects on the Lungs.   Marijuana smoke is toxic to the lungs, containing more carcinogens than cigarette smoke. Lethal pulmonary disease develops in laboratory animals tested with marijuana. In humans, asthma, bronchitis, and emphysema can follow hashish use. Studies demonstrate decreased pulmonary function in healthy volunteers after several weeks of heavy marijuana smoking. Burning and stinging of the mouth and throat, accompanied by a heavy cough, can occur even with infrequent use.

Effects on the Cardiovascular System.   Effects of marijuana on the heart are mild, usually related to an increase in heart rate. Blood pressure rises slightly when lying down; it decreases if a person often stands and smokes. Dizziness and loss of consciousness may occur.

Effects on the Eye.   Impact on the visual system usually consists of redness of the conjunctiva and a decrease in intraocular pressure (the pressure behind the eyes). This effect has led some to suggest that marijuana be used to treat glaucoma, a condition in which the increased pressure can cause blindness.

Other Effects. Miscellaneous effects relating to marijuana use include a "hangover," experienced the morning after smoking, a dry throat, and an increased appetite. In various experiments, marijuana has been shown to impair immune function, cause infertility in laboratory animals, and decrease sperm counts and blood testosterone levels in men. Disrupted menstrual cycles and complications with labor and delivery have been reported in women. These experiments have been faulted because they were done in laboratory settings using much higher doses of marijuana than usual, or on people prone to using other mood-altering drugs. So the practical value of the findings is unconfirmed.

Administering marijuana by intravenous injection is rare, but the practice has been reported. It produces a severe toxic-allergic reaction, which can include nausea, vomiting, and diarrhea. These symptoms are frequently accompanied by shock, kidney failure, and alterations in the blood clotting mechanism. Almost all such effects can be traced to the numerous unsterile substances found in the marijuana.

MOVING TO STRONGER DRUGS

Researchers studying marijuana use in adolescents say that experimentation with the drug sometimes leads from occasional social use, to continued regular use, and finally on to cocaine, heroin, or hallucinogens. Almost every such study, however, has shown that alcohol and nicotine consistently preceded that kind of progression as well. So it's curious that many who are quick to claim marijuana as a "cause" of subsequent illicit drug use are reluctant to see a causal link with alcohol and tobacco. Marijuana is neither benign nor harmless, but applying the same severe sanctions against its use as those against cocaine and heroin is unwarranted.

MEDICAL USES

Those who argue for legalization of marijuana say that, at the very least, it should be available by prescription for disorders that can't be treated effectively with existing medications. Delta-9-THC has been proposed for a number of medical conditions (Table 9.1). Its adverse effects when smoked, however, make it preferable to use a pure form of THC, or one of the several synthetic cannabinoids now being studied. The latter would provide the desired outcome without the side effects that even pure THC can produce.

The two most promising benefits appear to be marijuana's ability to alleviate nausea and pain. These effects, combined with the drug's mood-altering action, make it particularly valuable for cancer patients. As noted early in this chapter, dronabinol (Marinol) and nabilone (Cesamet) are now commercially available.

Studies of marijuana as a pain reliever, however, have not been consistently positive. When used as an analgesic under well-observed conditions, side effects are common. Furthermore, the actual degree of pain relief is low. The synthesis of delta-9-THC analgesics has yielded drugs that act well against pain and produce relatively few side effects, but their effectiveness doesn't appear to be greater than available analgesics.

TREATMENT ISSUES

Marijuana is considered a benign illicit drug with few or no withdrawal symptoms and minimal physical dependency, so no specific treatments have been developed. Surveys have revealed that marijuana users begin to taper off beginning in their early twenties; this decrease probably continues for the vast majority of smokers and so leads into a natural "maturing out" process. But marijuana's increasing potency and frequent association with other mood-altering drugs (predominantly alcohol) have verified its ability to cause psychological impairment and difficulty in functioning. Dealing with the antimotivational syndrome, especially among young users, has made both treatment and general counseling programs much more attuned to the problem.

Marijuana dependency is far less dramatic and obvious than dependency on cocaine, heroin, or amphetamines. But its effects on the daily functioning of those seriously involved with the drug are no less severe. One response has been the development of Marijuana Anonymous groups on the West Coast.

Chapter 10

Opiates and Opioids

Cultivation of the poppy plant dates back to 4500 B.C. The Sumerians, in what is now Iraq, cultivated the plant to extract its opium as early as 4000 B.C. Derived from the Greek work for "onion," opium was the name subsequently given to the juice of the poppy.

The first recorded reference to poppy juice was by the Greek philosopher Theophrastus in the third century B.C., but the medicinal value of opium was first described by Hippocrates, who praised it as a cathartic, styptic, and narcotic. By the seventeenth century, opium was being used throughout Europe; by the eighteenth century, it was being traded on a large scale. Increasing quantities were exported to the Far East, bringing prosperity to the many European countries that actively traded with China.

Profits from opium were so huge that the Opium Wars erupted in 1834 when China tried to stop importation of the drug. The Treaty of Nanking in 1842 legalized the Chinese opium trade. United States ships played a major role in transporting opium, but U.S. involvement with the drug wasn't limited to passive conveyance. During the nineteenth century, opiates were available in American grocery stores and pharmacies. They were dispensed freely by physicians and were consumed in numerous patent medicines. Invention of the hypodermic in the 1850s added injection as another way of taking opium, but smoking remained the prevalent method.

A German chemist isolated morphine from the alkaline base of opium in 1805, and several years later codeine was isolated in France. As concern about opium smoking escalated in the late 1800s, injectable morphine was touted as a cure for opium dependency.

This "solution" had just the opposite effect: the number of people dependent on morphine increased dramatically and the term "Soldiers' Disease" was coined during the American Civil War. Opium smoking began to decrease in the United States early in the twentieth century—about the time heroin was synthesized in England.

Early in this century an estimated 400,000 Americans were dependent on narcotics—roughly the same estimate as today. Despite many local, state, and federal efforts to restrict importation and use of opium and heroin, consumption didn't slack off until America's entry into World War II, when international drug traffic was severely limited. Toward the end of the war, fewer than 20,000 Americans were heroin-dependent. When international shipping routes opened again at war's end, heroin traffic flourished.

The demographics of heroin users have changed somewhat over the years. In the early 1900s, it was used primarily by Caucasians and Asians in brothels and opium parlors. After World War II, heroin use became common in the inner cities. In the 1950s it began to be seen more often in the young and in the suburbs. Heroin use peaked in the late 1960s and early 1970s and for several years during that time was the single leading cause of death of 20- to 35-year-old men in New York City. Heroin use has leveled off, but 1990 estimates put the number who are still dependent on it at 400,000 to 700,000, with concern being expressed that these numbers may increase.

OPIUM PREPARATIONS

Opium is derived by cutting the pod of the poppy plant to obtain a milky fluid. When air-dried, the fluid forms a thick brown mass that eventually becomes opium powder. The powder contains alkaloids, including morphine and codeine. Several legal opium preparations are still available today (Table 10.1). Morphine approximates 10 percent and codeine 0.5 percent of dry opium, by weight. Originally, these naturally occurring substances and their derivatives were called opiates. Substances made through synthetic processes were termed opioids. But currently, owing to common usage, both "opiate" and "opioid" are interchangeable and are also used to refer to

TABLE 10.1
Licit Opium Preparations

Name	Contents
Brown's mixture	12% paregoric, alcohol, antimony, potassium tartrate, glycyrrhiza extract
Pantopan	Opium alkaloids; slightly less potent than morphine
Paregoric*	Camphorated tincture of opium, 45% alcohol
Tincture of opium	10% opium, 19% alcohol

*Used by mixing with an antihistamine and injecting (street name Blue Velvet)

receptors in the brain specific for these drugs as well as to those drugs that mimic and oppose their action.

The natural opiates, the semisynthetic derivatives, and the synthetic opioids are all considered narcotics, defined as "a drug that in moderate doses dulls the senses, relieves pain and induces profound sleep, but in excessive doses, causes stupor, coma or convulsions." In a broader sense, however, "narcotic" refers to any drug that produces dependency; consequently, it has been used to describe cocaine, marijuana, alcohol, and amphetamines, depending on the locale.

It's misleading to use "narcotic" to encompass all dependency-producing drugs. In this chapter, the word refers only to the opiate and opioid drugs or their antagonists.

OPIATE ACTION ON THE BRAIN

Among the narcotic drugs, morphine, the original derivative of opium, is considered the standard or prototype when discussing dependency, tolerance, and withdrawal. Its actions are relatively consistent and have been studied extensively. But all narcotics in equivalent doses can have similar effects, varying only in intensity and duration of action.

TABLE 10.2
Commonly Used Licit Narcotics

Common or Brand Name	Generic Name	Street Name	Potency*
Morphine and related opioids			
Duramorph PF, MSIR, RMS, Roxanol, Uniserts, Mscontin	Morphine	Big M, Micro Dots, Miss Emma	1
Codeine			(0.3)
Dilaudid	Hydromorphone	First Line, Fours	6
Hycodan	Hydrocodone		No data
Levo-Dromoran	Levorphanol		5
Percocet**, Tylox**, Roxiprin**	Oxycodone	Morph, Percolators	2
Codoxy**, Percodan, Roxicet**, Roxicodone		Morphine	2
Numorphan	Oxymorphone	Goma	1

Demerol and related drugs			
Demerol	Meperidine	Cube	0.13
Lomotil	Diphenoxylate, atropine sulfate		
Nisentel	Alphaprodine		0.2
Fentanyl, Sublimaze	Fentanyl	China White	80–100
Methadone and related drugs			
Dolophine	Methadone	Disks, Dollies, Wafers	1
Darvon, Darvon N, Darvocet**, Doxaphene**, Dolene, Genagesic**, Profene 65, SK65, Propacet**, Wygesic**, E-Lor**, Bexophene**	Propoxyphene	Pinks and Grays	0.5

*Compared with 10 mg morphine (injected), except for Percocet, Tylox, Percodan, Codoxy, and Doxaphene, which are taken orally

**Contains acetaminophen or aspirin

Common effects on the central nervous system include pain relief without loss of consciousness (analgesia), mood changes, drowsiness, nausea, and vomiting. Constriction of the pupils and respiratory depression can occur, depending on dose. With chronic or high-dosage use, hormones secreted from the pituitary gland may be affected.

Opiate Receptors.   In 1973 scientists in three different laboratories identified certain nervous system receptors believed to be sites for opiate binding. Those findings have helped us better understand how opiates act on the brain and why people go on taking them even when there's no pleasurable effect (Chapter 3). Eight receptors have already been identified, but many more are known to exist. The four considered most closely associated with opiate activity are the mu, kappa, delta, and sigma receptors.

The mu and, to a lesser extent, the kappa receptors are considered primarily responsible for the classic opiate effect of pain relief. Delta receptors are probably involved with the pleasurable or unpleasurable reactions. Sigma receptors are thought to relieve depression and may be the sites for such mood-altering drugs as PCP. The kappa receptors also moderate the sedative effects of the opiates.

Opiatelike substances in the brain, pituitary gland, and other parts of the body were isolated several years after discovery of the opiate receptors. These substances, called endogenous peptides, are classified in three major groups: enkephalins, endorphins, and dynorphins. Although their exact roles have yet to be determined, they're being closely examined in connection with an individual's predilection for pain, their effect in producing dependency, and even in maintaining emotional well-being.

Agonists and Antagonists.   Three major groups of drugs have been identified on the basis of opiate action on the receptors:

- those that primarily alter mood and relieve pain (agonists)
- those that displace or block opiates from receptors and have no mood-altering effects (antagonists)
- those that have both agonist and antagonist actions

If agonist effects in the third group predominate, the drugs can alter mood and are susceptible to nonmedical use. That is important because, as discussed below, a number of agonist-antagonist "pain-killers" are on the market. They've been touted as being able to provide effective pain relief with little or no risk of dependency. That is not the case.

EFFECTS ON THE BODY

Except for its depressant effect on the brain and potential for overdose, the physical effects of morphine and other opiates are mild—probably less harmful physically than other drugs. Common effects of opiates include:

- decreased secretion of stomach acid
- decreased activity in the large and small intestines, resulting in constipation—one of the reasons opium and morphine are used to treat diarrhea
- probable constriction of the gallbladder ducts
- somewhat decreased urine flow as a result of action on muscles of the urethra and bladder
- slowed labor and depressed fetal respiration when given to control predelivery pain

All these manifestations vary, depending on individual suscepti-bility and the specific opiate.

The liver metabolizes morphine but is minimally affected by it. In the presence of liver disease, however, increased levels of mor-phine may exist in the blood and brain—posing a risk for respiratory depression and an overdose reaction.

TOLERANCE, DEPENDENCY, AND WITHDRAWAL

Tolerance.   Morphine tolerance develops at different rates, de-pending on the receptor involved. Tolerance to the analgesic or eu-phoric effects develops quickly, but tolerance to respiratory depression may remain unchanged. That makes opiate dependent people more susceptible to respiratory depression when they take increasing quantities to get high.

Subtle physiologic changes produced by opiates persist long after use is discontinued. Laboratory animals can have altered responses to pain up to 12 months after morphine withdrawal. Morphine-induced changes in the respiratory center can also persist in humans for prolonged periods. These changes can be measured in a laboratory setting but are not chemically important.

Dependency.   Morphine and its related compounds can cause high degrees of dependency, tolerance, and withdrawal (Chapter 2). When used inappropriately, addiction can develop quickly in both laboratory animals and humans. In humans, withdrawal can be brought on by a narcotic antagonist after taking only four to six pain-relieving doses of morphine or comparable drug a day for as few as three days. But when such drugs are used to control acute pain, the level of dependency isn't great enough to outweigh the primary objective—relief of pain.

The reinforcing effects of morphine are not necessarily related to physical dependency. Rats that become dependent by drinking bitter-tasting morphine solutions will consume greater quantities of quinine solutions (also bitter) than other rats. By the same token, people who inject heroin cut with quinine often experience a high from quinine alone if they think the substance contains heroin. As with other mood-altering substances, expectations and the environment in which heroin is taken often greatly influence the pleasurable effects (Chapter 3).

Withdrawal.   Physical signs of opiate withdrawal consist of early and late phases, with the time of appearance of each phase depending on the duration of action of the specific opiate. The user who realizes that another dose is unobtainable can develop anxiety considerably earlier than actual physiological symptoms. The resulting behavior is called "purposive," focused on obtaining the drug. Symptoms that can be objectively evaluated, independent of environment or other people, are "nonpurposive" (see Chapter 11).

OPIATES SUSCEPTIBLE TO NONMEDICAL USE

Almost all medically prescribed opiates can be used inappropriately, either to get high or to substitute for heroin or other opiates (Table 10.2). Many medically prescribed opiates may be combined with other analgesics such as aspirin or acetaminophen in order to enhance pain relief. One solution used for many years, "Brompton's Cocktail," contained cocaine in addition to heroin (or morphine), alcohol, and syrup. Originally used quite successfully for persons with severe pain due to cancer treatment, it has undergone numerous "recipe" changes over the years and has now finally given way to newer drug combinations.

Opium.   Opium is commercially available in a variety of medications. One method of using these medications inappropriately occurred some years ago and involved paregoric, a camphorated tincture of opium. Before the development of the synthetic opiate diphenoxylate (Lomotil), now commonly used for diarrhea, paregoric was the common treatment.

When paregoric was sold as an over-the-counter medication in the 1960s, heroin addicts regularly boiled it with the antihistamine tripelennamine. The mixture, sold on the street as "Blue Velvet," was injected. It was first believed that addition of the antihistamine reduced allergic reactions and gave the substance its distinctive smooth consistency. The understanding now is that the antihistamine probably allows greater uptake of opium in the brain. The mixture was so thick that peripheral veins quickly became clotted, and the larger veins in the neck were used. Scarring of the skin over the jugular veins became a sign of Blue Velvet use.

Morphine and Related Opioids
Codeine.   A naturally occurring alkaloid of opium, codeine is found in raw opium in concentrations of 0.7 to 2.5 percent. It's a mild analgesic widely available in combination with acetaminophen (Tylenol), aspirin, and many commercial cough medicines. Codeine used appropriately is an extremely effective analgesic. Codeine used inappropriately in high doses is not.

Hydromorphone (Dilaudid).   Dilaudid is a semisynthetic derivative of morphine, approximately six to eight times more potent. It's
an effective analgesic and can produce a high with a dependency
similar to that of morphine when taken either orally or by injection.
   Oxycodone combinations.   Percodan, Percocet, Roxicet, Roxi-
prin, Tylox, and Codoxy are oral analgesics that contain oxycodone,
plus homatropine, aspirin, or acetaminophen (Tylenol). These commonly prescribed semisynthetic opiates produce a dependency similar to that of morphine when used continuously. Dependency occurs
by rapidly escalating the oral dose or by dissolving the tablet in water
and injecting the solution. A large amount of oxycodone and aspirin
taken orally can cause gastric upset and bleeding, primarily a side
effect of the aspirin.

Demerol and Related Drugs

Meperidine (Demerol).   Demerol is one of the prototype synthetic opiates called phenylpiperidines. It's similar to morphine, but
as an analgesic is only one-quarter as effective and has a much shorter
duration of action. Unlike morphine, Demerol in large doses may
result in central nervous system toxicity, ranging from tremors to
seizures. These toxic effects are primarily due to the accumulation
of normeperidine, a Demerol metabolite. Normeperidine is further
metabolized in the liver and excreted in the urine by the kidneys, so
individuals with liver or kidney disease may be particularly susceptible to its toxicity. The general belief that Demerol is a ''mild''
narcotic has made it one of the most widely prescribed narcotic analgesics. It can be taken orally or by injection. Chronic use several
times a day can result in considerable dependency and tolerance.
   Lomotil.   Frequently used to treat diarrhea, Lomotil is a derivative of the group of drugs that contain meperidine (Demerol) and
fentanyl (China White). It also contains atropine sulfate. Its potential
to produce dependency is far less than morphine's, and it was once
mistakenly thought not to be a narcotic. In that guise, Lomotil was
briefly used as a maintenance agent to treat heroin dependency
(Chapter 11).
   Fentanyl (China White).   Fentanyl, another synthetic opiate in the
phenylpiperidine group, is approximately 80 times more potent as a

pain reliever than morphine. The drug is used mainly during anesthesia and in the immediate postoperative period. In the early 1980s a fentanyl analogue, China White, was being sold on the street, primarily in Southern California. It is 50 to 2,000 times more potent than street heroin. Extremely small amounts provide a high. Compared with heroin, Fentanyl provides, according to users, a subtler initial "rush," a longer period of sleepiness following injection, and a more gradual "come down" (Chapter 11). However, it is far more deadly because of the possibility of overdosing.

Methadone and Derivatives

Methadone.   Methadone, one of the phenylheptylamine group of synthetic opiates, was originally synthesized in Germany at the end of World War II when morphine supplies were not readily available. Through the next several decades it received considerable attention in the United States and became the drug of choice for treating chronic, unremitting pain. It was taken off the market soon after first being used as maintenance therapy for heroin addiction (Chapter 11) but became available again for pain relief in 1975.

Methadone is about equal to morphine in actions and potency, but much more effective when taken orally and slightly more potent when injected. Unlike morphine, methadone provides consistent analgesia without the need to rapidly increase the dose because it's widely distributed to body tissues and then slowly released into the bloodstream. These properties are most beneficial to patients in need of continuing pain relief and/or maintenance therapy (Chapter 11). They also allow detoxification from opiates to proceed smoothly. Methadone is rarely used inappropriately when prescribed for pain relief. Its use in maintenance therapy, however, has created a street market, where it's sold to those who don't want to enter heroin treatment programs or who want to "boost" their highs.

L-Acetylmethadol (LAAM).   LAAM is a long-acting methadone preparation developed specifically for use in maintenance therapy. It suppresses withdrawal symptoms for up to 96 hours on a single dose. LAAM is no longer available, however; it was found to be associated with adverse side effects and fetal toxicity in laboratory animals.

Propoxyphene (Darvon).   Propoxyphene is a derivative of methadone. The drug, which like other opiates produces analgesia, is manufactured in various forms by more than 35 companies. Shortly after propoxyphene was introduced, more than 31 million prescriptions were written, making it the third most commonly prescribed drug. Alone, or in combination with aspirin, phenacetin, or caffeine, in 1987, it ranked approximately fifteenth among the most commonly prescribed drugs in the United States. The analgesic effect is similar to codeine's but its potency is not as great. Propoxyphene is available as both a short-acting and long-acting agent; Darvon-N is the brand name for the latter.

Most physicians consider propoxyphene a relatively safe, nondependency-producing analgesic. But it is an opioid and can lead to dependency, tolerance, and withdrawal when taken in large doses. Dependency on the drug has become well recognized; it was the eighth most frequently used mood-altering substance in the United States in 1987. In 1979 the Food and Drug Administration required that a warning of risks be placed on the labels of all products containing propoxyphene, and that printed information be made available to patients.

Both toxic reactions and treatment of overdose reactions are similar to those seen with other opiates. Respiratory depressant effects of propoxyphene are also enhanced by alcohol or any other CNS depressant.

Opiate Agonists-Antagonists. Opiate antagonists displace opiates from the receptors in the brain. That action is extremely helpful in treating a pharmacologic overdose and can be useful in diagnosing subtle opiate dependency by producing withdrawal symptoms. Efforts to develop an opiate analgesic that produces pain relief without dependency resulted in a new series of drugs with both agonist and antagonist properties (Table 10.3). Although these drugs can displace pure opiate agonists from receptor sites and produce withdrawal, they also have dependency-producing potential.

Pentazocine (Talwin). Talwin was initially promoted as a nonnarcotic analgesic with low risk of dependency. For a time, it was one of the most frequently prescribed analgesics. But its dependency-producing power was amply demonstrated in laboratories and in clin-

TABLE 10.3
Opiate Agonists-Antagonists

Brand Name	Generic Name	Potency*
Nubain	Nalbuphine	1
Stadol	Butorphanol	5
Talwin	Pentazocine	0.3
Buprenex	Buprenorphine	25–30

*Compared with 10 mg morphine (injected)

ical studies among people for whom it was prescribed, and in some physicians and other professionals who had access to it.

The drug quickly became available on the street. It was either injected as a mixture with the antihistamine tripelennamine (street name Ts and Blues) or injected alone as a heroin substitute. Typical illicit use is to crush one or two 50-milligram tablets with a tripelennamine tablet, dissolve the powder in water, strain it through cotton, and inject it intravenously.

The rush is indistinguishable from that of heroin. But it is followed by dysphoria, or a low, and a repeat injection is needed to experience a high. Several injections may be needed. Frequent use can lead to withdrawal similar to that seen with pure opiates. Frequent injections of Talwin have caused seizures, apparently the result of tripelennamine's stimulation of the central nervous system.

Talwin is now a Schedule IV drug, which limits prescriptions to six months and requires accurate record keeping.

Newer agonists-antagonists. Some of these drugs have potencies 5 to 40 times greater than that of morphine. They are promoted as having low levels of dependency and therefore can be prescribed without any of the restrictions usually applied to dependency-producing drugs. But since all these drugs have a mood-altering effect, dependency and subsequent addiction can follow. In fact, heroin addicts report that buprenorphine (Buprenex) has essentially the same effects as heroin. Inappropriate use of this drug has already been reported in Ireland. Another brand of the same agent, Stadol, has been diverted from pharmacies in the United States as well.

Chapter 11

Heroin Addiction

Heroin (diacetylmorphine) is a morphine derivative with three to five times the potency of morphine. The pharmacological effects of heroin and morphine are almost identical. Heroin is transformed into morphine within five minutes of being injected; after 40 minutes concentrations of morphine in the blood may exceed those of heroin. The one major difference between injecting pure heroin and pure morphine is the greater speed at which heroin enters the brain, perhaps precipitating an overdose. Heroin is legally available by prescription in England and several other countries but classified as a Schedule I drug in the United States. As an illegal drug, it is supplied only by the street trade.

HEROIN FROM OPIUM: THE STREET TRADE

Preparing heroin from opium is a relatively simple process requiring little sophistication. Raw opium is dissolved in water and "purified" by adding lime salts, ammonium chloride, alcohol, and ether. The mixture is filtered to extract organic wastes, leaving "pure" morphine. This solution is combined with hydrochloric and sulphuric acids, charcoal dust, and water. It's filtered, heated, filtered again, then mixed with ammonia to facilitate separation of morphine. The process yields a brown morphine base, reduced about one-tenth in volume, ready for conversion to heroin.

Producing the morphine base requires only minimal laboratory equipment. Synthesis of heroin is more complicated, taking up to 24 hours to pass the base through cycles of mixing with acetic acid anhydride and chloroform to remove impurities. The resulting brown heroin is sold as is, or bleached and treated with hydrochloric acid. Baked and sifted, it becomes a white powder up to 90 percent pure.

Heroin may be sold at any point in the process (Table 11.1). Heroin Number 1 is the crude morphine base used in producing more refined products. Heroin Number 2 is used for smoking and injection, Number 3 mainly for smoking. Many variations exist, and the composition of a specific heroin preparation may change with locality.

Once the dealer gets the heroin, all pretense of quality control ceases. The drug passes through several more levels of distribution and quality consistently decreases as it's "cut" with a variety of adulterants (Table 11.2), many of them poisonous. The most common are sugar (lactose) and quinine. Lactose gives the heroin mixture a white color to suggest greater purity. Quinine's bitter taste is similar to heroin's and can confuse the buyer about the mixture's quality and actual heroin content. Dealers may also add coloring to identify their own particular brand or may mix in other mood-altering drugs, such as amphetamines (Bombitas) and cocaine (Speedballs). Adding such stimulants provides an immediate rush and may also decrease the period of sleepiness that immediately follows a heroin injection.

Once heroin reaches the dealer on the street, its concentration is unpredictable. A substance supposedly containing heroin might have none at all or 20 to 30 percent. Consequently, the user always risks a pharmacologic overdose.

Many street names are given to heroin itself (Table 11.3) and to heroin preparations and combinations (Table 11.1). Some are simply slang; others may refer to a particular type of heroin produced in a particular place. Names are changed regularly to promote sales. A newer form of heroin, Black Tar, originated in Mexico and contains much higher proportions of heroin (40 to 80 percent) than the usual samples of street heroin (2 to 6 percent). Black Tar is difficult to dilute because of its gummy consistency, giving it a greater potential for overdose. It also attracts moisture from the air to form acetic acid, which can cause severe scarring when injected.

Some substances sold as heroin may really be designer drugs made by modifying a synthetic narcotic (Chapter 2). Derivatives of fentanyl (China White, Tango and Cash) are 3,000 times more potent

TABLE 11.1
Types of Heroin

Street Name	Composition and/or Color	Method of Administration
Heroin preparations		
Number 1	Crude morphine base; tan/brown	Smoking
Number 2	White/gray	Injection and smoking
Number 3—White	May contain caffeine (30–50%) or small dose of strychnine (rarely); tan/gray	Smoking
Number 4	White to yellow	Injection
Black Tar	Higher-quality heroin	Injection
Iranian Heroin (Dava, Rufus, Persian Brown)	Heroin with adulterants, becoming dark, reddish brown powder	Injection
Red Chicken	Heroin and red dye, Fentanyl	Smoking, injection

Heroin combinations		
Mexican Brown	Heroin and coffee	Injection
Bombitas	Heroin and amphetamines	Injection
Speedball	Heroin and cocaine	Injection
Designer "heroin"		
China White	Fentanyl analogues	Injection
Tango and Cash	Fentanyl analogues	Injection
MPPP, MPTP	Meperidine analogues	Injection
*Other illicit opiate preparations**		
Blue Velvet, Ts and Blues	Pentazocine, tripelennamine	Injection
Loads (Setups)	Codeine, glutethimide (Doriden)	Injection

* Used when heroin is unavailable

TABLE 11.2
Contaminants and Adulterants in Heroin

Amphetamine	Cotton fibers	Nicotine
Baking soda	Fuel oils	Parathion
Barbiturates	Gum resin	Procaine
Battery acid	Lactose	Quinine
Caffeine	Mannite (Mannitol)	Starch
Cocaine	Methapyriline	Strychnine

TABLE 11.3
Street Names for Heroin

Bing	Dynamite	Mud
Boy Jive	Estuffan	Scat
Brown	Foolish Pleasure	Shit
Caballo	Funk	Skag
Chivo	H	Smack
Crap	Hombre	Sugar
Dead on Arrival	Horse	Sweet Jesus
Dope	Jive	Tango and
Doo Doo	Junk	Cash
Duke	La Bamba	

than morphine and produce a high indistinguishable from that of heroin. Analogues of meperidine (MPPP and MPTP) are also sold on the street as synthetic heroin. They may cause a syndrome resembling Parkinson's disease, that destroys neurons in the brain.

PATTERNS OF USE

Heroin can be taken several ways: smoking, snorting or sniffing, injecting under the skin (skin popping), and injecting intravenously (mainlining)—the most common method. Frequent use of any of these techniques can result in dependency. Many heroin addicts began by sniffing the drug when they were teenagers.

Mainlining causes the greatest degree of dependency and addiction. The heroin is usually dissolved in water, boiled in a futile effort to remove impurities, and then injected. Shooting up is often a group activity, where a set of works may be used by dozens of people in one day without being cleaned between uses. This, of course, exposes the user to a wide variety of communicable diseases, including hepatitis and the human immunodeficiency virus (HIV), the cause of AIDS (Chapter 17).

GETTING HIGH AND COMING DOWN

Several seconds after injection, a flush and warmth are felt throughout the body, followed by drowsiness. The user appears to be asleep at that point but can be aroused and will respond to questions. Next comes a high that can last for several hours, followed by a feeling of relaxation, when the user may function normally. Except for constriction of the pupils, it's not always apparent that the user is on opiates.

Frequent injections are necessary once dependency has developed, or withdrawal symptoms appear. How long it takes for dependency to develop depends on many factors, including frequency, quantity, and user's expectations. Dependency can show up after several days of frequent injection. Early signs of withdrawal may be due to increasing anxiety over obtaining another dose of heroin (purposive behavior). Later signs may result from physiologic changes that occur after heroin use has stopped (nonpurposive behavior).

Purposive behavior includes extreme nervousness or anxiety, demands for money and/or drugs, and an increased level of activity. This type of behavior peaks within 24 hours and can be modified greatly by a sympathetic observer and a calm environment.

Nonpurposive symptoms range from mild to severe (Table 11.4) and generally appear eight to 12 hours after the last injection. Untreated, the symptoms become intense within 36 to 48 hours, then gradually subside over the next week. Late signs and symptoms of

TABLE 11.4
Heroin Withdrawal Signs and Symptoms

Mild	Moderate	Marked	Severe
Yawning	Loss of appetite	Deep breathing	Vomiting
Tearing of eyes	Dilated pupils	Fever	Abdominal cramps
Running nose	Tremors	Restlessness	Diarrhea
Sneezing	Gooseflesh (termed	Agitation	Muscle spasms
Sweating	"cold turkey")	Elevated blood pressure	(termed "kicking the habit")

withdrawal, however, have been observed for up to two years in prisoners who have stopped using drugs.

Withdrawal symptoms can be eliminated at any time by administering an opiate.

ADVERSE EFFECTS

Many severe and often life-threatening complications result from heroin use (Table 11.5). Almost all are related entirely to impurities in the drug, unsterile injection, and injection of unknown strength of heroin.

Acute Fatal Reaction. At one time, the acute fatal reaction accounted for 80 percent of heroin addict deaths in New York City. Death strikes so fast that the user is found with the needle still stuck in a vein and a hand on the syringe. For many years such deaths were believed to result from true pharmacologic overdose, an understandable conclusion since a bag of heroin might contain from zero to 10 milligrams of the pure drug. An accumulation of evidence,

---

TABLE 11.5
Complications from Heroin Use

Acute fatal reaction

Allergic and febrile reactions

Cardiovascular system
Rhythm disturbances, infarction of heart valves (endocarditis),
inflammation of small arteries (vasculitis), inflammation and
clotting of veins (thrombophlebitis)

Dermatologic problems
Abscesses, ulcers, hyperpigmented areas, track marks, scarring,
swelling

Endocrine system
Low blood sugar, sexual dysfunction

Gastrointestinal tract
Decreased stomach-emptying, bile secretion, and intestinal
activity; constipation

Hematologic and immunological abnormalities

Liver
Hepatitis, chronic liver disease

Infections in multiple organ systems

Respiratory system
Increased susceptibility to pulmonary infections; increased
pressure in pulmonary vessels

---

however, failed to support pharmacologic overdose as the major
cause of death.

For one thing, postmortem toxicology reports were positive for
morphine or heroin in only half the cases. And when those drugs
were detected, their levels were quite low, and other drugs were also
found. The Medical Examiner's Office in New York City found that

half of those who died from acute fatal reactions had detectable levels of blood alcohol—greater than 0.1 percent in 25 percent of the cases.

Even when a group of people had shared heroin, only one might have experienced an overdose. The inferior quality of the heroin on the street, or in bags surrounding the deceased, also made it unlikely that pharmacologic overdose would occur in someone with high tolerance.

Many factors unrelated to actual heroin concentrations may contribute to a death (Table 11.6). One of the most common is use of multiple drugs, including alcohol and other CNS depressants (Chapter 6, Chapter 7). Several postmortem studies of heroin addicts have shown alcoholic cirrhosis to be the most common form of liver disease, a finding that implicates multiple drug use in overdose reactions.

The suddenness of the death is associated with marked fluid accumulation in the lungs and brain, similar to severe allergic reactions from such drugs as penicillin. Considering the various adulterants and contaminants in heroin, allergic reactions might be expected. Another cause is suppression of the gag reflex and aspiration of stomach contents into the lungs. This can happen when heroin is injected after a full meal and the user becomes sleepy. Suffocation and death follow.

In some cases contaminants (Table 11.2), notably quinine, can affect cardiac rhythm. When combined with a depressant effect on the central nervous system and a drop in oxygen level, abnormal heart rhythms may be fatal.

Of course, a true pharmacologic overdose may sometimes be the cause of death. And it may become more prevalent as more potent forms of heroin, including designer drugs, appear on the street.

Treating the acute fatal reaction. Someone who is undergoing an acute reaction to heroin must be taken to a medical facility as quickly as possible. An open airway must be maintained, artificial respiration applied, and oxygen given if needed. At the medical facility, an opiate antagonist should be administered immediately. If the problem *is* overdose, the drug will reverse the action of the heroin.

TABLE 11.6
Causes of Acute Fatal Reaction
Alcohol and multiple drug use
Allergic reaction
Aspiration of stomach contents
Changes in cardiac rhythms
Pharmacologic overdose

Unfortunately, that scenario is rarely followed. Typically, home-made remedies—never appropriate—are tried first. Coffee is urged on the person to provide a stimulant. He or she may be slapped or doused under a cold shower. Fluids are forced down the throat to induce vomiting. Salt may be injected under the skin in an effort to "draw out" the heroin. Such measures serve only to seriously delay proper treatment and to worsen the situation if vomiting is induced.

The acute fatal reaction needn't cause death if prompt and correct measures are taken.

Infections. Infections are the most common complications of heroin use because contaminated material is often injected into the body under unsterile conditions. Almost every organ system can be affected.

Infection of the heart valves (endocarditis) often results in significant destruction of the valve with a progressive impairment of heart function. Surgical replacement of the damaged valve is often required.

Multiple pulmonary infections are frequent. They can range from pneumonia to lung abscesses, formed when pieces of contaminated material travel from the veins through the right side of the heart and into the lungs.

Infections can also occur in the muscles, bones, and brain. All have chronic, often disastrous complications.

Localized infections at the injection site are particularly common. Abscesses beneath the skin from skin popping, track marks (veins clotted from infections), and puffiness of the arms and hands from old infections are all signs of injecting contaminated material and/or using unsterile needles.

Liver Disease.   Hepatitis, a viral infection of the liver, is regularly transmitted through shared needles. Laboratory evidence of liver dysfunction due to hepatitis exists in up to 75 percent of users. The illness may subside or become chronic and ultimately lead to cirrhosis. Since many heroin addicts also drink large quantities of alcohol, the role of alcohol in chronic liver disease must also be considered.

Effects on the Immune System.   Heroin use also affects the immune system; enlargement of the lymph nodes is a routine finding in users. The many immunological abnormalities also identified in heroin users are highly likely to increase susceptibility to all infections, including AIDS (Chapter 17). Transmission of the human immunodeficiency virus (HIV) by shared needles is the most recent in a long line of complications associated with heroin dependency.

Effects on the Central Nervous System.   Multiple and sometimes deadly effects of heroin use involve the central nervous system: overdose reactions with depression and coma, paralysis caused by destruction of the spinal cord lining (demyelination), local nerve impairment, and extensive muscle damage following injection of contaminated mixtures. Some of those complications can be severe enough to cause considerable disability, impairing use of the arms or legs.

Effects on the Cardiovascular System.   In addition to endocarditis, abnormal cardiac rhythms and acute inflammation of the blood vessels (vasculitis) may be attributed to heroin. Even after a valve is replaced surgically, the compulsive use of heroin may destroy the prosthetic valve and create the need for a heart bypass operation.

Kidney Disease.   Chronic heroin use shows up in the kidneys by persistent blood in the urine and disease of the kidney cells causing renal shutdown. Long-term hemodialysis is a real possibility for addicts.

Endocrinologic Disturbances. Disturbances in the endocrine system range from lowered blood sugar to difficulty with sexual functioning in men.

Women who use heroin are especially prone to complications of childbirth and the reproductive system (Chapter 18). Menstrual irregularities include amenorrhea (failed periods), and infertility from disruption of normal ovarian function. The increased sexual activity of women heroin addicts who need money to support their habit results in frequent exposure to venereal disease. This may lead to pelvic infections that cause scarring of the fallopian tubes and subsequent infertility. Scarring of the fallopian tubes also places women at additional risk during conception and childbirth.

THE CHALLENGE OF TREATING HEROIN ADDICTION

Just as with other addictive behaviors, treating heroin addiction is filled with frustration. Understanding why someone turns to drugs in general, and to heroin in particular, is a valuable point of departure. As described in Chapter 4, successful treatment must address psychological, physiological, and sociological problems (Table 11.7).

Several treatment approaches are available for treating heroin addicts (Table 11.8). Despite considerable effort, no one has been able to define a single treatment profile that works for everyone. So no one form of therapy is clearly better than any other. Each approach can prove effective under a specific circumstance. A melding or integration of several approaches is needed to come up with the best plan for each person.

Detoxification. Short of just stopping drug use (cold turkey), detoxification is the simplest and quickest way to become abstinent (Chapter 5). It slowly lowers the blood level of heroin (morphine), gradually decreasing the tolerance threshold to prevent withdrawal symptoms. This is best accomplished with decreasing doses of an

---

TABLE 11.7
Principles for Treating Heroin Addiction

Address reasons for starting heroin use

Address physiologic changes produced by heroin dependency

Address both short- and long-term changes produced by abstinence and withdrawal

Decrease reinforcement associated with heroin use

Eliminate conditioning or environmental effects that promote use

Change long-term behavior to maximize chance of remaining abstinent

Provide training and help develop skills needed for productive participation in society (when necessary, retrain to accomplish)

TABLE 11.8
Approaches for Treating Heroin Addiction

Detoxification
  Methadone
  Clonidine

Psychotherapy and other outpatient programs

Therapeutic communities

Maintenance therapy

Opiate antagonists

Narcotics Anonymous and other self-help groups

Acupuncture

---

oral opiate, usually methadone. Oral methadone is given daily in decreasing doses for seven to 14 days, until the person is drug-free. Detoxification from methadone maintenance (discussed later in this chapter) can take considerably longer and is usually accompanied by counseling sessions.

Abstinence can be achieved solely by discontinuing heroin use, but withdrawal symptoms will occur in varying intensity depending on the level of dependency. These symptoms are uncomfortable and usually lead to drug-seeking behavior within hours of withdrawal. Withdrawal symptoms should never be allowed to develop in someone dependent on heroin or other opiates, unless this negative effect is part of conditioned-behavior therapy (aversion therapy). Even then, permitting withdrawal to occur is controversial.

Detoxification clinics. To combat the perceived heroin epidemic of the 1970s, many cities developed clinics that could provide detoxification services on relatively short notice. Referral was then made to a treatment facility. Such clinics gave immediate relief to those on long waiting lists to enter programs, and to others who believed they could remain drug-free if they could avoid withdrawal without entering a formal treatment program. Many successfully completed the detoxification process, but just as many returned to heroin use after several days.

Clonidine in detoxification. Withdrawal symptoms are largely due to secretion of norepinephrine (Chapter 3) by neuronal cells in the brain. The brain cells involved are located in the nucleus locus coeruleus (LC). Opiates inhibit secretion of norepinephrine by depressing the activity of LC cells. When these cells become tolerant to chronic opiate exposure, they must work harder to produce the body's normal quota of norepinephrine. And to maintain an equilibrium, the number of binding sites in the LC also increases. When heroin is suddenly discontinued, the "restraints" are removed; the cells become hyperactive and greatly increase the secretion of norepinephrine. Clinical signs of withdrawal follow.

Clonidine (Catapres), used to treat high blood pressure, is effective in blocking norepinephrine release. By thus decreasing norepinephrine activity, clonidine suppresses the signs and symptoms of opiate withdrawal, allowing a relatively quick detoxification without opiates. The drug was considered to be particularly valuable to people on low-dose methadone therapy, because methadone detoxification and withdrawal can take weeks or months. Similarly, clonidine can provide rapid detoxification, allowing earlier treatment with an opiate antagonist (see discussion later in this chapter).

When clonidine was first used in detoxification, the medical community had great hopes that it might be given to anyone who didn't want further treatment or a prolonged detoxification. But side effects and complications quickly appeared. Most common was substantially lowered blood pressure. Managing that hypotension requires a medical setting. Feelings of sedation, depression, insomnia, and muscle pains were also reported. Since some of these symptoms are the same as those seen during withdrawal, the precise role played by clonidine is unclear. Using clonidine on an ambulatory basis without appropriate monitoring is now considered hazardous.

Other drugs with similar capabilities of suppressing norepinephrine secretion are being studied. They include lofexidine, guanfacine, and guanabenz (Wytensin).

Psychotherapeutic Approaches.   Because intense depression and anxiety are often seen in heroin addicts, early treatment efforts focused on the reasons for starting drug use. These attempts at psychotherapy were less than successful. Freud noted that addicts were poor candidates for psychoanalysis because they lacked the necessary character and discipline. Psychiatrists and psychologists have certainly been discouraged by the antisocial personality traits of addicts and in general have avoided treating those who are dependent on heroin. Heroin users often have difficulty forming meaningful relationships and not infrequently are aggressive and manipulative. So it's easy to understand the lack of enthusiasm when it comes to treating heroin addiction with a purely psychotherapeutic approach.

Many heroin addicts have antisocial characteristics; just as many are depressed and anxious. The latter inject heroin as much to relieve their pain as to obtain a high. For that reason, they can benefit from psychotherapy, in combination with other approaches.

Another approach is the minimal counseling provided at drug-free outpatient units. These facilities sometimes use former heroin addicts as counselors or employ trained therapists. These settings have little structure, and whether meaningful, ongoing relationships can be established in such a brief time frame remains to be demonstrated.

Residential (Therapeutic) Communities. Probably the best-known treatment approaches for heroin addiction are therapeutic communities, or TCs (Chapter 5). Their great appeal lies in their effort to establish a drug-free environment while helping a person achieve abstinence. Heroin addiction is seen not as the primary problem but as a symptom. The problem is the person, not the drug. The focus is on letting the individual develop a socially productive, drug-free life-style.

According to TC philosophy, that kind of substantive life change can take place only in a live-in environment that provides a social, learning context through role modeling and identification with others. Those others may be staff or peers, almost all of whom have overcome a similar problem. The addict is helped to examine the reasons he or she started taking drugs and the kinds of stresses to expect on returning to the former environment. Outside influences are minimized during residency; they're dealt with when the person in treatment is better prepared to cope with them.

The induction phase at most therapeutic communities lasts up to two months, followed by the primary treatment phase of up to 12 months and a reentry phase of up to two years. The induction phase, which orients a person to the rules and regulations of the community, is probably the most difficult to accept. It's when relationships are formed within the community, and specific duties are assigned.

In the primary treatment phase, the person gets a full and varied schedule, including educational and vocational chores. Understanding the conditions surrounding heroin use is part of the educational objective. An orderly, regimented environment is provided for those whose search for drugs made chaos of their lives. Part of the treatment is the confrontation technique, a process that challenges those who are not living up to the standards of the community. It's an emotionally draining process that is difficult for most people. Individual changes are carefully monitored, with feedback and support constantly provided.

The reentry phase prepares the person to rejoin the community at large. Appropriate educational and vocational counseling tries to pinpoint the stresses and frustrations likely to be encountered. During the early reentry phase, the individual remains mainly within the TC as discharge plans are developed. In the late reentry phase, residents are allowed to move freely in the outside community in full-time jobs or educational activities.

Approximately 14 percent of all patients in federally funded facilities for drug dependency are admitted to TCs. The success rates of TCs are comparable to those of other programs. Of those who complete the process, about 70 percent achieve favorable outcomes, with 30 percent able to remain drug-free. The drop-out rate, especially in the early stages of therapy, is high, however, with successful abstinence related to time spent in treatment. After treatment is completed, people are encouraged to participate in networks that strengthen the resolve to remain abstinent.

Maintenance Therapy. The concept of maintenance therapy for heroin addiction is far from new. In the late 1800s and early 1900s physicians freely prescribed morphine, and opium preparations were widely available in a variety of over-the-counter preparations. But the 1914 Harrison Act suddenly diminished the availability of opium preparations, and physicians became wary of prescribing opiates. In 1919 physicians were prevented from prescribing opiates solely to maintain a dependency.

To provide relief for the unknown number of addicts, at least 44 clinics were opened in cities across the United States to dispense heroin or provide prescriptions for heroin or morphine. The precise number of people treated at these facilities nationwide is unknown, but in New York City about 7,000 people were registered in one year. The effectiveness of legal distribution of heroin or morphine in preventing crime and allowing addicts to engage in socially productive activities was never documented. But the public considered the legal maintenance of these addicts immoral, and outrage over such activity led to the closing of all the clinics by 1924.

Maintenance therapy—demonstrated to be effective in treating heroin dependency—is no less controversial today. Supporters pro-

---

TABLE 11.9
Rationale for Maintenance Therapy in Heroin Addiction

Heroin-produced biochemical changes in the body make abstinence difficult to achieve and maintain.

Therapy facilitates normal functioning by providing doses at tolerance threshold. Maintaining tolerance prevents discomfort of withdrawal.

Slow elevation of tolerance threshold prevents a high from injection of street heroin.

With drug-seeking behavior eliminated and comfort level maintained, rehabilitative effort can begin.

Slow detoxification from maintenance therapy, accompanied by supportive services, can result in prolonged abstinence.

---

mote maintenance as a way to help people become functioning members of society. Critics say that, at best, it's another form of opiate dependency. Much of the controversy comes from ignorance of maintenance therapy's rationale, effectiveness, and limitations.

Basis for maintenance therapy. The lessons learned from laboratory models (Chapter 3) and observation of heroin addicts provide the rationale behind maintenance therapy (Table 11.9). Five premises are involved.

Premise 1. Dependency produces biochemical and physiologic changes that make it difficult for a formerly dependent person to remain abstinent. The changes involve the body's tolerance to opiates and are responsible for the severe distress of withdrawal. In the nontolerant, nonopiate user, the opiate receptors control the body's response to stress by synthesizing and releasing endorphins and enkephalins. Used repeatedly, heroin occupies the receptor sites, decreasing synthesis of the natural opiates.

As tolerance develops, a fixed dose of heroin has less and less effect on the system. But at the same time, the cells that secrete the neurotransmitter norepinephrine become less active, requiring more cells to work at the task of maintaining constant levels of norepinephrine in the body. So long as heroin is injected, the system is regulated by the "outside" influence. But the equilibrium is disturbed when blood- and brain-heroin levels drop. The natural opiates that regulate secretion of norepinephrine are gone, as is the inhibiting effect of the heroin, and norepinephrine pours out of the cells. The increased levels are responsible for withdrawal symptoms, narcotic craving, and, most often, a rapid return to heroin use.

Premise 2. A conditioning effect makes it difficult to remain drug-free. Placing someone who has been drug-free back in an environment where he or she previously used heroin can lead to craving for the drug, withdrawal symptoms, and a return to heroin use.

Premise 3. A heroin user can function normally when doses don't exceed the tolerance threshold (Chapter 3). Indeed, many people seemingly lead functional lives even when they are dependent. Function is impaired only when the threshold is passed, resulting in a high, or not reached, resulting in withdrawal. Thus, maintaining the individual at the tolerance threshold avoids withdrawal and decreases drug-seeking behavior due to physiologic changes or the conditioning effect.

Premise 4. Slowly raising the tolerance threshold of appropriately administered opiates produces neither a high nor an overdose. A threshold can be raised enough in that way to prevent a high from injection of street heroin. Without the high, the conditioning and reinforcement of injection begin to disappear, since the individual is disinclined to spend money on something that doesn't produce the desired effects.

Premise 5. With heroin-seeking behavior eliminated and the individual maintained at a comfortable tolerance threshold, it is possible to examine the reasons that prompted initial drug use, to isolate the steps that must be taken to prevent relapse, and to identify the kind of training required to help the person become a functioning member of society. Once the life-style has changed and heroin is no longer being used, the tolerance threshold can be slowly lowered through detoxification, with abstinence being maintained.

Choice of opiate in maintenance therapy. All opiates (narcotics) can be interchanged if given in equivalent doses. So theoretically, any opiate can be used in maintenance therapy. The ideal drug, however, would have to fulfill certain criteria. It would have to be:

- in a form that can be taken orally to break the behavior associated with injection
- relatively long-acting, so the receptor-neurotransmitter system is regulated correctly and can return to a state of equilibrium
- readily absorbed to provide consistent serum levels with a specific dose
- taken up by body tissues and released in the blood at a constant level to prolong both time and intensity of withdrawal—if it were abruptly discontinued

Use of heroin and/or morphine for maintenance therapy has some advocates. However, that approach is impractical; to be effective, those drugs would have to be injected several times a day. And when injected frequently, they can cause wide fluctuations of mental states because of their constantly changing levels in the brain.

This effect is seen when patients are given injectable opiates for pain control. Shortly after the injection, they become sleepy, high, or even anxious. And even when tolerance increases, the peaking levels of morphine or similar drugs alter mental activity—at least temporarily. That was the case in England when government-approved maintenance programs were established in the late 1960s. Heroin was the drug first prescribed. But as the problems of heroin as a maintenance drug became apparent, most programs switched to methadone—initially by injection but later in oral form.

With one exception, all medically available oral opiates have to be given every four to six hours. What's more, their absorption from the gastrointestinal tract varies. The exception is oral methadone.

Methadone (Chapter 10) is about equal in potency to morphine but is much longer-acting. When taken by mouth, it sustains plasma levels for approximately 24 to 48 hours. It's rapidly absorbed from the gastrointestinal tract, 99 percent is bound in the tissues, and levels in the tissues and the blood are quickly equalized. As the methadone blood level falls, more is released from the tissues to sustain a steady supply in the blood. The methadone keeps the opiate receptor occupied, allowing behavior to normalize and receptor-neurotransmitter functions to continue at consistant levels. That's why methadone works in maintenance therapy.

Before its use in maintenance therapy, methadone was the drug of choice for controlling such chronic painful conditions as severe deforming arthritis and cancer, and in detoxification from opiate dependency. Its effectiveness in detoxification was demonstrated at the U.S. Public Health Service Hospital in Lexington, Kentucky, in 1946.

Ironically, for a number of years after methadone was approved for maintenance, physicians weren't permitted to use it for pain control. Why? Because of public concern about its potential for inappropriate use. Reason finally prevailed, and methadone can once again be prescribed for chronic pain control.

Effectiveness of methadone maintenance.   The pilot program for methadone maintenance was initiated at Rockefeller University, using volunteer "hardcore" criminals over the age of 21 who had been addicted for at least four years and had been unable to kick their habits. Methadone was administered in an orange-flavored commercial drink, Tang, in slowly increasing amounts up to a daily maintenance dose of 80 to 100 milligrams. The subjects consistently said they had no need to seek out heroin, and felt rather normal throughout the day.

The group reported that, for the first time since becoming heroin addicts, they were able to focus on nonheroin-related activities such as seeking educational or vocational training, establishing social relationships. Arrest rates dropped significantly, and the medical complications of heroin use were no longer seen. Essential parts of treatment were careful monitoring of urine for use of heroin and other mood-altering drugs, frequent clinic visits, medical evaluations, and counseling services.

Minimal standards for methadone programs were established by the Food and Drug Administration and the National Institute on Drug Abuse in keeping with the Narcotics Treatment Act of 1974.

A slow but steady increase in use of methadone programs peaked in 1977, with 80,000 persons enrolling. The number of people in treatment declined through the 1980s for a variety of reasons, including failure of funding to keep pace with increasing costs of living, availability of other treatment approaches, and a persistent public opinion that maintenance therapy is morally wrong. About 25 to 30 percent of those now in opiate dependency treatment are receiving methadone maintenance.

Success rates are directly linked to the amount of time spent in treatment. Of all available approaches, methadone maintenance consistently retains the most people in treatment for the greatest period of time; 65 to 90 percent of those admitted stay for at least one year.

Adverse effects of methadone. As is the case with any drug, people who take methadone regularly may experience a variety of feelings—some based on the drug's pharmacologic properties, but most due to the individual's sensitivity. Like other opiates, methadone frequently causes slowing of bowel activity and constipation. A proportion of methadone is excreted in sweat and is sometimes the cause of excessive sweating on hot days.

Other side effects include difficulty in sexual function in both men and women, weight gain, insomnia, and bone pain. But those symptoms are present to varying degrees in many persons before and during heroin use. Any reactions to methadone must be specifically assessed. In the original methadone maintenance study at Rockefeller University in 1964, 214 persons were on maintenance for three years. Not one was discharged because of methadone side effects.

When combined with other mood-altering drugs in the alcohol-barbiturate-tranquilizer group, methadone can produce a depressant effect on the central nervous system—that is, sedation. Sedation may also result when methadone is taken irregularly or in doses greatly above tolerance level.

Misconceptions about methadone maintenance. Hundreds of thousands of addicts have gone through methadone maintenance programs. Some do extremely well and go on to lead drug-free, productive lives. Others can't tolerate requirements of the program, or have adverse effects and drop out of treatment. Still others can't easily become detoxified and prefer long-term maintenance.

The continuing bad public image of methadone maintenance leads many of those in therapy to hide this fact. As a result, successes are not always visible, while failures are well publicized.

Methadone maintenance has obvious limitations. Methadone allows development of tolerance to other opiates, but not to nonopiate mood-altering drugs. So people on maintenance use and misuse substances such as alcohol, sedatives, and cocaine, just as others do.

The success of methadone maintenance is often judged on the basis of abstinence from all drugs. But persons on methadone have the same stresses and anxieties as those who are not. The only difference is that they can no longer relieve those stresses by injecting heroin. So without accompanying supportive services, people on methadone act much like those who never took heroin: they may turn to other mood-altering drugs. Some individuals in government want to provide methadone maintenance without appropriate rehabilitative services. Their thinking is that methadone will decrease spread of the HIV and AIDS by cutting the number of heroin injections, and that cutting off the services will save money. But cocaine by injection is a preferred method of administration by heroin users and will spread AIDS as effectively as mainlining heroin (Chapter 17).

To prevent heroin highs, the daily methadone dose must be at least 60 to 80 milligrams. But such doses aren't always given. A study by the National Institute on Drug Abuse revealed that in 69 percent of the programs surveyed, the methadone dose was less than 30 milligrams—despite awareness that low dose is commonly associated with poor retention rates and doesn't prevent heroin use. The institute has shown that at a daily dose of 34 milligrams or less, 35 percent use heroin at least once a week, but at a dose of 80 milligrams or more there is virtually no heroin use.

Why are inadequate doses prescribed? Partly because of fear that ''potent doses'' of methadone will be diverted to the street; mainly because of ignorance of methadone pharmacology combined with the belief—even of those in the field—that less is better.

Some patients clear methadone from their systems more rapidly than usual, thus exposing them to varying degrees of abstinence during each day. The result is drug-seeking behavior and the perception that methadone is not working. The simple solution is to increase doses needed on a case-by-case basis.

Heroin users with severe psychological problems will continue to have them while on methadone. So, while methadone is helpful in treating borderline patients, other psychotropic medications are often needed as well.

Careful medical follow-up has revealed no serious consequences of long-term methadone administration. (By the same token, chronic use of opiates under sterile conditions has never been associated with significant adverse physical effects.)

Methadone does pose certain problems. It's sold illegally on the street; children may take a parent's dose; a nontolerant person may accidentally overdose; and someone detoxified from methadone may return to heroin. But a program that has worked for tens of thousands of people should not be condemned.

Methadone maintenance is not the only realistic answer to rehabilitation. But for many people it's the most practical, whether alone or in combination with other services.

Narcotic Antagonists. As noted earlier, an opiate with purely antagonist properties can displace such opiates as heroin from the brain receptor sites, thus preventing a "high" from injected heroin. Until the early 1980s, there was no pure narcotic antagonist safe enough to make testing feasible. Opiates with mixed agonist-antagonist properties displace heroin from the brain binding sites, but are themselves associated with a high and thus can be misused (Chapter 10).

Naltrexone. After considerable research, the National Institute on Drug Abuse approved naltrexone (Trexan) for treatment of opiate dependency. Before administering naltrexone, the person must be detoxified with either methadone or clonidine. Detoxifying with clonidine allows naltrexone to be taken much sooner, because several days must pass after the last dose of methadone before naltrexone can be used.

Administered orally, naltrexone has been consistently effective in preventing the high associated with heroin injection for up to 72 hours. But it must continue to be taken to be effective, and long-term therapy of up to a year may be required. If naltrexone is stopped and heroin is injected, a high will result. Consequently, many studies evaluating naltrexone have documented a high attrition rate—

sometimes no different from that of a placebo. As many as 40 percent of those treated stop the drug after one month in order to experience the heroin high.

Widespread use of naltrexone poses some difficulties:

- Detoxification and subsequent abstinence must precede treatment, not easy tasks for someone craving heroin.
- The blocking action is easily overcome by an extremely large dose of heroin or by omitting one or more doses of naltrexone.
- Unless accompanied by intensive support, use of naltrexone fails to address the other principles involved in successful rehabilitation.
- High doses may induce liver injury.
- It may deplete naturally produced opiates, increasing heroin sensitivity if injections are resumed.
- It may block the craving for heroin more effectively than it can prevent heroin from depressing the respiratory center.

The last two possibilities are theoretical, but if correct can lead to an overdose reaction when heroin is injected. Moreover, blocking effects of the body's natural opiates may prevent the receptor-neurotransmitter system from returning to normal, something that can perpetuate persistent feelings of discomfort.

Naltrexone appears to be most valuable for the limited number of people who are highly motivated to remain abstinent.

Buprenorphine. A synthetic opiate agonist-antagonist (Chapter 10) developed for control of pain, buprenorphine, has been suggested for use as a preliminary to naltrexone. Studies to determine its potential for street use by heroin-dependent people remain to be performed. Caution is warranted, however, because those given the drug reported a feeling of contentment, and the history of inappropriate use of pentazocine (Talwin) by those dependent on heroin is well known.

Self-Help Groups. Narcotics Anonymous (NA), like Alcoholics Anonymous and similar self-help groups, is a valuable resource. It offers group support for heroin addicts and people dependent on medically prescribed opiates. Groups are also available to help family members better understand addiction and ways of coping with those who are addicted. A fair degree of commitment is required for those who wish to remain drug-free immediately after detoxifying from opiates, so NA, when combined with other modalities, can be extremely useful in promoting abstinence. The number of persons participating in NA was estimated to be 14,000 in 1988 and will undoubtably increase as more family members of those dependent on drugs and at risk for AIDS look for additional support.

Acupuncture. Acupuncture, the insertion of needles into critical parts of the body, has been a mainstay of medicine in China for more than 2000 years. A variety of ailments are believed to be effectively treated when the needles are placed in specific sites. The effectiveness of many of these procedures hasn't been consistently demonstrated, however.

In the early 1970s, doctors in Hong Kong found acupuncture effective in relieving withdrawal symptoms in opium addicts undergoing surgical procedures. Subsequently, a number of physicians have been using acupuncture needles with electrical stimulation to detoxify individuals from heroin without medication, and to keep them heroin-free after detoxification. In most programs needles are placed at specific points in the ear and stimulated with electrical pulses for approximately 30 minutes a day. The treatment period varies but usually lasts at least several weeks.

The exact mechanism that makes acupuncture effective in decreasing withdrawal symptoms is unknown. But several limited studies have shown it to be associated with an increase in the body's secretion of endorphin (met-enkephalin). That phenomenon is believed to compensate for the lack of heroin once injection has ceased, as well as for the suppressed levels of naturally occurring met-enkephalin during heroin use.

To date, probably thousands of people have been treated with acupuncture. Its supporters are convinced of its ability to diminish craving and withdrawal, and to help maintain abstinence. But there have been few rigorous studies assessing the clinical effectiveness of acupuncture. Support for such studies should be provided.

MEASURING TREATMENT EFFECTIVENESS

Much has been published about treatments for heroin addiction, but most evaluations have been descriptive. Still to be done are carefully designed studies that incorporate control groups and sufficient follow-up. Outcomes are often obtained by users' self-reporting; and prior socioeconomic status bears on the ability to engage in productive activity. Both these facts can skew results. What's more, some programs that focus on treating heroin addiction may have many clients who use or are dependent on other mood-altering drugs.

With such cautions in mind, most large-scale evaluations of different treatment approaches yield similar results, with time spent in treatment being the most important predictor of success. An exception are detoxification programs, which usually end with a quick return to heroin use. After appropriate time in treatment, however, heroin use and criminal activity decrease, and social productivity increases. Evaluation of opiate-antagonist therapies, however, often shows high attrition rates.

By two or three years after discharge from a treatment program, heroin use may be infrequent. But use of other mood-altering drugs, mostly alcohol, can take its place. Excessive alcohol use remains the most common form of drug use in society today, so it's difficult to attribute to program failure the former heroin addict's turning to alcohol.

Much more investigation is needed to explore the biology of heroin addiction and effective treatments. In that regard, basic research and clinical evaluation make good partners. As succinctly stated by Dr. Vincent P. Dole, one of the methadone maintenance pioneers at Rockefeller University, "It is not necessary to await an ultimate reduction of addictive behaviors to molecular terms before effective treatment can be provided. On the contrary, effective treatment, empirically found, can lead to a better understanding of molecular processes."

Chapter 12

Amphetamines, Amphetamine-like Drugs, and Caffeine

Stimulants have been in wide use by all societies from the beginning of organized cultures, being described by the Chinese 5100 years ago. They're taken to increase wakefulness and ability to concentrate; to become more alert, decrease fatigue, and elevate mood. Their effects vary from a mild feeling of well-being to intense exhilaration and euphoria.

The intensity depends on the specific drug, how it's taken, and the user's psychologic status at time of consumption. Stimulants consistently reduce appetite and give one the perception of being able to take on Herculean tasks. Continued intense use, however, results in irritability, depression, and physical and mental deterioration. Ultimately, paranoid behavior may appear.

Stimulants are among the easiest drugs to obtain: they're legally prescribed for medical reasons, then purposely misused; they're manufactured in clandestine laboratories and become an integral part of the street-drug trade; and they're purchased over-the-counter as diet aids or as inhalers for asthma.

Current inappropriate use of these licit "pharmacologic agents" is not high. According to the 1988 National Household Survey on Drug Abuse, among the population at greatest risk for stimulant use—those between the ages of 18 and 25—only 2 percent currently use stimulants and 11 percent have ever used such drugs. Stimulants used in our daily lives—coffee, tea, soft drinks, and cigarettes—are consumed far more frequently by the majority of people in the United States.

Almost all stimulants, including those legally available, have a potential for dependency and inappropriate use. The degree to which this can happen varies greatly (Table 12.1).

AMPHETAMINES

The first amphetamine was synthesized in 1887 and appeared in physicians' practices in the late 1920s. When marketed in 1932, it was known as benzedrine and produced as tablets, inhalers, and injectables. Since then, amphetamines and related substances have come to market on a regular basis. Initially, they were prescribed for narcolepsy, a condition that causes sleep without warning at any time. Their positive stimulant effects led to their use in treating depression and suppressing appetite. They're still used for narcolepsy and a relatively small number of other medical problems, including obesity and attention-deficit disorder, a condition of early childhood and adolescence marked by hyperactivity, impulsive behavior, and inability to focus on a subject (Table 12.2).

In the 1950s and early 1960s, amphetamines were widely used by people who needed to stay awake or to exhibit a "peak performance" for long periods, such as long-distance truck drivers, athletes, servicemen on extended tours of duty, and students studying for examinations. In 1962 the Food and Drug Administration estimated that enough amphetamines were produced that year to supply everyone in the United States with one 250-milligram tablet. Because there were no appropriate controls, about half of that quantity was believed to be for illicit use. At that time, 19 companies manufactured these drugs, nine of them not requiring proof or proper FDA registration of buyers. Most of the amphetamines on the street came from these legitimate manufacturers.

Others, of course, took amphetamines specifically for their mood-altering effects. Initial users swallowed the pills, but soon many people began experimenting with intravenous use. Early on, amphetamines were mixed with heroin (Speedballs or Splash), but young people soon began using them alone. When taking high doses

TABLE 12.1
Common Licit Stimulants

Substance	Illicit Use	Rx Required	Dependency Potential	Dependency Potential Psychological	Physical	Frequent Daily Use
Amphetamines	+	+	+	++++	+++	+
Caffeine	−	−	−	+	−	+
Cocaine	+	−	+	++++	++	+
Nicotine	−	−	+	+++	++	+
Stimulants for weight loss	−/+	varies with drug	+	+++	++	+

Key
− = No association
+ = Association
+ + = Moderate association
+ + + = Marked association
+ + + + = Severe dependency

TABLE 12.2
Medical Uses of Stimulants

Severe depression unresponsive to antidepressant drugs

Pain relief, in conjunction with narcotic drugs

Hyperactivity in children

Motion sickness

Parkinsonism unresponsive to other drugs

Weight loss

Narcolepsy

Urinary incontinence

---

of pills, or mainlining for several days at a stretch, the user would virtually go without sleep or food until becoming unable to function.

By the late 1960s, recognition of amphetamines' severe adverse effects led to them being placed in Schedule II, markedly restricting their availability. With the 1970 Controlled Substances Act, mandatory quotas on production were imposed. By 1972, most of the amphetamines in the street trade were being obtained through smuggling or by synthesis in clandestine laboratories.

Street Preparations. By 1975, only 10 percent of street samples sold as amphetamines actually contained the drug. The rest were mixtures of caffeine and amphetamine-like substances, such as ephedrine, pseudoephedrine, or phenethylamine, used for weight loss or treatment of asthma or coughs. These products were marketed under such names as Black Beauty, Penthouse, and Hustler, and some were advertised openly in counterculture magazines.

Speed's negative publicity came just when the young were becoming increasingly disillusioned with the government's inability or unwillingness to provide accurate information concerning U.S. involvement in Southeast Asia. This probably accounted for a certain amount of disbelief over amphetamines' adverse effects and an acting out through increased experimentation. Other legitimate stimulants also began finding their way to the street (Table 12.3). Use of amphetamines and amphetamine-like drugs decreased considerably through the 1980s. Nevertheless, in a 1987 survey 12 percent of high school seniors admitted using such drugs the preceding year. The overall decrease in amphetamine use was accompanied by a rise in cocaine use (Chapter 13).

There are a number of amphetamine "look-alike" drugs on the street (Table 12.3). These are not real amphetamines but when taken in large doses can produce serious adverse reactions.

One of the newer street drugs, smokable methamphetamine crystals (Ice, LA Ice, Crank), first appeared in Hawaii and on the West Coast. In Honolulu its use has now surpassed that of cocaine. Although methamphetamine use is far from new, prior street trade had been in either oral or injectable forms.

Unlike Crack, Ice can be produced at extremely low cost using relatively unsophisticated equipment and common chemicals such as ephedrine or phenylacetone. The cost of producing one pound of methamphetamine has been estimated at $700, with a street yield of $225,000. It is obvious why Ice is more attractive to the drug dealer than Crack.

Much like Crack, smoking methamphetamine crystals allows the drug to reach the brain even more rapidly than through injection. Since methamphetamine's half-life is 12 hours and its metabolism is associated with the production of pharmacologically active metabolites, its effects last much longer than Crack's, with a high persisting up to 14 hours or more. Acute psychotic behavior, severe paranoia, incoherent speech, hallucinations, and uncontrollable behavior lasting up to 48 hours are frequent side effects.

Absorption and Distribution. Amphetamines are thought to exert their mood-altering effects by acting on the neurotransmitter system in the brain (Chapter 3). Amphetamines cause increased release of dopamine and neuroepinephrine from brain cells, and block both their uptake and the activity of the enzyme responsible for metabolizing them. It's the increased levels of those neurotransmitters that result in many of the behavioral effects peculiar to this type of drug.

TABLE 12.3
Commonly Used Amphetamine and Amphetamine-like Drugs

Drug	Trade Name	Street Name
Amphetamines	Benzedrine, Delcobese, Fetamine, Obetrol	Bennies, Blue Angels, Crank, Crisscross, Crossroads, Hearts, Lip Poppers, Peaches, Pep Pills, Pinks, Rosas, Roses, Speed, Splash, Thrusters, Truck Drivers, Uppers, Ups, Wake-ups, Whites
	Desbutal	
	Dexedrine, Ferndex, Oxydess, Spancap	Caplets, Dexies, Oranges
	Biphetamine, Diphetamine	Footballs
	Curban*, Dexamyl*, Eskatrol*	
	Desoxyn, Methadrene	Crystal, Mets, Water, Minibennies, Mollies, Chris/ Christine
Methamphetamine crystal	—	Crystal, Crank, Ice, LA Ice
Methylphenidate	Ritalin	

Catha edulis Forsk (Khat)	—	Kitty Kat
Phenmetrazine	Preludin	Pocket Rockets, Ludies
Other commonly prescribed pills for weight loss**	Adipex, Bacarate, Cyclort, Didrex, Ionamin, Plegine, Pondimin, Pre-sate, Sandrex, Tenuate, Tepanil, Voranil	
Drugs used to prevent sleep	Ban, Drowz, Kirkaffeine, NoDoz, Stim-250, Tireno, Vivarin	
Ephedrine, phenyl-propanolamine	Variety of decongestant medications and anti-asthmatic drugs	Usually sold on the street as Speed

*No longer available
**Many other weight-reduction pills are available. Although they are not structurally similar to amphetamines, they still have varying degrees of stimulant effects.

Amphetamines also stimulate the reward system of the brain (Chapter 3), which in turn intensifies the need to continue taking them. Amphetamines are readily absorbed from the intestinal tract and distributed to the tissues. Their affinity for lipid-containing tissues allows them to rapidly enter the brain as well as other organs. When amphetamines are injected directly into the bloodstream or inhaled, effects can be seen within seconds. Metabolism occurs in the liver, however much of the drug may be eliminated unchanged. As a result, the effects of the amphetamines may last from eight to 12 hours, depending on the specific drug. When amphetamines are taken frequently and intravenously, extremely high levels can accumulate.

Effects on the Body. The major effects of amphetamines stem from their action on the central nervous system, heart, and blood vessels (Table 12.4). An oral dose of 10 to 15 milligrams daily makes an individual more alert and able to perform mental or physical tasks with a greater degree of self-confidence and a higher level of activity. Whether tasks are performed more accurately remains unclear. Perfectly clear, however, is that one can work longer without fatigue or quickly recover from fatigue. Respiration is stimulated and the appetite depressed—more from not wanting food than from an increased body metabolism. Cardiovascular consequences include a rise in blood pressure and rapid, sometimes irregular, heart rates.

Intravenous use is characterized by a quick onset of euphoria, described as an immediate "rush" or "flash" sensation. That's followed by a feeling that anything can be accomplished and a perception of physical, mental, and sexual prowess. The perception usually greatly exceeds the reality. Desire for food or sleep is absent.

Mainlining the drug in runs can ultimately lead to extreme paranoid behavior. In that state, depending on the setting and the mainliner's personality, aggressive behavior may be directed at those perceived as threatening. Runs can continue for several days, usually ending in exhaustion. Next come prolonged periods of sleep, followed by bouts of eating and depression ("crashing"), which may last several days, accompanied by increasing craving for the drug until the cycle begins again.

Runs can also develop with oral use of amphetamines when taken

---

TABLE 12.4
Temporary Effects of Amphetamines on Mental Functioning
Increased wakefulness
Decreased fatigue
Increased ability to concentrate
Decreased appetite
Sense of exhilaration, euphoria

---

in high doses (1,000 milligrams or more, every few hours). Sometimes depressants such as alcohol or sleeping pills are taken to counteract the hyperactivity generated by amphetamines.

Tolerance, Dependency, and Addiction.   The effects of intravenous amphetamine use are similar to those of cocaine. In research settings, cocaine addicts are frequently unable to distinguish intravenous cocaine from intravenous amphetamine (Chapter 13).

Not all the effects of amphetamines are subject to tolerance, but initial weight loss and the mood alterations are. So an impressive increase in dosage is necessary to achieve the same effect. Psychological dependency also develops. Once self-administration has been established in laboratory animals, for example, they choose the drug over food and water until seizures and death occur.

Withdrawal appears after a high degree of dependency. It usually consists of restlessness, anxiety, and depression accompanied by prolonged periods of sleep.

Adverse Effects.   Toxic effects of amphetamines depend on patterns of use, how they're taken, use of other mood-altering drugs, degree of tolerance developed, underlying medical disorders, and sometimes the conditions under which they're taken (Table 12.5).

The most severe effects come from large intravenous doses. Symptoms of acute intoxication are restlessness, hyperactivity, delirium, acute psychotic reactions, a significant rise in temperature, and intermittent seizures and convulsions. Because amphetamines can cause rises in body temperature, a particular risk exists when the drug is taken during hot weather. Effects on the heart can result in

TABLE 12.5
Toxic Effects of Amphetamines

Acute
Behavioral
　Hyperactivity
　Euphoria
　Impaired judgment
　Delirium
　Acute psychotic reactions: paranoid reactions, hallucinations,
　　suicidal or homicidal behavior; convulsions
Nausea or vomiting
Rise in body temperature
Marked rise in blood pressure
Irregularities in cardiac rhythm
Hemorrhages in brain or skull
Shock

Chronic
Weight loss
Chronic skin lesions
Psychotic states, especially paranoia
Heart disease
When used intravenously: hepatitis; infections of skin, HIV
　infection, subcutaneous tissue, heart valves, and lungs;
　hemolytic anemia; clotting of veins and small arteries of brain
　and retina; allergic reactions; emboli to lungs; and destruction of
　muscle tissue

a marked rise in blood pressure, sometimes accompanied by rupture
and hemorrhage of small arteries in the brain. Irregular heartbeats
may develop, sometimes causing fatal arrhythmias. People with heart
disease are at greater risk.

Amphetamines are often taken with depressant drugs to modify
the stimulant effect. Among them are alcohol, barbiturates, and ben-

zodiazepines—each associated with specific effects. Combinations with heroin (Splash, Speedball) are also common (Chapter 11).

Massive doses of amphetamines are rarely taken intentionally. But large quantities can be taken unknowingly in various street drugs that contain pure amphetamines or other stimulants. Bleeding in the brain can result from the extreme increase in pressure in the cerebral arteries. Alternatively, the system may be so stimulated as to result in complete loss of blood pressure (shock), extreme elevation of temperature, convulsions, coma, and death. Chronic amphetamine use produces significant weight loss, skin lesions, and psychotic reactions similar to schizophrenia. Psychotic reactions with oral amphetamine use don't usually appear until the drugs have been taken for several months or as a manifestation of an intense "run." Once they do, however, they reappear quickly with recurrent use. Acute psychotic behavior, at times uncontrollable, can be seen following the ingestion of Ice, even after a single dose.

Damage to blood vessels in the brain and heart with intravenous injection has been reported. Intravenous use of amphetamines, with its likely contaminants, adulterants, and unsterile needles, subjects the user to all the complications that accompany heroin use, including: hepatitis; skin, lung, and heart valve infections; destruction of blood vessels; and transmission of the human immunodeficiency virus (HIV).

Treatment.   Treatment of acute amphetamine reactions is usually directed toward preventing seizures, controlling body temperature, and quieting the person while the acute behavioral changes subside over several days. Appropriate tranquilizers are given for psychotic reactions or when behavior can't be controlled, resulting in violence. Depression and lethargy once the drug has been eliminated from the body are common and must be addressed to prevent an early return to the drug. Long-term treatment is more difficult to manage than just dealing with the acute effects of the drug, but it's of utmost importance to maintain abstinence. An uncommon sequel to amphetamine use is the appearance and subsequent persistence of a previously unrecognized psychologic disorder such as manic depression.

AMPHETAMINE-LIKE DRUGS

Ritalin. Methylphenidate (Ritalin) has been used for several decades to treat children and adults with hyperactivity disorders manifested by difficulty in maintaining attention (attention deficit disorders). Its pharmacologic effects are similar to those of amphetamines, although it is believed to have a greater effect on mental than on motor activity. It's generally used in conjunction with behavioral therapy and dietary regimens.

Methylphenidate, a Schedule II controlled substance, is taken orally or dissolved in water and injected when used inappropriately. Although considered a reasonable treatment for hyperactivity, with an estimated 800,000 children taking it, its safety and efficacy over long-term use according to some have not been demonstrated. Moreover, complications are possible and the potential for misuse exists, just as with continued use of any stimulant. So tolerance, psychological dependence, and abnormal behavior may occur in some users. Psychotic reactions have been reported with intravenous use. However, when supervised medically, its effects on hyperactivity and attention deficit disorders can be beneficial, and it has helped many children with this disorder to function normally.

Ephedrine. Far less potent than amphetamine, ephedrine is a stimulant in a large variety of decongestants and antiasthmatic medications. Its easy availability has resulted in its being sold as amphetamine on the street.

Khat. Grown in the highlands of East Africa and the Middle East, khat (*Catha edulis Forsk*) is a shrub whose leaves when chewed produce an effect somewhat less intense than but similar to that of amphetamine. Its use is well accepted as a traditional social activity in areas of North Yemen, Somalia, and parts of Ethiopia. Reports of its use have appeared in England and in the United States; use is extremely limited, however.

The usual method of consumption is chewing the shoots or leaves of the plant within four days of harvesting. Of the plant's chemical substances, the phenylalkylamine cathinone is believed to be primarily responsible for the mood-altering effect, which is described as euphoria, anorexia, heightened libido, increased socialization, and enhancement of concentration. Khat can induce craving and a certain degree of tolerance; physical dependence has not been reported. On the day following Khat use, drowsiness and dysphoria can occur. The most common adverse effects are esophageal and gastric irritation accompanied by constipation.

Phenylpropanolamine.   Phenylpropanolamine is commonly used as a nasal decongestant and appetite suppressant in over-the-counter and some prescription medications. It first appeared on the street as an ''illicit amphetamine'' but is now available mainly through legal purchase. It has minimal stimulant properties in the dosages recommended for treatment of congestion, but some sensitive people do report feeling high. If used in large doses, it causes a definite amphetamine-like effect, though usually not as pronounced.

Appetite suppressants.   Other stimulant drugs used mostly for weight reduction have the potential for inappropriate use, but far less so than the amphetamines. Some, such as phenmetrazine (Preludin) tablets, have considerable potential for inappropriate use; these can be taken orally, or crushed, mixed with liquid, and injected. The tablet contains talc, which presents a particular problem when injected: it can block the small blood vessels in the eyes, lungs, and brain.

Inappropriate use of phenmetrazine is well known; users describe the effects as similar to those of amphetamines. Other appetite suppressants (Table 12.3), although associated with a low potential for dependency, can still be misused. In some instances, people taking appetite suppressants do become dependent because of their mood-altering effects. Because of their availability, appetite suppressants can initiate drug use in young people.

CAFFEINE

Caffeine is consumed in some form by more than 90 percent of the U.S. population. Most who drink caffeine-containing beverages

experience minimal deleterious effects, but those who consume unusually large quantities are prone to adverse effects and reactions
similar to those produced by amphetamines and cocaine.

Caffeine exists in many natural substances (Table 12.6). It's one
of three drugs classified as methylated xanthines. The others are
theophylline, found in smaller concentrations in tea, and theobro-
mine, found in chocolate and cocoa. All three are stimulants, but
caffeine is the most potent. Caffeine is in coffee, tea, chocolate,
some soft drinks, and many over-the-counter medications used for
pain relief or central nervous system stimulants. The amount of caffeine consumed in such beverages as coffee or tea varies with strength
of the brew and amount consumed (Table 12.7).

Effects on the Body.   Caffeine is easily absorbed; peak concentrations appear in the blood within 15 to 45 minutes. It's quickly
distributed to the central nervous system, subsequently metabolized
in the liver, and excreted in the urine. Caffeine elimination is enhanced by smoking, but its metabolism is inhibited by oral contra-
ceptives or the antiulcer drug cimetidine (Tagamet).

The popularity of caffeine results from its positive effects on the
central nervous system (Table 12.8). These effects are variable, depending on a person's susceptibility and the quantity of caffeine
consumed. Nevertheless, one to three cups of coffee can produce an
elevation of mood, decreased fatigue, increased mental and physical
work capacity, ability to think more clearly, and occasional relief of
headaches and anxiety.

Caffeine, however, affects other parts of the central nervous system and other organ systems. It constricts blood vessels in the brain.
It increases the heart rate, raises blood pressure slightly, dilates arteries in the lung, relaxes smooth muscles in the respiratory tract,
induces acid secretion in the stomach (perhaps causing heartburn),
and increases urine flow through its diuretic action.

Whether caffeine can be considered a dependency-producing drug
capable of inducing withdrawal symptoms is unclear. But there's no
question that caffeine is habituating. Millions of people feel they
can't "get going" without their morning cup of coffee. That need

TABLE 12.6
Natural Sources of Caffeine

Source	Location
Cocoa tree	North and South America
Coffee beans	North and South America, Ethiopia, Arabia, Turkey
Tea leaves	China, Japan, India
Kola nuts	West Africa
Ilex plant	South America
Cassina	North America

TABLE 12.7
Caffeine Content of Common Beverages, Chocolate, and Over-the-Counter Medications

Product	Unit of Measure	Caffeine (mg/unit)
Coffee*		
Ground	cup (8 oz)	80–190
Instant	cup	30–100
Decaffeinated	cup	3–5
Tea*	cup	20–90
Cocoa	cup	6–42
Colas	12 oz	40–50
Chocolate	bar	25
Medications		
Analgesics	tablet	15–100
Stimulants	tablet	100–200

*Caffeine content depends on the strength of brew

TABLE 12.8
Positive Effects of Caffeine on the Central Nervous System

Elevates mood
Decreases fatigue
Increases psychological and physical work capacity
Enhances rapid, clearer thought
Relieves headache
Stimulates respiration

---

is sometimes work-related, and the desire for coffee during recreational hours is not as great.

Dependency and accompanying withdrawal is quite unusual, however. In one study, chronic coffee drinkers were given the beverage containing caffeine doses of 25, 50, and 100 milligrams. Those who drank the lower-dosed coffee quickly increased consumption to reach 100 milligrams.

Other studies involving coffee drinkers who consume large quantities of caffeine have shown that withdrawal reactions occur when caffeine is replaced with a placebo. The subjects experienced anxiety, headaches, increasing irritability, decreased alertness.

Adverse Effects of Caffeine.   Determining what is an excessive level of caffeine is difficult. Toxic effects may appear after consumption of 500 milligrams (approximately four cups of coffee) or after as little as 250 milligrams in susceptible persons. Symptoms of caffeinism are restlessness, flushing, gastrointestinal disturbances, increased rapidity of speech, nervousness, insomnia, confusion, and irritability.

Severe toxic effects (caffeine poisoning) is rare, but can cause abnormalities in cardiac rhythm, extreme agitation, seizures, and death. Such reactions may follow ingestion of five to 10 grams of caffeine (approximately 25 to 50 cups of coffee). But severe effects have been reported from as little as one gram. Even 500 milligrams can be toxic, especially in children who, with their low body weights, may consume excessive amounts in soft drinks or chocolate. Adverse effects appear quickly in such cases.

Individual susceptibilities vary greatly, so it has not been possible to establish a precise relationship between the particular effect and the amount of caffeine consumed. Underlying medical disorders or personality traits can accentuate the appearance of such effects.

Increased irritability, difficulty sleeping, and increased gastric secretions are the most common manifestations of excessive caffeine. But even low doses can have an impact on muscle coordination. More than five cups of coffee (or equivalent) a day can lead to difficulty concentrating.

Heartburn—the symptoms of gastric secretion—can be so severe in those who drink many cups of coffee that a heart condition may be suspected. Current popular thinking is that decaffeinated coffee prevents such symptoms. But decaffeinated coffee is only slightly less potent than regular coffee in stimulating gastric secretions. Coffee can also be particularly hazardous for those with, or prone to, peptic ulcer disease. The symptoms diminish or disappear when caffeine consumption is decreased or stopped.

The effects of caffeine on the heart and blood vessels have been studied extensively, but with varied and contradictory findings:

- People who drink excessive amounts of coffee tend to be smokers, drink alcohol, and, often, are high-powered, hard-driving individuals, all of whom tend to have a high incidence of cardiovascular problems. At present, no reliable evidence exists that proves caffeine is a significant risk factor in coronary artery disease. Excessive caffeine may perhaps elevate cholesterol levels. However, studies have shown that moderate coffee consumption has no adverse effect on serum cholesterol.
- Caffeine doesn't appear to cause persistent elevation of blood pressure or increase frequency of hypertension. In reasonable amounts, it doesn't interfere with treatment of hypertension.

Even if a positive relationship between caffeine and coronary heart disease is identified, a question will remain: is caffeine an independent risk factor, or does its excessive use simply accompany high-risk behavior?

A prudent recommendation for those with, or at high risk for, serious heart disease, and who wish to drink coffee, is to consume only moderate amounts.

Caffeine has also been suggested, but not confirmed, as a risk factor in certain cancers of the kidney, urinary tract, esophagus, and larynx. Also controversial is the relationship between caffeine and the ability of a woman to conceive easily and have an uncomplicated pregnancy and delivery (Chapter 18).

Chapter 13

Cocaine

I expect it [cocaine] will earn its place in therapeutics by the side of morphine and superior to it. I have other hopes and intentions about it. I take very small doses of it regularly against depression and against indigestion and with the most brilliant success.

—Sigmund Freud

Cocaine is obtained from leaves of the Erythroxylon Coca shrub. Evidence of coca leaf use dates back to Ecuador in 3000 B.C. In the Inca Empire, dating from the thirteenth century A.D., the emperor acknowledged the right of his subjects to choose the coca leaf above silver or gold.

Cocaine was isolated in 1844, with its pharmacological effects first studied in 1880. A subsequent study provided a comprehensive review of cocaine's action in the central nervous system. Sigmund Freud was a cocaine enthusiast who promoted its use for a wide variety of disorders, including those of the digestive tract and respiratory system, as well as for sexual dysfunction, treatment of opium and alcohol addiction, and as a local anesthetic.

The enthusiasm for cocaine continued into the early twentieth century, when it was widely available in over-the-counter preparations and elixirs. Cocaine was being used in more than 60 cola drinks at the time. The makers of Coca-Cola removed cocaine from the drink around 1906 and replaced it with caffeine. It is alleged that today's Coca-Cola is still flavored with a ''nonnarcotic'' extract of the coca plant.

Over the next two decades the adverse effects of cocaine became increasingly well known. It was one of the proscribed drugs included in the Harrison Narcotic Act of 1914, which levied a tax on those who compounded such drugs as opium and cocaine. The result was a noticeable decrease in availability.

Until the 1970s, cocaine use was generally concentrated among people in the arts and those who could afford it. And because cocaine was believed to be neither physically addictive nor capable of causing serious physical complications, aside from irritation and ulcers of the nasal passages, even medical opinion was tolerant. The combined use of cocaine and heroin was an exception, but that was also deemed insignificant when compared to heroin use alone.

Use of cocaine increased at a truly remarkable rate in the late 1970s, in part because of new restrictions on amphetamines and their decreased availability. In 1972, 14 percent of adolescents and 48 percent of young adults reported having tried marijuana. But less than 2 percent of adolescents and only 9 percent of young adults had tried cocaine. From 1976 to 1986 the National Institute on Drug Abuse reported a 15-fold increase in emergency room visits for cocaine use, in cocaine-related deaths, and in admissions to treatment facilities. In 1986 more than 3 million people were using cocaine regularly, and 15 percent of the U.S. population had tried it. Of those, 40 percent were between the ages of 25 and 30. In 1987 data from the National Institute on Drug Abuse suggested that as many as 6 million Americans may be using cocaine regularly, with 1 million dependent on this drug.

USER PROFILES

The 800 National Cocaine Hotline for helping cocaine users and their families received over 1 million calls between 1980 and 1985, sometimes totaling more than 1,200 a day, from every state in the nation. A more detailed follow-up survey of hotline callers helped draw a profile of the cocaine user.

In 1985, 64 percent were white, 36 percent black or Hispanic; women represented 42 percent. Seventy-two percent had annual incomes under $25,000; 27 percent had incomes above $25,000; approximately 1 percent earned more than $50,000. Seventy-four percent admitted they used cocaine at work. Because only hotline callers were surveyed, this study might be biased. Nevertheless, it demonstrated the magnitude of use.

Another survey tracked 739 young adults between the ages of 19 and 24. Its findings:

- 37 percent of the males and 32 percent of the females had used cocaine within the previous six months.
- Users were more likely than nonusers to have dropped out of high school, collected welfare, not attended college, and engaged in deviant behavior, including use of other mood-altering drugs.
- 99 percent of cocaine users combined it with alcohol; 82 percent with marijuana. 87 percent of nonusers drank alcohol; 16 percent used marijuana.
- 70 percent of users took other drugs, compared with 2 percent of nonusers.
- 18 percent of users drank alcohol to excess, compared with 6 percent of nonusers.
- 26 percent of users took cocaine at work.
- Users were more likely than nonusers to have been arrested for drug-related crimes (26 percent versus 8 percent).

Two of the more recent surveys show that regular use of cocaine among teenagers has decreased. One notes a drop from 13 percent in 1986 to 5 percent in 1990, and that the surge of crack use that appeared in 1986 has leveled off. Only 2 percent of seniors reported any use of crack in the past year, compared to 4 percent in 1987. The other survey found a drop in cocaine use among 12- to 17-year-olds from 4 percent in 1985 to 2.9 percent in 1988.

In 1989, the National Institute on Drug Abuse report on Epidemiologic Trends in Drug Abuse noted an increase in cocaine-related deaths in cities across the United States, with cocaine ranking highest of drugs mentioned in emergency rooms (increasing by 27 percent to 132 percent between 1987 and 1988).

The overall prevalence of cocaine use, however, varies greatly, depending on location and age group. In some cities, up to 40 percent may have experimented with cocaine use as early as junior high school. And the 1988 National Household Survey on Drug Abuse estimated that approximately 21 million Americans had tried cocaine at some time in their lives, and 2,923,000 were using it that year.

Although the number of cocaine users has decreased, the amount of cocaine consumed by those who use it has increased dramatically. According to the 1988 National Household Survey on Drug Abuse almost 10 percent of cocaine users have used it 100 or more times. This represents approximately 2 million past or present long-term users. This may explain why the number of cocaine-related deaths between 1988 and 1989 increased by 11 percent.

Increased efforts by law enforcement agencies to halt the distribution of cocaine accompanied by large seizures of the drug may have finally affected availability. Reports from the U.S. Drug Enforcement Agency indicate the wholesale price of cocaine to have increased considerably between 1988 and 1990, accompanied by a decrease in purity from 70 to 90 percent to 55 percent.

PATTERNS OF USE

The earliest form of cocaine use was chewing coca leaves, still a common method in countries where the coca plant is grown. Cocaine shows up in the blood within five to 10 minutes after chewing coca leaves, along with a considerable mood-altering effect (Table 13.1).

Cocaine sold on the street was initially prepared from cocoa paste and cut with adulterants (Table 13.2). Cocaine in powder form (with purity ranging from 30 to 90 percent) can be sniffed (snorted) or dissolved in water and injected. But it can't be smoked directly because heat quickly destroys it. When sniffed, it's absorbed through the blood vessels in the nose, transmitted through the veins to the heart and lungs, and carried by the arteries to the rest of the body. This process takes only two to three minutes to produce an effect. When cocaine is taken orally, the absorption process occurs in seven to 15 minutes. And when it is injected directly into the veins (mainlining), effects are apparent within 15 to 30 seconds.

TABLE 13.1
Time Lag Between Cocaine Consumption
and Onset of Effects

Method of Administration	Time (Seconds)
Chewing leaves or swallowing	300–600
Sniffing	120–180
Mainlining (intravenous)	15–30
Smoking (free-base cocaine or crack only)	6–8

TABLE 13.2
Cocaine Adulterants

Ascorbic acid
Aspirin
Benzocaine
Butacaine
Caffeine
Cornstarch
Herbicides
Heroin
Lactose
Lidocaine
Manganese carbonate
Magnesium sulfate
Mannitol
Procaine
Quinine
Stimulants: ephedrine, diet pills, amphetamines,
    phenylpropanolamine
Talc
Tetracaine

TABLE 13.3
Street Names for Cocaine

Type of Cocaine	Street Name
Cocaine hydrochloride	Blanco, Blow, C., Caine, Coca, Coke, Cola, Flake, Girl, Gold Dust, Heaven Dust, Lady Line Muser, Nose Candy, Paradise, Perico, Peruvian Flake, Polvo, Snow, Toot, White
Crack (free base)	Bazooka, Crack, Crystal, French Fries, Fry Daddie, Ready Rock, Rock, Space Base
Crack and heroin	Moonrock, Tar
Crack and PCP	Space Cadet, Tragic Magic

FREE BASING AND CRACK

Waiting two or three minutes for a drug to take effect doesn't seem burdensome. Yet free-base cocaine was developed to produce a higher-intensity high and to cut the time necessary to reach it. In about the time it takes to finish this page a reader can be on a "crack" high (Table 13.1).

Initially, free-base cocaine was processed by using ether, a highly flammable solvent, to produce a relatively heat-resistant, smokable substance. Free-base kits rapidly became available on the streets and in Head Shops, with total sales estimated in the tens of millions of dollars. But the ether caused a number of explosions, and it was taken out of the production process.

The resulting product was crack, so called because of the cracking sound it made during both processing and smoking. Other names include Rock, Ready Rock, and Crystal (Table 13.3).

Crack is almost—but not quite—a pure cocaine, prepared by heating ammonia with baking soda in a liquid solution of cocaine hydrochloride. The cocaine precipitates out and is sold in lumps (rocks, slabs, or caps) or in three-inch sticks (French Fries). Crack is "purer" than street cocaine but still contains impurities, including varying amounts of baking soda.

Crack can be smoked in a pipe or crushed and mixed with tobacco and smoked in cigarette form. Inhaling the smoke introduces the cocaine directly into the lungs and subsequently into the left side of the heart, bypassing the veins. An effect is produced within six to eight seconds (Table 13.1). The high is intense but lasts only minutes; by comparison, the effect of snorting peaks between 15 and 40 minutes. Crack is easy and inexpensive to manufacture. The result has been a significant drop in the street price of cocaine since the late 1980s. In 1990 the cost of one gram of cocaine was $40 to $100; when it was cut and sold as crack, each smoking unit cost $5 to $20, depending on location of the supplier. Because crack's extremely short-lived, intensely pleasurable high results in a constant craving, the compulsive user can easily spend $500 a day on the drug.

COCA PASTE

An intermediate product in the production of cocaine is coca paste. The paste, though impure, can contain 40 to 85 percent cocaine, plus a number of solvents used in the extraction process. Coca paste can produce behavioral effects identical to those seen with other forms of cocaine. Coca paste smokers are uncommon in the United States, but increased availability of the substance could lead to a subset of users with a tendency to progress to free base.

STAGES OF COCAINE USE

A cocaine rush is followed by a stimulation phase of increased alertness, feelings of sexual prowess, and euphoria (Table 13.4). The high associated with cocaine or crack is so pleasurable and so distorts perceptions that the user quickly feels that anything can be accomplished. Social or recreational users tend to take the drug sporadically and may not escalate their use. However, the pleasurable effects of the drug may result in a progression to its use in order to cope with a stressful situation. Relief in such settings may result in

TABLE 13.4
Stages of Cocaine Use

Intoxication
    Rush-euphoria
    Increased alertness, energy, confidence, intellectual functioning,
        sexual performance

Restlessness, anxiety

Repeat use to relieve negative feelings and regain high

Binge behavior

Crash
    Despair, anxiety, increased appetite, depression, desire—but
        inability—to sleep

Withdrawal
    Decreased energy, impaired intellectual functioning, muscle
        pains, tremors

Return to use
    At risk when in environment of prior use

more frequent use. When the drug is taken in other than social or recreational settings, the initial effects may give way to dysphoria (unhappiness or sadness), restlessness, and irritability within 30 minutes. That state often leads to depression, which produces enough discomfort to necessitate a rapid return to the drug.

The Runs.   Recurrent cocaine use results in binges of constant sniffing, smoking, or injecting. Binges can last from hours to days, with cocaine being taken as frequently as every 10 minutes. Similar runs are seen with amphetamines, but their effects last much longer; cocaine must be taken far more often.

The Crash.   For a recurrent user, the inevitable ''crash'' comes at the point where judgment is virtually destroyed and the body is run down from the consistent, repetitive use of cocaine. A crash manifests itself as despair, anxiety, a tremendous desire to sleep, severe depressive symptoms, and a huge appetite. Sedatives or alcohol are sometimes taken to facilitate sleep, which is not easily achieved.

Withdrawal. Decreased energy, impaired intellectual functioning, muscle pains, and tremors appear 12 to 96 hours after the crash. These and other withdrawal symptoms can last several weeks. Behavior becomes more normal during this time, but the craving for cocaine can resurface. The depression accompanying the crash quickly brings the user back to the realities of life, including all its frustrations and unfulfilled needs. Nothing seems right; everything is a burden. For some, the reality becomes overwhelming.

Following that second stage, even those who are drug-free can succumb to the lures (positive-reinforcement effects) of cocaine. Despite the will to abstain, they often quickly return to the drug if they meet former fellow users or find themselves in an environment associated with cocaine use.

COCAINE METABOLISM

Once in the body cocaine is rapidly broken down mainly by enzymes in the plasma (esterases), although metabolism in the liver may also occur. These breakdown (metabolic) products are mainly inactive and are excreted in the urine. They do, however, provide a basis for the laboratory detection of cocaine use by urine testing.

DEPENDENCY, TOLERANCE, AND ADDICTION

Cocaine increases energy, restores confidence, makes one able to face any task, increases intellectual functioning, relieves boredom, and increases sexual performance. In the mid-1970s, a presidential drug adviser wrote that cocaine "is probably the most benign of the illicit drugs currently in widespread use." So why shouldn't it be legalized and made available to everyone?

The pleasurable mood-altering effects are extremely short-lived, often leading to binge behavior. And use often progresses from occasional to daily to compulsive. That's well documented in several 1988 and 1989 surveys, which reveal that although the prevalence of cocaine use among teenagers and adults appears to be decreasing compared to prior years, those who are still using cocaine are increasing the frequency and the amount of cocaine or crack used.

Most of those who try cocaine once or twice don't become compulsive users. But the dependency potential of cocaine is great. Use can begin (as with a cocktail) simply as a means of deriving some pleasure and relaxation after a long day. Soon, however, use can become more frequent and more expensive. Rather than using cocaine just to relax after work, it may be taken to get started in the morning, and then to make the day more tolerable. Wide mood swings become noticeable. The user may be devoting all of his or her energies to getting more of the drug.

The Craving for Cocaine.   A number of hypotheses have been advanced concerning cocaine's mode of action (Chapter 3). Like other stimulants, cocaine affects neurotransmitters in areas of the brain believed to be responsible for behavior. These neurotransmitters include norepinephrine, epinephrine, serotonin, and dopamine. The release of dopamine is thought to stimulate the brain's reward mechanisms, or pleasure centers.

As part of a normal cycle, the released dopamine is reabsorbed or metabolized. But cocaine blocks dopamine's reabsorption, thus preventing a feedback mechanism from stopping dopamine production. The result is first an increase in dopamine transmission, but ultimately a depletion of its stores in the brain.

The initial increase of dopamine surrounding the brain results in overstimulation, manifested as euphoria, or the cocaine high. As the dopamine supply becomes depleted, depression sets in, followed by a craving for the drug. Thus stimulation of the pleasure centers in laboratory animals results in continual self-administration of the drug until death. As a result, the addictive potential for cocaine is exceptional.

On that basis, it's believed that since chronic cocaine use inhibits dopamine activity, activating dopamine can mediate the cocaine high. By depleting both dopamine and norepinephrine, long-term cocaine use results in an increased sensitivity of the neurons to those neurotransmitters. This increased sensitivity (to the now increased levels of norepinephrine and dopamine) causes withdrawal symptoms when cocaine use suddenly stops.

Long-term use also increases sensitivity of the brain to cocaine's nonmood-altering effects. Termed reverse tolerance, this phenomenon, brought on by even small amounts of cocaine in chronic users, shows up as hyperactivity and even convulsions.

ADVERSE EFFECTS OF COCAINE

Adverse effects of cocaine may occur during acute use (Table 13.5), with cocaine withdrawal, or with chronic use. They are common and at times may be fatal. They can develop at any time, depending on how the cocaine is taken, the dose used, the presence of underlying medical disorders, and the contaminants or adulterants with which the cocaine may be mixed.

Acute Reactions
Behavioral effects.   Acute adverse effects of cocaine on behavior include increasing irritability, aggression, delirium progressing to hallucinations such as bugs under the skin (coke bugs), flashing lights (snow lights), extreme agitation or paranoia, impaired judgment, and loss of conditional reflexes (disinhibition). The user is quick to argue and quick to fight. A perceived slight can result in acting out behavior against those who are often unaware and uninvolved. Judgment can be severely impaired without the user realizing it. Inappropriate decisions are made. The user may be impossible to relate to in any meaningful way, and at times anger may be excessive.

Such a stimulant effect is sought out by those engaged in antisocial behavior. According to data from the National Institute of Justice on male and female arrests in Washington, D.C., in May 1989, 65 percent of those arrested tested positive for cocaine. By comparison, in a similar survey in May 1984, the rate was 18 percent. Adverse behavioral effects of cocaine are common and can result in harm to

TABLE 13.5
Acute Toxic Effects

Behavioral effects: irritability, aggressive behavior, delirium, hallucinations, psychosis (including paranoid behavior)

Increased blood pressure and heart rate

Irregular heart rhythms, sometimes fatal

Anginal pain, potential for heart attacks

Increased potential for stroke

Elevated body temperature (malignant hyperthermia)

Rupture of brain aneurysms

Brain hemorrhage

Seizures and convulsions

Loss of consciousness

Coma

Respiratory and circulatory collapse

Death

others even in the absence of criminal intent. According to the Cocaine 800 Hot Line Survey, 19 percent of the respondents had been in auto accidents while using cocaine. In New York City from 1984 through 1987, cocaine or its metabolites was detected in 18 percent of autopsies in motor vehicle fatalities. Drivers between the ages of 16 and 45 were 13 times more likely to use cocaine. Statistically, this means that at least one of four drivers in this age group who were killed in such accidents in the city had used cocaine within 48 hours of death.

Effects of cocaine on the heart and vascular system. Acute use of cocaine can result in severe and even fatal effects on the cardiovascular system. Cocaine has long been known to cause an increase in blood pressure and heart rate. Frequent use, or even sporadic use with high doses, can result in irregular heart rhythms, including that of ventricular fibrillation, which without immediate intervention is fatal. The ability of cocaine to constrict the arteries leading to the heart muscle can result in decrease of blood flow associated with heart attacks, especially in those with underlying heart disease. A number of cases of myocardial infarction in young individuals subsequent to use of cocaine has been reported. The sudden increase in blood pressure in the arterial system can cause an increase in pressure in the vessels of the brain, resulting in hemorrhage and stroke.

Effects on the central nervous system. A direct effect of cocaine on the central nervous system can be a marked increase in body temperature, producing what is termed "malignant hypothermia." Increases in blood pressure, accompanied by constriction of the arteries to the brain, may also result in seizures, convulsions, and coma.

Effects on the respiratory system. Complications of the lungs resulting from cocaine's effects on blood vessels or from an allergic reaction to the contaminants in the cocaine can result in the lung tissue filling with fluid (pulmonary edema) and death by lack of oxygen (anoxia). If injected, infected material may remain in the lungs, causing pneumonia or a condition termed septic pulmonary emboli.

Unusual Effects of Cocaine Use. Among the more unusual effects of cocaine use are impaired blood circulation to the bowels, resulting in a severe impairment to the intestinal circulation and in gangrene; sudden death during sexual activity from rapid absorption of large amounts of cocaine applied directly to the penis or the vagina; gangrene from injection directly into the urethra of the penis, and a condition called "body packer syndrome" seen in cocaine smugglers.

The "body packer syndrome" is a consequence of swallowing large amounts of cocaine in rubber containers or condoms to escape detection. Once the smuggler successfully enters the country, a mild laxative is taken and the packs are excreted. This method of transport can result in blockage of the intestines and/or acute cocaine overdose and death, if the packets leak or rupture.

Adverse Effects During Withdrawal. Adverse and even fatal reactions have been reported hours and days after using cocaine or during withdrawal. In one study of young, presumably healthy young men being withdrawn from cocaine, up to 38 percent revealed decreased blood flow to the heart muscle. The relationship between myocardial infarctions and withdrawal from cocaine has been the subject of an increasing number of articles. In one study of men who developed chest pain between one and a half to 18 hours following cocaine use, approximately 30 percent developed actual heart attacks. The reasons for myocardial infarctions developing in the absence of cocaine in the body need to be more clearly determined. However, it is believed that two factors may play a role. The first hypothesis involves a sudden replenishment by the body of neurotransmitters depleted by cocaine, more specifically catecholamines. This results in a marked stimulation of the heart and vascular system. The second hypothesis involves the metabolite benzoylecgonine, produced when cocaine is broken down in the body. This substance can be detected in the body days after cocaine has been eliminated. It may also explain the lingering effects of cocaine on the brain, such as headaches, seizure, or strokes, which also can occur hours or days later.

Effects on Users with Underlying Medical Disorders. Even relatively small amounts of cocaine can have adverse effects on this category of users (Table 13.6). People with epilepsy, coronary artery disease, liver disease, diseases of the heart valves, rhythm disturbances, or psychological disorders are most susceptible. In one study of people undergoing coronary angiograms, very low doses of cocaine decreased the diameter of the left coronary artery—which supplies blood to most of the heart—by 8 to 12 percent.

People are often unaware that they have such conditions. For example, more than 500,000 people have silent coronary artery disease, and many of them would experience a cardiac complication if they took cocaine. Mitral valve prolapse, a condition seen in up to 10

TABLE 13.6
At-Risk Conditions

Medical Disorder	Risk
Abnormalities in blood vessels in brain	Brain hemorrhage, stroke
High blood pressure	Brain hemorrhage, stroke
Epilepsy or potential for seizure disorders	Convulsions
Coronary heart disease	Heart attacks (often fatal), serious disturbances in heart rhythm
Disease of heart valves, including mitral valve prolapse	Serious disturbances in heart rhythm, infection of valves (endocarditis) if cocaine injected
Psychological disorders	Psychotic reactions

percent of the population, may also predispose someone to irregular heart rhythms when cocaine is used. The drug has also been responsible for psychotic reactions in people not known to have prior psychologic disturbances. Whether such psychotic behavior results from cocaine alone, or would have appeared eventually without cocaine use, has not been clearly determined.

Effects of Adulterants and Substitutes. Adulterants in cocaine mixtures cause many adverse effects. Quinine, when injected, causes increased tissue destruction and abscess formation. Manganese carbonate can cause Parkinson-like symptoms, and such stimulants as antiasthmatic medications, amphetamines, and diet pills can increase toxicity to the central nervous system. A herbicide used to curtail growth of the coca leaf was found in one batch of cocaine and caused eye irritation and gastrointestinal disturbances. Other substances mixed with cocaine include all those found in heroin mixtures (Table

13.2). Allergic reactions to a number of such adulterants can occur quite easily, often with fatal results.

Sometimes a substance sold as cocaine may contain no cocaine, but instead a substitute capable of producing similar effects. The most potent are the amphetamines, particularly Ice, the methamphetamine derivative (Chapter 12). Other substitutes include such less potent stimulants as ephedrine and phenylpropanolamine, and the anesthetics lidocaine, benzacaine, procaine, and tetracaine. These anesthetic drugs, especially lidocaine, may be associated with seizures when larger doses are injected.

Chronic Adverse Effects of Cocaine Use. Consistent use of cocaine may produce a variety of local complications, depending on the way the cocaine is taken. These may range in intensity from a runny nose and sinusitis resulting from snorting, to severe lung and heart valve infections, to hepatitis and the transmission of the AIDS virus from intravenous use (Table 13.7). Use of coca paste has been associated with psychotic behavior, including hallucinations and suicidal or homicidal attempts. Complications to the heart and lungs from inhaling the solvents used to make the paste may also occur. Cocaine taken in any form has considerable effects on pregnancy and the newborn (Chapter 18). General nonspecific symptoms reported by cocaine users include chronic insomnia, fatigue, headaches, sinus infections, disrupted sexual function, nausea and vomiting, depression, anxiety and irritability, paranoia, loss of interest in all but drug-related activities, and marked difficulty in function (Table 13.8). One recent study of brain damage in chronic cocaine users found that 50 percent have a condition called cerebral atrophy, a shrinkage of brain tissue.

Effects of Cocaine in Combination with Other Drugs. Cocaine may also be used with other drugs to reduce its stimulant effect or to offset the sedative effect of another drug. Using cocaine with alcohol, especially when driving, is particularly dangerous, for the depressant effect of alcohol lasts much longer than the stimulant effect of cocaine. Since both substances can reduce awareness, judg-

Table 13.7
Adverse Effects of Cocaine, by Route

Intranasal (Snorting or Sniffing)	Intravenous (Mainlining)	Free Basing or Crack
Sinusitis	AIDS	Pulmonary infections
Running nose	Hepatitis	Coughing up blood
Upper respiratory infections	Infection of heart valves	Asthma
	Multiple skin infections	Voice loss
	Pulmonary infections	Chest pains
Ulceration of nasal septum	Acute allergic reactions	Burns*
		Eye irritation

*Free basing only

TABLE 13.8
Effects of Chronic Cocaine Use

Depression	Nausea and vomiting	Panic attacks
Insomnia		Postcocaine dysphoria
Fatigue	Disruption in sexual function	Cocaine psychosis
Severe headaches		Malnutrition
Loss of consciousness	Increased anxiety, irritability	
	Inability to function	

ment, and reaction time, they represent a particularly dangerous combination.

Effects of Cocaine on Others. As the need for more and more cocaine escalates, so does the user's need for money. Discretionary personal funds are the first to go, followed by depletion of money necessary for family responsibilities. And when pleas to family and friends eventually fail, the user often turns to illicit activities to get money.

Even the unborn are affected. The fetus is at risk, both from the effects of cocaine and from complications of sexually transmitted diseases if a woman engages in sex to support her habit (Chapter 18).

The safety of entire neighborhoods is severely compromised when the sale and use of cocaine and other drugs become prevalent. Residents are afraid of venturing out of their apartments. Complaints to the police can bring reprisals from dealers. And warfare between dealers for distribution rights can turn neighborhoods into battlegrounds.

To evade the law, dealers recruit children into the distribution chain. Lured by the relatively risk-free quick money, many youngsters begin to deal crack and soon find themselves users who are dependent on and bound to their supplier.

To many readers, this may seem overly dramatic, an updated version of a Dickens novel. But it's bitter reality to the many people who have seen their children's emotional and physical lives destroyed by crack. The added misfortune is that this drama is played out in economically depressed areas, where residents struggling simply to survive also have to face the overwhelming drug burden. Worse yet, their plight is accompanied by much outside sympathy but little actual support.

TREATMENT OF COCAINE DEPENDENCY

Treatment of Acute Toxic Reactions. The treatment of acute toxic reactions to cocaine varies with the specific manifestations. In many cases, just keeping the person in a quiet environment and providing reassurance suffices. For acute psychosis and/or hallucinations, a major tranquilizer and neuroleptic agent such as haloperidol (Haldol) can be used. Seizures can be controlled with benzodiazepines. But it is important to take the person to a hospital as quickly as possible.

The Phases of Rehabilitation.   Treating the chronic cocaine user physiologically, psychologically, and behaviorally is highly challenging, but far from impossible. As described by Arnold Washton, Ph.D., to achieve long-term abstinence usually requires passage through five distinct phases.

Phase 1 consists of withdrawal—usually lasting two to four days, but sometimes two weeks—accompanied by irritability and urgent craving for cocaine.

Phase 2, lasting one to four weeks, finds the person feeling quite well and convinced that the problem has been resolved. Only a minimal craving for cocaine is present.

Phase 3 may last for two months and shows up as depression, anxiety, inability to concentrate, and a sharp escalation of craving for the drug. One authority, Richard Rawson, Ph.D., terms this phase "the Wall" because it's where the person is at greatest risk of returning to the drug, especially in social settings of prior use where alcohol, cocaine, and other drugs are being consumed.

Phase 4 begins three to four months after abstinence starts and is marked by a return to normal functioning with only occasional cravings for cocaine, unless the person is in high-risk settings.

Phase 5 sees almost complete normalization of behavior or development of another addictive behavior such as excessive drinking.

Treatment Options.   A variety of forms of treatment are available. There are therapeutic communities (Chapter 5) and programs that offer a 28-day inpatient stay followed by outpatient care. Patients may be offered a shorter inpatient time plus the outpatient care, or perhaps a program of outpatient care exclusively. Each form of treatment has advantages and risks. But the treatment most cost-effective and acceptable to the greatest number of those seeking treatment is outpatient care preceded by a brief inpatient stay.

A variety of pharmacologic therapies also exist, but none has yet been vigorously evaluated.

Inpatient care.   Inpatient treatment is recommended for management of cocaine addiction when:

- the person can't stop using cocaine even for short periods

- dependencies to other mood-altering drugs exist, requiring detoxification
- a severe psychologic or medical problem exists (psychotic paranoid behavior, suicidal or homicidal thoughts, or severe heart, liver, or lung disease); or
- there are accompanying problems such as lack of a support system whereby the person can provide self-care, lack of motivation to attend any outpatient therapy, or a history of failed outpatient therapy

Inpatient treatment specifically for cocaine use is similar to outpatient treatment, except that it also allows other problems requiring hospitalization to be treated. Preexisting psychological disturbances should be recognized and treated. Mood disorders, which increase susceptibility to inappropriate cocaine use, have been found in up to half of those who do use it excessively, as well as infections, nutritional deficiencies, and other physical disorders. Most important, and often the most difficult problem to address, is the development of adequate support systems; unless the person can be kept from returning to the environment in which he or she used cocaine, successful rehabilitation is rare. Therapeutic communities, which provide a readily available residence phase and then continuous support on an outpatient basis, can also be effective.

Outpatient treatment.   The three stages of outpatient treatment begin with the immediate and complete cessation of cocaine and other drug use. Gradually decreasing the quantity of cocaine doesn't work because the mood-altering effects and reinforcement continue and use will resume at its prior level. Use of other mood-altering drugs must be stopped as well because they, too, provide a positive conditioning effect and a desire to continue using cocaine. They also lower inhibitions, thus increasing susceptibility to returning to cocaine. Frequent urine testing is often necessary for effective monitoring. Several therapy or counseling sessions a week help provide support and encouragement, and can address the craving and reasons for having started cocaine use. To be most successful, these sessions should be part of a structured program that includes instruction in stress management and relaxation techniques. That can be provided as part of individual or group therapy run by professional therapists, or through such self-help groups as Cocaine Anonymous and Narcotics Anonymous.

The second stage focuses on prevention of relapse. It requires a change in life-style: learning to avoid the factors associated with cocaine use, detecting the early warning signs of craving, and handling the feelings of defeat after instances of sporadic use. Building self-esteem and coping with unavoidable situations linked to prior cocaine use are some of the other problems that are tackled.

The final stage is consolidation, usually beginning after a year of treatment. It consists largely of continuing individual, group, or self-help therapy. How long this stage lasts depends on a person's needs and personality. As with other drug dependencies, relapse is almost certain if drug use was initiated because of inability to function in society. So sufficient supports, such as retraining and vocational and family counseling, must also be part of the consolidation stage.

Pharmacologic Therapies. Directed primarily toward relieving acute symptoms in the early phase of withdrawal, as well as depression, pharmacologic therapies also help block the brain effects that may be responsible for the craving for cocaine.

Many of cocaine's effects are probably the result of increased levels in the brain of the neurotransmitter dopamine, which chronic cocaine use depletes. Selective drug therapy tries to block those effects with a "nonaddicting" drug, and then to replenish the depleted neurotransmitters. Other drugs are prescribed to block the cocaine high or to prevent the depression that accompanies withdrawal. Such drugs may well decrease the reinforcing effects of cocaine and therefore lessen the craving for it.

Increasing dopamine effects. Both bromocriptine (Parlodel) and amantadine (Symmetrel) have been effective in relieving the craving and dysphoria in the first phase of cocaine withdrawal. Bromocriptine, a dopamine agonist, significantly increases energy and relieves depression. Side effects may include headaches, dizziness, and sedation. Amantadine can cause release of dopamine and norepinephrine from neuronal pleasure centers and may be effective in treating acute symptoms of withdrawal.

In efforts to directly influence production of dopamine, the substance from which dopamine is made, L-tyrosine, has been administered in a preparation (Tropamine) that also contains L-tryptophan, L-glutamine, L-phenylalanine, and a variety of vitamins and minerals. One study suggests that Tropamine can reduce withdrawal symptoms and help put patients remaining in treatment at ease.

L-tryptophan food supplements have been associated with Eosinophilia Myalgia Syndrome, a rare disorder manifested by a variety of symptoms, including itching, fatigue, muscle pains, tenderness and cramps, joint pains, weakness, and, at times, shortness of breath. The Food and Drug Administration ordered a recall of all such products in November 1989, followed by a warning to the public in March 1990 not to use them.

So far, the effectiveness of bromocriptine, amantadine, and Tropamine has not been proven on a widespread basis. They should never be the sole method of therapy.

Antipsychotic drugs.   Neuroleptics, a group of drugs classed as major tranquilizers, are believed to block the euphoria of cocaine and amphetamines through their dopamine-inhibiting effects, and to reduce self-administration of cocaine in laboratory animals. Two such drugs are chlorpromazine (Thorazine, Promaz, Sonaz) and fluphenazine (Prolixin, Permitil). But their side effects make it unlikely that people will take them voluntarily for any period, and the unpleasant feeling they produce may even promote cocaine use.

Under study is another drug in this group, flupenthixol, which may turn out to be more successful. At low doses it acts as an antidepressant and can be administered as a slow-release, long-acting injectable. Haloperidol (Haldol), an antipsychotic drug with fewer side effects than the other major tranquilizers, has been used with apparent success in Japan to prevent a return to cocaine use. Much more research is needed in this area.

Antidepressants.   Certain tricyclic antidepressants have been used both to treat depression and to reduce the craving for cocaine. They include desipramine (Norpramin, Pertofrane) and imipramine (Tofranil, Janimine, Pramine). They've been especially effective during the second phase of withdrawal. Their use in treatment, however, requires careful monitoring because some—notably amitriptyline (Elavil)—have a well-known history of inappropriate use. The antidepressants trazodone (Desyrel, Trazon, Trialododine) and buspirone (BuSpar) may also be helpful in relieving withdrawal and promoting abstinence.

Miscellaneous drugs. A variety of other drugs are in various stages of evaluation for treatment of cocaine dependency. They include lithium, pemoline, and several stimulants. One of the stimulants, methylphenidate (Ritalin), has known potential for inappropriate use and so carries its own risks. As noted previously, this is an extremely effective drug for hyperactivity and when recommended by a physician should not be withheld for fear of dependency. Buprenorphine (Buprenex), an agonist-antagonist marketed to control pain (Chapter 10), has decreased cocaine self-administration in animals. Mazindol (Mazanor, Sanorex), a dopamine blocker used to treat compulsive eaters, has also been suggested for cocaine addiction. None of those drugs has been proven successful and some may be associated with dependency risks of their own.

Chapter 14

Nicotine

Smoking Causes Lung Cancer, Heart Disease, Emphysema, and May Complicate Pregnancy.

Quitting Smoking Now Greatly Reduces Serious Risks to Your Health.

Smoking By Pregnant Women May Result in Fetal Injury, Premature Birth, and Low Birth Weight.

Cigarette Smoke Contains Carbon Monoxide.
　　—surgeon general's warnings on cigarette packages

Evidence of tobacco use appears in Mayan stone carvings from 600 to 900 A.D. Explorers to the New World found the Native Americans inhaling smoke from pipes or rolls of leaves to produce mood-altering effects. After the tobacco was brought to Europe and elsewhere, it was either smoked, chewed, or ground to be used as snuff. No matter how it was consumed, tobacco's positive-reinforcing—and even addicting—qualities became well known.

Papal bulls prohibiting its use were issued by Popes Urban VIII and Innocent X between 1640 and 1650. Also in the 1600s, Bavaria, Saxony, Zurich, and Japan initiated measures first to restrict and then to prohibit its use. The prohibitions were unsuccessful, so severe penalties, including mutilation, were imposed. In Russia and Constantinople, the penalty was death. Ultimately, all those efforts proved futile.

Chewing tobacco and snuff were popular in the United States through the early 1900s. The social stigma of spitting, and the transmission of tuberculosis through this route, soon led to decline of the practice. The decline was accompanied by a significant increase in cigarette smoking. At first, people rolled their own by hand, but went on to use an 1884 invention—the mechanical cigarette rolling machine. Cigarettes soon became widely available to both adults and children. By 1921, reaction was so strong that 14 states had enacted legislation prohibiting cigarettes. As with Prohibition, it soon became evident that smoking habits couldn't be legislated and all such legislation was repealed by 1927.

In 1964 the first of many reports on smoking and health was released by the surgeon general's Advisory Committee on the Health Consequences of Smoking. It can probably be credited as the first major contributor in reducing cigarette consumption. The report detailed many of the unpublicized effects of smoking and was followed by a definite but short-lived decrease in cigarette consumption. But smoking gradually increased again over the next decade.

Tobacco manufacturers began developing filter-tip cigarettes that contained less tar and nicotine and again touted the use of smokeless tobacco.

Since the late 1960s, the surgeon general's office has been joined by all major health-related organizations in trying to limit smoking. Many government agencies have funded education and prevention programs as part of the effort.

The 1985 Comprehensive Smoking Education Act unequivocally emphasized the need and obligation of tobacco manufacturers to inform the public of the hazards of smoking. That warning, plus identification of chemical substances in cigarettes, was displayed on each package. To emphasize those facts, the Department of Health and Human Services legislated a mandatory public education program monitored by the Interagency Committee on Smoking and Health.

The committee included representatives from the public sector, major health organizations active in promoting a nonsmoking theme, and research agencies dealing with the adverse effects of smoking. The National Cancer Institute and the National Institute on Drug Abuse were among this latter group.

A report of the surgeon general in 1989 recognized smoking as an addiction and clearly identified tobacco as another addictive drug—albeit a legal one.

CIGARETTE SMOKERS TODAY

From 1976 to 1987, the population of cigarette smokers in the United States decreased from 37 percent to 29 percent—the lowest ever recorded. As of 1989, an estimated 49 million Americans—still 29 percent of the population age 18 or older—were smokers. About 40 million, nearly half of adults who have ever smoked, identified themselves as former smokers, a clear indication of the impact of education on smoking habits.

The 1989 surgeon general's report estimated that without the educational efforts there might have been 91 million smokers in 1985 instead of 50 million. That success, however, seems related to educational background and socioeconomic status. People with a high school education account for 35 percent of smokers; those with postgraduate college education account for only 17 percent.

A study projecting trends in cigarette smoking to the year 2000 suggests that 22 percent of the adult population, or 40 million people, will be smokers at that time. But those with a high school education or less will account for 30 percent of the smokers, compared with 10 percent among college graduates.

Smoking habits are also sex-related. The 1988 National High School Survey found that women were only slightly more likely than males to smoke in high school, but much more likely than men to do so in college. And fewer women than men stop smoking later on. The number of male smokers decreased from 50 to 31 percent between 1965 and 1987, whereas the decrease among women was from 32 to 26 percent. Female deaths from lung cancer are increasing steadily.

In the overall population, the highest proportion of smokers (33 percent) was found among those between the ages of 25 and 44; the lowest (9 percent) among those 75 or older.

A 1987 survey of more than 4,000 students in Pennsylvania found that 12 percent of boys and 10 percent of girls had experimented with cigarettes by the third grade. The percentages increased to 79 percent of boys and 74 percent of girls by the twelfth grade.

Daily use of one or more cigarettes by adolescents decreased 35 percent between 1975 and 1986, but 18 percent of high school seniors reported daily use of cigarettes in 1988—a greater proportion than with any other group of drugs—with 11 percent smoking at least 10 a day.

Estimates put at 3,000 the number of American teenagers who start smoking each day. One researcher observed that one-third to two-thirds of adolescents who smoke two or more cigarettes become habitual smokers. That's about 1 million young people per year.

Although cigarette smoking continues to abate, the United States still has an extremely high per capita rate of cigarette consumption. Sales from tobacco products in 1990 were more than double those of the early 1960s, when the adverse effects of smoking first began to be publicized. More important, however, are the findings of the 1990 national high school survey, which indicated that smoking among high school seniors has remained virtually unchanged over the last decade.

AVAILABLE NICOTINE PRODUCTS

Low-Nicotine Cigarettes.   Efforts to meet public demand for a "safer cigarette" have greatly reduced the tar and nicotine content of cigarettes since the 1950s. Between 1955 and 1987, average tar yield per cigarette fell from 34 to 13 milligrams; the average nicotine yield from two to 0.9 milligrams. The most recent efforts have included cigarettes containing 0.1 milligrams nicotine or less, with tar levels as low as one milligram. Other cigarettes contain perfumed paper and have less visible sidestream smoke.

The preliminary data suggesting that the new type of cigarettes may be less hazardous assume that smokers won't change their smoking patterns. The fact is, to get the same amount of nicotine, many who use low-yield cigarettes take more frequent puffs, inhale more deeply, and smoke a greater number of cigarettes. The use of additives to enhance flavor may attract more smokers, especially adolescents. And the inability to see sidestream smoke may give the impression that smoking is less dangerous. Such gimmicks may mislead heavy smokers into thinking that switching to the low-yield nicotine and tar cigarettes is safe.

However, even determining the actual tar and nicotine yields of a specific brand may not be easy. Ronald Davis, M.D., and associates in a survey of 160 cigarette brands found tar yield listed on only 14 percent and nicotine yield on only 11 percent. As the tar yield of a brand increased, it was less likely to be shown. No cigarette yielding 11 mg. or more of tar had this disclosed on the package.

SMOKELESS TOBACCO

The popularity of smokeless tobacco among the young is also increasing. Even when general use of this product declined in the 1920s, athletes continued to use it over the next two decades. It was particularly popular with baseball players, who appreciated chewing tobacco's ability to produce saliva to keep their mouths moist and their gloves soft. By the 1950s, smoking had pretty much replaced chewing and was, in fact, advocated by many athletes in cigarette advertisements.

In the early 1970s, smokeless tobacco began to appear again with some frequency on the ball fields, both as a chew and as a snuff (dip). Snuff is a ground tobacco product placed between the gum and the cheek. Pluck is a chewing tobacco sold loose in a container or as a solid chunk. These products are advertised as alternative methods of nicotine use, and a number of brands have appeared on the market.

A survey of male college baseball players revealed that 40 percent used smokeless tobacco regularly, compared with 3 percent who smoked cigarettes. In a survey of 265 players on seven major league teams, 34 percent were current users of smokeless tobacco; 17 percent past users. Of the current users, 93 percent took snuff, either alone or in combination with chewing tobacco, and 8 percent used chewing tobacco alone. Of the current users, 15 percent were also smoking approximately 10 cigarettes per day.

Twenty-eight percent of the players admitted that smokeless tobacco was very harmful, and 65 percent believed it was somewhat harmful. Twenty-eight percent said they couldn't stop because they were "hooked."

Tobacco companies aggressively promote smokeless tobacco. Their campaigns work: use of snuff increased by 55 percent between 1978 and 1985, a time when cigarette sales were decreasing. By 1985, men under age 19 were the heaviest users of smokeless tobacco, compared with 1970, when men over age 55 were the greatest users. In the younger group, the proportion of men between the ages of 17 and 19 who used oral snuff rose from 0.3 to 2.9 percent; the proportion for chewing tobacco rose from 1.2 to 3 percent—a 10-fold and three-fold increase, respectively.

In 1988, an estimated 29 million people in the United States, or 15 percent of the household population, used smokeless tobacco, 8 million within the last month. The greatest proportion of use is in the 18 to 25 years age group; however, since household surveys may tend to underestimate the number of children using this product, individual surveys of young people provide more relevant information.

One survey of elementary and high school students found that 7 percent of girls and 22 percent of boys had chewed tobacco by the third grade. For the boys, that was twice the number that had tried smoking. By the tenth grade, 70 percent of the boys reported such experimentation. In the third grade, more than 90 percent of the children believed smokeless tobacco was harmful; by the twelfth grade, only 45 percent of the boys and 65 percent of the girls believed it harmful.

Other surveys confirm the widespread use of smokeless tobacco. A survey of 1,180 ninth and eleventh graders in the state of Washington found that smokeless tobacco was being used by 34 percent of male Native Americans and 20 percent of other males; by 24 percent of female Native Americans and 4 percent of other females. In Connecticut, random samplings of seventh to twelfth graders revealed that 37 percent of boys had used smokeless tobacco, with 8 percent using it daily by the twelfth grade.

Use of smokeless tobacco by Native American adolescents is unusually high, with surveys reporting 24 to 64 percent of boys to be using it. The evidence is compelling that smokeless tobacco produces nicotine levels in the body comparable to those produced by smoking and carries additional risk of cancer of the mouth.

Other Products.   Although the major emphasis has been on the harmful effects of cigarettes and chewing tobacco, pipe and cigar smoking are far from risk free.

TOBACCO ECONOMICS

The direct and indirect public costs of tobacco use are staggering. Health-related costs alone reached $55.5 billion in 1985, decreasing somewhat in 1990 to an estimated $52 billion. That doesn't include the federal price-support system in which the government buys tobacco leaves not bought by tobacco companies. More than 13 billion pounds of blue-cured tobacco or barley are stored in government warehouses. If sold through a "discount buyout," the cost would be $500 million to $1 billion in failed subsidy loans.

But tobacco sales (mainly cigarettes) are quite profitable, easily justifying the more than $3.27 billion spent in advertising each year by the tobacco companies. In 1983 tobacco and related industries employed more than 700,000 workers, accounting for $31.5 billion of the Gross National Product (GNP), and $13.5 billion in tax revenues.

Although many tobacco companies have diversified and tobacco no longer constitutes a major portion of their activities, profits from tobacco sales continue to represent a disproportionate amount of total income. The financial stakes in maintaining tobacco use are obvious.

INGREDIENTS IN TOBACCO

More than 3,000 substances are generated by the combustion of tobacco, and at least 43 are believed to be able to cause cancer. Of most concern are nicotine, carbon monoxide, and "tar" (the material remaining after water and nicotine are removed).

Nicotine, the active ingredient in tobacco, was first isolated in 1828 at the University of Heidelberg, in Germany. Its chemical formula was determined in the 1840s, and it was synthesized before the 1890s. By the early 1900s, nicotine was considered the reason for tobacco's popularity.

The nicotine content of a cigarette can vary from 0.2 to 5 percent. When smoked, a cigarette delivers from 0.1 to two milligrams of nicotine. Pipe and cigar tobacco smoke contain greater amounts of nicotine; but the smoke is usually not inhaled, and absorption of nicotine occurs mainly through the mucous membranes of the mouth.

Some cigarette manufacturers identify the nicotine, tar, and carbon monoxide content, but relating these figures to individual clinical patterns of smoking is difficult, if not impossible. The amounts of tar, nicotine, and carbon monoxide inhaled depend on the number of puffs, depth of inhalation, and number of cigarettes smoked. Filters can trap a small quantity of gas and particles, but neither low-tar nor low-nicotine cigarettes actively reduce the amount of carbon monoxide that is produced. Traps near the top of the cigarette are designed to reduce tar and carbon monoxide, and appear to be effective in laboratory settings. But they're far less so during actual smoking.

Nicotine in Cigarette Smoke.   A cigarette emits three types of smoke:

- mainstream, inhaled directly by the smoker
- sidestream, produced by the tobacco burning between puffs
- environmental, the combination of sidestream and exhaled mainstream smoke

Sidestream smoke has the same constituency as mainstream smoke but has higher concentrations of carbon monoxide. And because it's produced at lower combustion temperatures, it contains more of smoke's organic constituents, including those considered carcinogenic.

Environmental smoke is largely diluted by air and aged to varying degrees before it's inhaled by nonsmokers (passive smokers) and smokers. About 85 percent of environmental smoke consists of sidestream smoke.

Each puff of a cigarette contains about 0.25 milligrams of nicotine, and each cigarette lasts an average of 10 to 12 puffs. How much nicotine is absorbed through the mucous membranes of the mouth and pharynx depends on the pH (alkalinity/acidity) content of the material being smoked. Cigarette tobacco has a low pH (low alkalinity), so there's little absorption. But the air-cured tobaccos used in pipes, cigars, and smokeless products have a higher pH, so absorption through the membranes of the mouth, pharynx, and respiratory and gastrointestinal tracts is far greater. Regardless of pH, inhalation results in rapid absorption in the lungs; 90 percent of the nicotine is absorbed and begins to reach the brain in eight seconds. The absorption rate from swallowing or chewing is 25 to 50 percent. Because blood nicotine levels accumulate—but decline slowly— chronic smokers may have nicotine in their systems 24 hours a day.

Smokeless Nicotine.   Moist snuff contains 12 to 16 milligrams of nicotine per gram, and plug tobacco about 25 milligrams per gram. Blood nicotine levels produced with smokeless tobacco are equivalent to those from smoking, but they're reached more slowly and sustained longer. Typically, smokeless nicotine levels plateau at 30 minutes and decline over two hours. Snuff can deliver two to three times the nicotine of a cigarette; eight to 10 dips of snuff (or plugs of tobacco) delivers the same amount of nicotine as 30 to 40 cigarettes.

PHARMACOLOGIC EFFECTS OF SMOKING

Nicotine is an unusual stimulant; its mechanism of action is different from that of other drugs. It readily crosses the blood-brain barrier, acting on specific binding sites in the central nervous system, spinal cord, and autonomic nervous system.

Nicotine produces many effects on the body (Table 14.1). It decreases muscle tone; increases the concentration of several hormones, including acetylcholine, dopamine, norepinephrine, corticosteroids, and pituitary hormones. It increases blood pressure, heart rate, and serum levels of cholesterol (all considered risk factors for cardiac disease). The blood-pressure response varies. The higher blood pressures aren't long-term, and high doses of nicotine can

TABLE 14.1
Effects of Smoking

Cardiovascular system
  Increases blood pressure, heart rate;* constricts blood vessels*

Central nervous system
  Increases alertness
  Decreases skeletal muscle tone (relaxation)
  Facilitates mental processes
  Decreases appetite
  Decreases irritability
  Increases secretion of neurotransmitters, norepinephrine, dopamine
  Nausea and vomiting**

Hematologic
  Increases clotting ability of blood*
  Decreases capacity of hemoglobin to deliver oxygen to tissues*

Gastrointestinal
  Nausea, vomiting, diarrhea

Irritates linings of bronchial tissue and lungs; irritates olfactory receptor cells in a nasal lining, with diminished sense of smell***

Metabolic
  Increases free fatty acids,* glycerol, lactate
  Increases low-density cholesterol (LOL)*
  Decreases high-density cholesterol*
  In women: earlier menopause and increased risk of osteoporosis

Neurotransmitter and hormonal function
  Increases norepinephrine, epinephrine, vaso pressin, growth hormone, ALTH, cortisol, prolactin, endorphin
  Decreases prostaglandin release

Neuromuscular
  Relaxes some muscle groups

*Adds to risk of coronary heart disease and heart attacks
**Occurs with early exposure
***Hypothesis observed for decrease in sense of smell

result in decreased blood pressure and slower heart rates. The carbon monoxide in cigarettes causes formation of carboxy hemoglobin, cutting the amount of oxygen delivered to the tissues.

Nicotine is metabolized primarily in the liver, secondarily in the kidneys and lungs. Excretion in the urine varies depending on pH content. With regular use, nicotine levels accumulate and persist while the smoker is sleeping, though some decline occurs.

Heavy smoking also interferes with the action of many medications (Table 14.2). In some cases, nicotine's stimulant effect on enzymes in the liver causes increased metabolism of the other drugs. The stimulation may also result from the additive effect of nicotine and the other drugs.

Smoking provides many pleasures. It increases alertness, facilitates mental prowess, and is credited with maintaining a degree of calm and muscle relaxation even in stressful situations. Relief from stress is one of the most common reasons given for smoking. Nicotine improves mood and even improves performance. It can also reduce the pain threshold.

Weight loss is a secondary effect. The reason some women give for starting to smoke is to control their weight. In general, a smoker's weight is six to 10 pounds less than that of a nonsmoker of comparable age and height.

The thinking nowadays is that the weight loss in smokers reflects the increased expenditure of energy resulting from the effect of nicotine on the body's metabolism. One study showed that male smokers spent less energy accomplishing a fixed task when deprived of nicotine. So it may be that cutting off nicotine decreases the metabolic rate, which results in a weight gain. Part of the weight gain can also be attributed to increased eating, the alternative means for satisfying oral needs.

DEPENDENCY, TOLERANCE, ADDICTION, WITHDRAWAL

Dependency.   The dependency-producing effect of tobacco was first demonstrated in 1942, when injectable solutions of nicotine were found to suppress craving in smokers. The researcher, Dr. Lennox

TABLE 14.2
Interactions of Nicotine with Other Drugs

Drug	Effect with Nicotine
Aminophylline (Theophylline)	Diminished
Antidepressants Imipramine (Tofranil, Janimine, SK Pramine)	Diminished
Benzodiazepines (Librium, Lorazepam, Alzapam, Ativan, Valium)	Diminished
Warfarin (Coumadin)	Diminished
Estrogens	May increase viscosity of blood
Insulin	Slows absorption from subcutaneous site
Narcotic agents	Diminished
Nifedipine (Procardia)	Diminished
Oral contraceptives	Increase risk of stroke and premature myocardial infarction *in women*
Propranolol (Inderal)	Diminished

Johnston, concluded that "smoking tobacco is essentially a way of administering nicotine, just as smoking opium is a way of administering morphine." Tobacco dependency wasn't listed in the Diagnostic and Statistical Manual of Mental Disorders (DSMIII) until 1980. It was changed to "nicotine dependence" in 1987.

Nicotine meets the same criteria for dependency as narcotics (opiates), alcohol and other central nervous system depressants, and cocaine. But cross-dependency doesn't occur between nicotine and other mood-altering agents. Alcoholics can substitute minor tranquilizers or sedatives for alcohol, and people dependent on stimulants can substitute antidepressants. But smokers who use other drugs continue to smoke.

Tolerance. The acute and chronic effects of nicotine tolerance occur in some individuals, and dependency develops rapidly. The body apparently adjusts to its own nicotine level, with chronic smokers consuming fewer high-nicotine cigarettes and more low-nicotine cigarettes to be comfortable. Controlled use of some mood-altering substances such as alcohol is common, but less than 10 percent of chronic smokers can manage with fewer than five or six cigarettes a day.

Addiction. Tobacco smokers fulfill the definition of "addict" in the true sense of the word. They defy sanctions prohibiting its use, and when necessary spend all available resources to get it—even in the presence of illnesses clearly made worse by smoking. When tobacco supplies in post-World War II Germany were rationed (two packs per day for men, and one for women), heavy smokers bartered food for tobacco, searched the streets for cigarette butts, and begged passersby for a cigarette. In one study of 1,000 persons in treatment for alcohol or drug dependency, 57 percent said cigarettes would be harder to give up than their primary drug of abuse, even though they felt the pleasurable effects from that drug were greater than from smoking.

Despite all that's been known for decades about tobacco, its addictive qualities are often denied. Many consider it habituating, rather than dependency-producing. As discussed earlier (Chapter 3), habituation is but one step on the road to dependency. In its dependency-producing potential, nicotine is like the more commonly feared drugs, such as alcohol, heroin, and cocaine. The 1989 report of the surgeon general's Advisory Committee on the Health Consequences of Smoking appropriately recognized that fact. The report concluded that cigarettes and other forms of tobacco, due to their nicotine content, cause an addiction manifested by pharmacologic and behavioral changes similar to those of heroin and cocaine.

Withdrawal. Withdrawal syndromes vary greatly in intensity and are apparent in up to 80 percent of smokers who quit. They include irritability, anxiety, restlessness, sleep disturbances, headaches, cravings for cigarettes, increased appetite, and an assortment of nonspecific gastrointestinal complaints. Symptoms can start within 24 hours after smoking stops, peak in 48 hours, and persist for weeks to months.

As with other dependency-producing drugs, the symptoms can be rapidly suppressed by the administration of nicotine, either in solution or as tobacco. Abstinence is difficult but can be achieved. The relapse rate, however, is similar to that of such other addictive substances as alcohol and heroin.

ADVERSE EFFECTS OF SMOKING

As the chief cause of avoidable deaths in the United States, nicotine can be considered the most dangerous of all mood-altering drugs. Smoking is responsible for an estimated 390,000 deaths each year—more than the combined deaths from AIDS, cocaine, heroin, alcohol, fire, automobile accidents, homicides, and suicides. In 1985 the estimated 390,000 deaths caused by smoking accounted for approximately 936,000 years of potential life lost before age 65. If adjusted for average life expectancy, deaths caused by smoking would account for the loss of approximately 3.5 million years of potential life. Except for those related to fires and environmental smoke, 99 percent of those deaths occurred in those who started smoking before 1964.

Mortality is directly related to the number of cigarettes smoked over time. Overall mortality for males who smoke fewer than two packs per day is 1.7 times greater than for nonsmokers. Mortality in males who smoke two or more packs per day is two times greater. Those who inhale are at greater risk than those who don't.

The most common complaints of chronic smokers are coughing (worse in the morning); shortness of breath associated with decreased exercise tolerance; and sometimes a decrease in the sense of taste and smell. Smoking primarily affects the cardiovascular and pulmonary systems, but it harms other organ systems as well (Table 14.3).

Lung Disease. Smoking markedly increases the prevalence of such acute pulmonary infections as bronchitis and chronic lung disease (emphysema). Since the late 1960s, deaths from chronic lung disease increased two to three times in women age 57 or older. Smoking also greatly increases the risk of lung cancer. Of the 126,000 deaths from lung cancer in 1986, at least 80 percent were attributed to active cigarette smoking.

Among people over the age of 35, the relative risk of death from lung cancer to smokers compared with those who've never smoked is 22 times greater for men and 12 times for women. The relative-risk comparison for former smokers is nine times for men, five times for women, respectively.

Smokers also have an add-on risk of developing lung cancer from other cancer-causing agents. The risk associated with radon exposure in smokers is six to 11 times higher than in nonsmokers. A similar increase in risk has been seen with asbestos exposure and smoking.

Lung cancer appears to have reached a relative plateau in men, perhaps due to the decline in male smokers since 1970. But, as noted, the rate among women seems to be increasing. In 1986 lung cancer surpassed breast cancer as a leading cause of death in women. Epidemiologic studies have suggested that the risk of developing lung cancer is decreased in those who smoke cigarettes low in tar and nicotine. Nevertheless, the risk is still much greater than for nonsmokers.

Cardiovascular Disease. Smoking's adverse effects on the heart are related to the stimulant action of nicotine, an increase in cholesterol levels, norepinephrine release, the coagulability of the blood and a decrease in oxygen delivery.

Coronary artery disease. Most reports linking smoking to heart disease are based on studies of heart attack victims. One study documented in dynamic fashion the effect smoking may have on blood flow to the heart. Researchers in Boston used a Holter monitor to record electrical activity of the heart in 24 smokers and 41 non-

TABLE 14.3
Health Risks Associated with Tobacco

Coronary heart disease
  Heart attacks
  Increased chest pain in persons with heart disease
  Aneurisms of aorta

Increased disturbances in cardiac rhythm

Blood vessels
  Stroke due to narrowing of cerebral vessels
  Narrowing of large arteries in legs (Berger's disease)

Lungs
  Chronic cough
  Chronic bronchitis
  Chronic lung disease (emphysema)
  Cancer of lung

Various cancers
  Larynx, esophagus, pancreas, oral cavity, bladder

Other conditions
  Nonspecific chest pain
  Peptic ulcer
  Heartburn

Pregnancy and childbirth
  Miscarriage, prenatal mortality, low birth weight, Sudden Infant
    Death Syndrome

---

smokers with known but stable coronary artery disease. Even in the absence of symptoms, the monitor can detect signs of decreased blood flow to the heart (ischemia) during everyday activities. Smokers had signs of ischemic activity three times as often and lasting 12 times longer than in nonsmokers.

Deaths due to coronary artery disease increase two- to threefold in smokers compared with nonsmokers, with chances of dying from heart disease increasing in direct proportion to how heavily one smokes, the number of years one smokes, and the specific age range studied. Deaths due to coronary artery disease are five times greater in smokers than nonsmokers between the ages of 35 and 44; four times greater for those between 45 and 54.

Smokers with coronary artery disease experience angina more frequently. They exercise less and are at increased risk for serious heart-rhythm irregularities. These risks are independent of other risk factors, but the individual has a far greater chance of a heart attack if there is a family history of coronary disease and/or if the cholesterol level is elevated. In 1985 smoking accounted for 21 percent of deaths due to coronary artery disease, 40 percent of them in men and women under the age of 65.

A study of 113,404 women who were followed for six years found that those who smoked more than 25 cigarettes a day had 5.5 times the risk for fatal heart attack, 5.8 times the risk for nonfatal heart attack, and 2.6 times the risk for angina. Smoking even one to four cigarettes a day was associated with a twofold risk of heart attack. The figures were the same for regular and low-nicotine cigarettes.

Cessation of smoking reduces the risk of death from heart attack regardless of sex or age. One study of 1,893 men and women over the age of 55 with known coronary artery disease revealed that those who continued smoking had a relative risk of death 1.7 times greater than those who quit.

Other cardiovascular effects.   These effects of smoking include aortic aneurysms, peripheral arterial disease with leg pain when walking, shorter survival after arterial grafts are placed, and increased incidence of cerebral vascular disease, including stroke.

The risk of cerebral vascular disease is directly related to the intensity of smoking, up to 5.7 times greater in heavy smokers. Lower but still significant risks have been reported in former smokers as well as in those who live with smokers.

Smoking temporarily increases blood pressure but probably isn't responsible for sustained hypertension. In the presence of hypertension, however, smoking may interfere with the effectiveness of some antihypertensive medications. It may also be associated with an acceleration of the hypertension and with stroke.

Cancer of Other Organs. Cancers of the larynx, oral cavity, esophagus, bladder, pancreas, and penis have all been related to potential and real carcinogens in cigarette smoke. Although the direct effects of smoking or smokeless tobacco are believed related to some cancers, notably lung, larynx, oral cavity, and esophagus, controversy exists as to whether this holds true for other cancers, such as cancer of the cervix.

Smokeless tobacco is associated with oral cancer and gum disease, with oral lesions seen in up to 37 percent of regular users in the seventh to twelfth grades.

Pregnancy. Women smokers of childbearing age are at particular risk during pregnancy. Possible complications include increased risk of miscarriage, low birth-weight babies, increased perinatal mortality, and sudden death syndrome in the newborn (Chapter 18).

Acute Nicotine Intoxication. Acute intoxication, a rare event, can cause nausea, vomiting, abdominal pain, diarrhea, lightheadedness, headache, confusion, weakness, and tremors. In more severe stages, the pulse may be weak and rapid, blood pressure quite low, and convulsions and respiratory failure can occur. Nicotine intoxication has been reported in tobacco harvesters who absorb excessive nicotine from the dew on tobacco leaves. Accidental poisoning by ingestion of nicotine-containing pesticides is another possibility. The condition is treated by inducing vomiting to remove gastric contents and, if needed, respiratory assistance and intravenous fluids.

Passive Smoking. Most Americans don't smoke, yet the amount of cigarette smoke in the environment is considerable. In one survey, almost two-thirds of nonsmokers reported some daily exposure to cigarette smoke; 16 percent said they were exposed for a minimum of 40 hours each week. Equally important was the observation that

70 percent of children have at least one parent or immediate family member who smokes.

Most passive-smoking exposure is to sidestream smoke. It contains a greater concentration of carbon monoxide than mainstream smoke, and smaller particles that are more likely to reach the smallest and most distant portions of the lungs.

In 1986, the nineteenth surgeon general's Advisory Committee on the Health Consequences of Smoking concluded that passive smoking can cause disease in healthy nonsmokers. The most common and least severe are unpleasant odor, headaches, eye irritations, and such respiratory effects as cough and bronchitis in people who are particularly sensitive. Whether these discomforts can result in chronic disabilities is not yet clear.

More serious effects of passive smoking exist. One review of the world's literature on the consequences of smoking to healthy adults notes that an estimated 2,500 to 8,400 deaths from lung cancer in the United States may be attributed to environmental tobacco smoke. A majority of 18 published epidemiologic studies found passive smoking posed an increased risk for lung cancer. But because of differences in the populations examined and in the way the studies were designed, more and better studies are needed before the risk relationship between involuntary smoking and lung cancer can be quantified. The relationship between environmental smoke and cardiovascular disorders has also been studied, but the results are inconclusive.

Children. Compared with children of nonsmokers, children of parents who smoke appear to have an increased frequency of respiratory and middle ear infections. There is also an increase in hospitalizations for bronchitis and pneumonia in the first year of life. The rate of lung-function development is also slightly lower. In addition, a child whose mother smokes may run twice the risk of developing acute, upper-respiratory infections.

TREATMENT

Despite the overwhelming evidence of smoking's dangers, in 1986, 24 percent of smokers were not concerned about the effects of smoking, with up to 30 percent of them saying that smoking did not increase the risk of either lung or heart disease. Only 18 percent of smokers were highly concerned over the effects of smoking on their own health.

Even when the hazards of smoking are recognized, quitting isn't easy. Over a 12-month period ending in 1986, 70 percent of current smokers said that they'd made at least one attempt to quit during their smoking careers; one-third had stopped for at least a day that year. In 1987, 45 percent of all adults who had ever smoked had quit. Remaining abstinent, however, is not easy.

The most common ways of treating tobacco dependency are simple detoxification (cutting down until the habit is eliminated), nicotine gum or nasal spray, behavioral therapy, psychological counseling, and hypnosis. Formal smoking-cessation programs have also been shown to be helpful. Combining two or more of those methods has helped many people. However, more than 90 percent of smokers who quit do so without formal therapy. Fewer people who try to quit on their own remain abstinent on their first attempt. Under physician direction or encouragement, however, the success rate is higher. One survey reported that attempts to quit were twice as likely to occur among those smokers who received encouragement from their physician to stop than among those who did not. Those smokers who quit "cold turkey" were found to be more likely to be successful than those who attempt to detoxify, as were those who quit on their own. However, since heavy smokers and smokers who had been previously unsuccessful in quitting are more likely to join cessation programs, a valid comparison is not easily made.

Nicotine Preparations.   Nicotine gum, which contains approximately two milligrams of nicotine, is a valuable adjunct when stopping the smoking habit. According to some professionals, nicotine gum works best when used in conjunction with a counseling program, and is taken for three to six months after smoking stops. The gum should not be used to help decrease the number of cigarettes smoked, since a high level of blood nicotine can result. Nor should it be used until smoking has completely stopped. The nicotine is absorbed in the mouth rather than the stomach, so the gum should be chewed slowly for 20 to 30 minutes. Usually 10–15 pieces of the gum per day are chewed.

When the gum is chewed throughout the day, average nicotine levels are approximately one- to two-thirds of those seen with smoking. Some studies have recommended four-milligram gum, but increased effectiveness has not been demonstrated.

Long-term use may be associated with dependency. It is estimated that up to one-third of those who use the gum continue for more than a year, despite advice to the contrary.

To date, success rates with the gum have not been clearly documented. In smoking-cessation programs, 27 percent of the gum users stay off cigarettes, whereas only 18 percent of those given placebos manage to do so. Among those who are treated by medical practitioners, the percentages are 9 percent and 4 percent respectively. From those numbers, it appears that the gum is fairly helpful in promoting abstinence when used in special centers with appropriate counseling, but not nearly so successful in general medical practice.

Nicotine gum should not be used by those with coronary heart disease, especially after a recent heart attack. Pregnant women and people with tempromandibular joint disorder also should avoid it. The gum should be used cautiously in people suffering from peptic ulcer disease and hypertension.

Adverse effects of nicotine gum include nonspecific gastrointestinal symptoms, palpitations, sore throat or mouth, and occasional hiccups. Although acute nicotine intoxication is a possibility, nicotine's slow release in the stomach, and its local metabolism, make that unlikely unless extremely large amounts are consumed.

Other products include nicotine skin patches and nicotine nasal spray, both still in need of evaluation.

Other Pharmacologic Approaches. Researchers have recently reported that clonidine (Catapres), an antihypertensive drug, has been useful for smokers undergoing withdrawal. The success rate with clonidine appears to be twice that of a placebo: 64 percent of patients given the drug versus 29 percent of patients given a placebo stopped smoking in four weeks. The drug was found more effective in women (72 versus 15 percent) than in men (47 versus 50 percent).

People with a history of depression also had higher success rates.

After six months, only 27 percent of those on clonidine and 5 percent of those on placebos remained abstinent. Among clonidine's advantages is its ability to reduce smoking without perpetuating nicotine dependency, as nicotine gum can. But side effects, notably lowered blood pressure, limited clonidine's use in narcotic withdrawal (Chapter 11).

Mecamylamine (Inversine), a receptor antagonist that is also used to treat hypertension, lessens the satisfaction of cigarette smoking. In short-term trials, however, subjects smoked more cigarettes to try to overcome the blocking effect of the drug. It also may have many side effects.

Chapter 15

Volatile Solvents, Inhalants, Anesthetics

The use of inhalants to alter mood can be traced back to the mythology of ancient Greece. At Delphi, the Pythoness—the priestess of Apollo—sat on a tripod above the cliffs, inhaling cold vapors containing carbon dioxide. This aid to meditation was soon followed by divine inspiration. Inhalation of volatile, organic solvents, however, is a relatively recent phenomenon related to our high-tech society. It wasn't noted in the medical literature and the media until 1959. The practice became widespread from then until the 1970s, when it began to decline.

Substances that are inhaled can be grouped into four general categories:

- volatile solvents in antifreeze, gasoline, glue, hairspray, lighter fuel, and paint thinner
- volatile solvents in aerosols such as paint spray and deodorants
- general anesthetic agents including methylene chloride, trichlorethylene, tetrachloroethylene, and nitrous oxide
- volatile nitrites such as in the amylbutyl and isobutyl groups

VOLATILE SOLVENTS

Inappropriate use of volatile solvents originated with the inhalation of gasoline fumes. Airplane glue and aerosol were used next. Indeed, many substances found in hundreds of commercial products can be misused and produce mood-altering effects (Table 15.1).

Table 15-1
Volatile Solvents

Solvent	Ingredients
Adhesives	n-heptane, n-hexane, benzene, naphthalene, toluene, xylene
Aerosol sprays	Ethanol, freon, toluene, xylene
Antifreeze	Isopropanol, methanol
Degreasers	Isopropanol, methylene chloride, tetrachloroethylene, xylene, n-butyl acetate, methyl ethyl ketone, n-heptane, n-hexane, benzene, naphthalene, toluene, xylene
Gasoline	
Model cement	Ethanol, isopropanol, n-hexene, styrene, toluene, xylene, acetone
Paint thinners	Ethanol, isopropanol, methanol, n-heptane, n-hexane, methylene chloride, naphthalene, toluene, xylene, ethyl acetate, n-propylacetate, acetone, methylbutyl, ketone, methyl ethyl ketone
Rubber cement	n-heptane, n-hexane, benzene, naphthalene, styrene, toluene, xylene
Spray shoe polish	Isopropanol, toluene
Typewriter correction fluid	Trichloroethylene
Window washing fluids	Methanol

*Source: The Deliberate Inhalation of Volatile Substances, Report Series 30, No. 2 (NIDA, Rockville, Md., 1978).

Patterns of Use. Inhalant users can be grouped into four major categories: inhalant-dependent adults who usually use a volatile anesthetic agent, organic nitrite users, multiple drug users, and young inhalant users.

Surveys suggest that inhalants have been used at one time by 10 percent of youngsters between the ages of 12 and 17, by 17 percent of people between 18 and 25, and by 4 percent of those age 26 or more. Those figures may vary greatly depending on the population studied, specific availabilities of inhalants, and cultural norms. Since inhalant use is primarily a phenomenon among youth, the data provided by the surveys of drug use among high school students and young adults have been most helpful.

Annual inhalant use in high school seniors rose from 3 percent in 1976 to 5 percent in 1979, then declined. It started to rise again in the early 1980s, in part due to use of amyl and butyl nitrites, and reached 7 percent in 1988. The use of inhalants within one month of the summary that year was reported at 2.6 percent of adolescents.

The popularity of solvent use among young people is easy to understand. Its availability and low cost make it readily obtainable; the small containers can be hidden easily or left in such appropriate places as a closet or garage; possession is legal; and the high is achieved within a few minutes, is more pleasant than an alcohol high, and is usually over much more quickly.

Use may be sporadic and ultimately come to a halt because of unexpected or unpleasant effects. Repetitive or daily use poses the greatest risk for toxicity and psychological dysfunction. Chronic use of inhalants is seen mostly in lower socioeconomic groups, since it's the least costly way to become high.

Dependency, Tolerance, and Addiction. Although tolerance does develop, physical dependency has not been clearly defined. Symptoms of irritability and anxiety, which can appear during abstinence, may be related to preexisting personality disturbances rather than to withdrawal. Habituation, however, is fairly common.

Complications. Complications, even in healthy youngsters, do occur and are sometimes fatal (Table 15.2). Minutes after inhaling,

TABLE 15.2
Complications from Use of Solvents

Anemia

Bleeding from stomach

Chronic brain dysfunction

Coma, convulsions

Difficulty in walking

Hallucinations

Leukemia

Liver failure

Lung disease

Muscle damage

Nausea, vomiting

Neurologic damage

Night tremors

Paralysis

Renal failure

a person will become disoriented and exhilarated. When these solvents combine with body fats, they can be particularly toxic to tissues containing a high lipid concentration, such as the brain and spinal cord. The effects of many of these agents are similar to those from central nervous system depressants.

Acute toxic effects.   The initial high can be complicated by nausea, vomiting, sneezing, nosebleeds, coughing, salivation, and, on occasion, loss of coordination. Depression of the central nervous system follows the high. Loss of consciousness and respiratory arrest can occur with large doses. There's also risk of brain damage. Cardiac arrest, resulting from the production of fatal heart rhythm abnormalities, is common. Sudden sniffing death syndrome (SSD) is also associated with aerosol inhalation. Fluorocarbons in the aerosol can sensitize the heart to epinephrine, leading to this fatal rhythm disturbance (Table 15.3).

At lower levels of intoxication, there can be a general loss of inhibitions, with subsequent impulsive behavior. Muscular coordination is diminished, and reflexes are depressed.

Chronic effects. Other effects of volatile substances depend on which substance is used and how it's taken. These effects (Table 15.4) vary from an innocuous lowering of the blood count to severe depression of bone marrow, progressive neurologic dysfunction and paralysis, failure of the kidneys and liver, and even leukemia. Pulmonary function is also altered, sometimes without symptoms.

Treatment. The incidence of volatile dependency is quite low, and the medical complications rare. So there's little experience in dealing with large numbers of those who are dependent. Since most users are young, family support is essential; counseling and therapy are generally helpful.

ANESTHETIC AGENTS

Ether, chloroform, and nitrous oxide were first used because they produced a high, rather than for their anesthetic properties.

The use of ether for recreational purposes began as early as the 1790s and was prevalent in England when the government increased the tax on alcohol. It was first taken orally; one teaspoon could produce inebriation lasting 30 minutes to an hour. Inhalation was common in a number of prestigious medical institutions in the eighteenth century.

Chloroform came into use somewhat later in Europe and the United States. It was first used in 1849 as an anesthetic for childbirth. Because of their toxic effects on the liver and kidneys, both ether and chloroform were gradually replaced by newer, less harmful anesthetics.

TABLE 15.3
Causes of Sudden Death from Sniffing

Respiratory depression

Fatal irregular cardiac rhythms

Metabolic abnormalities

Nitrous oxide. Nitrous oxide has been used as an anesthetic since 1845 and is now commonly used as an adjunct to local anesthesia in dental procedures. By 1976 it was again being used to produce a high. Within 30 seconds nitrous oxide can produce an effect that lasts for several minutes. Because it has low potential for tolerance and doesn't produce a hangover, it was advocated as a good substitute for alcohol, especially when tolerance to alcohol existed.

When used appropriately as an analgesic, nitrous oxide offers rapid onset of action, rapid recovery from effects, and minimal risk of toxicity. A 20 percent concentration of nitrous oxide can provide the same degree of analgesia as morphine. Inhalation of a 30 percent concentration, however, can sometimes cause loss of consciousness. An 80 percent concentration virtually always causes loss of consciousness, and death from coma and brain damage can result from the lack of oxygen.

Nitrous oxide is easily obtained in aerosol cans and as a propellant in small metal tubes (whippets). It's usually used by direct inhalation or from a balloon filled with the gas. Although excessive use of nitrous oxide has not been well documented, its ready availability to dentists and dental assistants has made it a particular risk among those professionals.

Nitrous oxide has relatively few physical effects on the body, although there may be an increase in blood pressure and heart rate. When taken in low doses, it has no known toxic effects on the central nervous system or other organs. Because onset of action and recovery are both fairly rapid, one can inhale nitrous oxide for short periods and function well afterward. The high is described as "floating sensations" and may be accompanied by visual hallucinations.

TABLE 15.4
Toxic Effects of Solvent Use

Substance	Anemia	Leukemia	Cardiac Complications	Kidney Failure	Liver Failure	Neurologic Changes	Gastrointestinal Changes
Benzene	+	+	+		+		+
Carbon tetrachloride	+					+	+
Gasoline	+					+	+
Hexane	+					+	+
Trichlorethylene			+	+	+	+	
Toluene	+		+	+		+	
Ketones						+	
Xylene	+					+	

+ = positive correlation

Tolerance has occurred with chronic use. Dependency and withdrawal similar to that of morphine can be easily measured in laboratory animals. Morphine can decrease signs of withdrawal from nitrous oxide in these animals. The relationship between nitrous oxide and the opiates is still unclear. Occasional reports in the medical literature suggest that nitrous oxide is effective in detoxification from opiates and in treating withdrawal. But whenever a mood-altering drug with known potential for inappropriate use is recommended for the treatment of another dependency, it should be viewed with caution.

Chronic use of nitrous oxide is associated with several complications (Table 15.5). Memory loss, depression, and occasional hallucinations are the most common. Those changes improve with time and subside with abstinence. Such neurologic changes as numbness in the hands and feet, tingling sensations, loss in finger dexterity, and other findings compatible with degeneration may also occur.

THE ORGANIC NITRITES

Amyl nitrite, a highly volatile substance, was used as early as 1867 to relieve pain stemming from coronary artery obstruction (angina pectoris). It served as the primary drug for angina until nitroglycerine was found to be more effective. A similar drug, butyl nitrite, has been around since the 1880s but was never used in angina. Because it was considered safe, the FDA in 1960 ruled that it was unnecessary to have a prescription in order to obtain amyl nitrite. By 1986, street use of the drug was so widespread that the decision was reversed. Butyl nitrite, often used in room deodorizers, under no such restrictions, quickly replaced amyl nitrite as a more readily available drug of use.

Amyl nitrite, isobutyl nitrite, and isopentyl nitrite (Table 15.6) are alleged to provide a general high, increase creativity and artistic ability, and enhance the male orgasmic response. Among amyl nitrite's alleged effects on sexual function are prolonged and heightened erections, relaxation of smooth muscle tone of the rectal and anal areas, and prevention of premature ejaculation.

TABLE 15.5
Toxic Effects of Nitrous Oxide

Memory loss

Visual hallucinations

Tingling and numbness of hands and feet

Loss of finger dexterity

Weakness of muscles

Bowel and bladder symptoms

Disturbances of immune function

Patterns of Use.   The nitrites are generally used later in life than other mood-altering drugs, and often in combination with other agents. The average age for first use of nitrites is 25.6 years, compared with 13.9 years for alcohol, 14.6 years for glue, and 17.6 years for marijuana. But studies in 1986 revealed that about 9 percent of 3,000 high school seniors had at some time used amyl nitrite, with 1.6 percent having used it within three days of the surveys. A household survey of 12- to 17-year-olds found that 9 percent had used these drugs, and that 4 percent were current users. A large survey of 1.3 million students in the seventh to twelfth grades in New York State revealed that 6 percent had used these drugs at least once, 3 percent were current users, and 1 percent had used them at least 10 times.

Although the proportion of adolescents using nitrites is small, the 1 percent of extensive users in the survey equals 9,000 students. The 1988 National High School Survey found that one in 30 high school seniors (3.2 percent) had tried these drugs at some time.

The incidence of nitrite use is much higher in specific high-risk groups. A study of chemically dependent adolescents revealed that 43 percent had used nitrites, and 22 percent had used them 10 to 99 times—compared to a prevalence of 11 percent in adult polydrug

TABLE 15.6
Nitrite Inhalants

Inhalant	Street Names*
Amyl nitrite	Poppers, Snappers
Isobutyl nitrite	Banapple Gas, Bang, Bolt, Bullet, Climax, Crypt, Cum, Hard-on, Hardware, Highball
Isobutyl alcohol	Aroma, Joc, Kick, Liquid Increase, Locker Room
Isopentyl nitrite	Locker, Popper, Rush, Satan's Scout, Toilet Water, Vaporole

*Because commercial preparations may not contain a single nitrite, the street terminology is interchangeable.

users. Seventy percent of homosexual men said they used nitrites before they became concerned about the AIDS epidemic.

Adverse Effects. Smooth muscles relax after inhalation of nitrites, causing drop in blood pressure; increase in heart rate, accompanied by feelings of warmth; throbbing sensation or headache; and occasional symptoms related to heat loss. Depending on the dose, dizziness, fainting, and severe decrease in blood pressure may occur. Both the high and the headaches are probably related to widening of the blood vessels in the brain. Dilated blood vessels in the penis can cause increased engorgement and a prolonged erection.

As with any inhalant, lung irritation and acute allergic reactions are common. Contact with the skin can result in severe irritation and ulceration. When nitrites are combined with hemoglobin in the bloodstream, the oxygen-carrying capacity of the blood is impaired and there may be a profound loss of oxygen. Increases in pressure behind the eyes, accompanied by severe eye pain, have also been reported.

The effects of nitrites on the immune system have taken on greater importance as the complications of AIDS have become more familiar (Chapter 17). No immunotoxic effects have been seen in laboratory animals after administration of amyl nitrite. But there has been a decrease in the cells believed to ward off infections (helper T-cells) after 21 weeks of exposure. The same pattern is often seen in those at high risk for developing AIDS. When given amyl nitrite, volunteers who were negative for HIV showed no specific changes in immune function. However, acute use of amyl nitrite was associated with a decrease in blood lymphocytes and other protective elements. All returned to normal within 24 to 96 hours after discontinuing the drug. Whether this has any clinical relevance to increasing vulnerability to AIDS is uncertain. But use of nitrites by people with compromised immune systems should be avoided.

Nitrites used in combination with naturally occurring nitrogen compounds can form nitrosamines, among the most potent cancer-causing agents (carcinogens) known.

PART III

AREAS OF
SPECIAL CONCERN

Chapter 16

Multiple Drug Use

Dependency on a single drug is more the exception than the rule; multiple drug use has increased significantly since the late 1960s.

Several patterns of multiple drug use can be identified (Table 16.1). Probably the most common pattern is typified by the user of alcohol who also uses marijuana and other stimulant or depressant drugs. Another pattern results from unavailability of the primary drug, typical with regard to alcohol and other central nervous system depressants. Tranquilizers, barbiturates, or other sedatives are easily substituted for alcohol; heroin addicts who can't afford heroin may turn to such opiates as hydromorphone (Dilaudid), meperidine (Demerol), or street methadone. Multiple drugs are sometimes used to mask dependency to a person's primary drug. Alcoholics, for example, may take tranquilizers during the working day to maintain their equilibrium without smelling of alcohol. Other drugs are also used to prevent withdrawal when the primary drug is unavailable. Heroin addicts often drink excessive quantities of alcohol or take barbiturates or tranquilizers when they can't get heroin.

Certain drugs are also used to counteract particular effects of the primary drug (Table 16.2). One example is use of central nervous system depressants by cocaine or amphetamine users to terminate runs, or to decrease the stimulant effects. It's also common to mix cocaine or amphetamines with heroin to lessen the drowsiness caused by heroin.

Other drugs are often taken to enhance the effects of the primary drug. Marijuana in combination with alcohol contributes to a high, as does mixing antidepressants, tranquilizers, or other central nervous system depressants.

TABLE 16.1
Patterns of Multiple Drug Use

To maintain initial "social" drug-use behavior while progressing to illicit drugs

To substitute when primary drug isn't available

To mask signs of dependency on primary drug

To prevent withdrawal when primary drug isn't available

To diminish undesirable side effects of primary drug

To enhance effect of primary drug

To obtain a different kind of high (part of underlying psychopathology to consume whatever is available)

Other combinations produce highs totally different from those of the primary drug. Heroin addicts, or people on methadone maintenance, frequently consume excessive quantities of alcohol or central nervous system depressants to obtain a "depressant high," or use cocaine for its stimulant effect. Those on methadone maintenance who can't get high on an opiate often turn to cocaine, alcohol, other central nervous system depressants, and even antidepressants.

In a few people, multiple drug use represents an underlying psychopathology demonstrated by a need to use any drug that produces a mood-altering effect. Such experimentation is fairly common in adolescents, but adults who adopt this behavior are usually the most difficult to treat.

Many combinations of drugs are known (Table 16.2), but some are rarely used because they produce inferior highs and severe psychological side effects. The high obtained with heroin (introversion), for example, is very different from the high from LSD (mind-blowing). The combination results in hallucinations and paranoia, so most multiple drug users avoid it. Other combinations, however, have equally serious—but less recognized—effects.

ALCOHOL AND OTHER DRUGS

Most future drug users try alcohol or cigarettes as their first mood-altering drugs. Marijuana and other available drugs often follow. Susceptible people may then go on to sedatives, cocaine, or opiates, with alcohol use continuing throughout this period.

A 1988 National Household Survey reported 13 percent of the population (26 million people) to have used alcohol in combination with other mood-altering drugs. Alcohol and marijuana were the most common combination, with alcohol combined with a nonmedically prescribed psychotherapeutic drug second. Alcohol consumption in those with a history of drug dependency is much higher—approximately 50 to 60 percent. Other surveys show that up to 60 percent of those using alcohol excessively have a co-existing drug problem. They are generally the younger members of the population.

One study of United States servicemen stationed in Vietnam revealed the ease of exchanging alcohol and other drug consumption. Before enlistment, half the men were regular drinkers, another 25 percent had experienced some drinking problem, and still another 4 percent were classified as alcoholics. In Vietnam, alcohol consumption decreased significantly in 75 percent of the men. But that was accompanied by an increase in the use of opiates. Half said they had tried opiates, and 20 percent were opiate-dependent. In the post-Vietnam era, opiate use decreased; alcohol use increased. Thirty-three percent of the men became problem drinkers; 8 percent were considered alcoholic.

Alcohol is the drug most often involved in multiple drug use because it can be combined with other central nervous system depressants, such as barbiturates and tranquilizers, to potentiate a high or mask an alcohol problem. The combination also prevents withdrawal symptoms and facilitates sleep following alcoholic binges. Alcohol and sleeping pills form a particularly dangerous mixture because the combined depressant effect on the brain can result in overdose.

Narcotic (opiate) addicts often use alcohol and other central nervous system depressants to enhance a high or minimize withdrawal. One 1985 study showed that 41 percent of drug-related deaths in men

TABLE 16.2
Common Drug Combinations

Drug	Reason for Use	Adverse Effects
Alcohol, barbiturates, sedatives, tranquilizers	Potentiate high; prevent withdrawal; facilitate sleep following drinking binge	Depressed brain and respiratory function
Alcohol, heroin, methadone, barbiturates, sedatives, tranquilizers	Diminish narcotic withdrawal symptoms; add to narcotic high; get high when on methadone maintenance	Depressed brain and respiratory function
Alcohol, marijuana	Intensify high	Rapid heart rate; increased impaired behavior
Talwin, antihistamine	Make injection smoother; diminish irritation of veins	As with each drug
Heroin, methadone, cocaine, amphetamines	Get different type high; decrease period of drowsiness caused by heroin	Rapid heart rate; possible heart damage
Alcohol-cocaine	Get different highs (social settings)	As with each drug

Cocaine, amphetamines, barbiturates, tranquilizers	Diminish runs; facilitate sleep	As with each drug
Hallucinogens, amphetamines	Increased intensity of trip	Marked paranoia; self-injury
Marijuana-phencyclidine	Intensify high (user may be unaware)	Marked stimulation with hallucinations

were related to combinations of alcohol and other drugs. Other studies show that up to 50 percent of deaths stemming from acute fatal reactions to heroin involved alcohol.

Patients on methadone maintenance may take alcohol and tranquilizers to get high (Chapter 11). Alcohol and tranquilizers are in a different group from narcotics but are still central nervous system depressants. So the added depressant effect when taken together can cause coma and death. In almost all cases of overdose in patients on methadone, the responsible agent is either alcohol alone or in combination with minor tranquilizers—not the opiate.

Cocaine and alcohol are another frequent combination. Alcohol reduces inhibitions, so it facilitates cocaine use and intensifies the high. One study from Harvard Medical School found that 85 percent of cocaine addicts were problem drinkers. A nationwide survey of patients entering treatment programs found that 80 percent reported using cocaine in the preceding months along with alcohol. It is estimated that 12 million people will use both drugs in combination in a year.

The alcohol and cocaine combination affects liver function since it is well established that alcohol has a toxic effect on the liver. In addition, some cocaine-related deaths have been linked to massive liver damage. In one animal study, mice who were on a diet of alcohol were given a single dose of cocaine. Thirty percent died of severe liver damage. No serious adverse effects were seen in animals given either alcohol or cocaine alone.

A direct jump from mouse to human can't be made, but it's reasonable to suspect that the same toxic reaction would occur in people. The diagnosis might be difficult because liver damage from cocaine takes considerable time to develop.

Other potential toxic effects can occur as a result of using both cocaine and alcohol. Combined use stimulates the cardiovascular system more than either drug alone, so people with heart problems are at much greater risk. The combination of drugs may act synergistically to produce adverse effects on the brain and, if used heavily, can cause seizures.

Alcohol, of course, can't be considered a "cause" of drug use, but those who don't drink are less likely to take drugs. Drug users drink—and get drunk—more often than nondrug users. Alcohol is frequently used with other mood-altering drugs, in combinations that can potentiate the risks of alcohol alone. Such risks include accidents when driving or performing other tasks requiring muscular coordination, and antisocial behavior, including criminal acts. Pregnant women face increased risk of fetal death, complicated deliveries, and birth deformities (Chapter 18). Whereas minimal alcohol consumption may carry low risk, combining alcohol with other mood-altering drugs carries a very high-risk burden.

SMOKING AND DRUG USE

Use of some mood-altering drugs is strongly associated with smoking. One of the strongest associations is smoking and drinking, with smoking rates in excessive drinkers reported as high as 90 percent.

Cigarette use is rarely addressed in dealing with dependency on mood-altering drugs because the immediate adverse effects of the other drugs are considered far more severe and therefore deserve the full attention of patient and staff. Trying to get rid of two dependencies can dilute the effort to eliminate use of the primary drug. In addition, experiencing the intense pleasure and stress-alleviating effects of smoking while trying to abstain from alcohol, opiates, or cocaine goes a long way toward preventing a rapid return to use of the primary drug.

In a survey of smokers also dependent on alcohol or other drugs, 75 percent reported that cigarettes would be at least as difficult to give up as their primary drug. Studies dealing with smoking cessation report an extremely low success rate over two years following treatment.

Most staff in alcohol and drug treatment facilities are unskilled in smoking-cessation techniques and often have few resources to establish such programs. Only limited evidence exists that quitting smoking helps to maintain abstinence from other drugs, and it deals mainly with smoking and drinking. The studies found that those who quit smoking were more likely to maintain abstinence from alcohol than those who continued to smoke.

OPIATES

Heroin is frequently injected along with cocaine and amphetamines to provide an initial rush and lessen the time of drowsiness. Because former heroin addicts generally inject cocaine, the risk of contracting AIDS continues unabated, even though they're no longer injecting heroin.

People on methadone maintenance often use cocaine, as well as alcohol, since they can't get high from heroin or other narcotics. The combination of heroin (or methadone) and other central nervous system depressants such as diazepam (Valium) is also common. The combination is one of the more frequent causes of overdose among those on methadone maintenance. In the laboratory, diazepam can cut in half the amount of methadone required for an animal to overdose.

Amitriptyline (Elavil) also is often used inappropriately by those dependent on opiates. That can cause a particular problem because heroin dependency is frequently accompanied by depression, which can be relieved with amitriptyline. However, inappropriate use can produce a high independent of the antidepressant effect.

Such opiates as paregoric, tripelennamine (Blue Velvet), the opiate agonist-antagonist petazocine (Talwin), and tripelennamine (Ts and Blues) are also combined with other drugs.

COCAINE

Cocaine and central nervous system depressants are commonly used together to end "runs" and induce sleep in the presence of insomnia and exhaustion.

Injecting cocaine while smoking marijuana is another phenomenon. One study found that using both these drugs together markedly increases heart rate, a serious problem in someone with coronary heart disease.

MARIJUANA

Next to alcohol, and perhaps cigarettes, marijuana is the drug most often associated with multiple drug use. The overwhelming majority of marijuana smokers, however, don't use other mood-altering drugs, except for alcohol.

At times, marijuana users unknowingly take PCP, which has been mixed into marijuana cigarettes. The result may be a high degree of stimulation, hallucinations, and bizarre behavior not usually related to marijuana. Since the user doesn't expect such effects, they can be disturbing. Aftereffects may persist once the acute effects subside.

TREATMENT

When it comes to treatment, the multiple drug user presents many seemingly insurmountable problems. Most well-known treatment strategies are oriented toward a specific substance. Those patients with a second dependency may meet resistance from staff members, who are unable to manage a dual dependency. Worse yet, because many staff members take a strong position on primary treatment objectives in their own areas of expertise, they may even have difficulty agreeing where to refer people with dual dependencies.

Facilities funded to treat alcoholics aren't eager to treat patients also addicted to heroin. Primary, or "pure," alcoholics are viewed as passive-aggressive, depressed people who are contrite and have strong motivation to succeed in therapy. Heroin addicts are viewed as manipulative, aggressive, and demanding—therefore capable of destroying the successful inpatient alcohol program milieu.

Facilities focused on heroin dependency (methadone maintenance) are often ill-equipped to manage the alcoholic. Abstinence programs such as Alcoholics Anonymous (AA), which have successful track records, often won't accept alcoholics who are on methadone. Many facilities insist that a person discontinue methadone before being treated for alcoholism. That presents an untenable problem, both for the person and, ultimately, society. Return to heroin use when methadone is prematurely terminated has run as high as 80 percent; excessive drinking on maintenance programs up to 50 percent. Many AA units are now recognizing this problem and are accepting persons on methadone maintenance who have drinking problems.

Cocaine use in heroin addicts, or those on maintenance therapy, presents still different problems, particularly when antisocial personality traits exist. People in this situation need a highly structured setting during treatment, not always possible when funds are limited.

Programs (mostly residential facilities) that treat multiple drug users are in short supply. The attrition rate is also fairly high because these patients tend not to accept an inpatient facility for prolonged periods. Even time-limited, inpatient facilities are expensive, and treatment is often inadequately covered by insurance.

The situation isn't hopeless; much can be done to provide effective treatment for multiple users. Some steps require little additional funding but much greater flexibility. Others clearly require a funding initiative or recognition by third-party carriers that the medical and psychological problems of multiple drug use should be covered by insurance.

Suggested changes include:

- admission by alcohol treatment facilities of patients who are on maintenance or other prescription drug therapy
- recognition by single-dependency treatment facilities that resources must be developed to manage ''secondary'' dependencies
- provision of sufficient funding for federal- or state-run programs to offer adequate resources for treating multiple drug use
- open communication between facilities providing different forms of treatment
- increased coverage by insurers to pay for outpatient as well as short-term inpatient therapy
- establishment of effective monitoring systems to evaluate treatments and chances for successful rehabilitation

Chapter 17

AIDS and Drug Use

More than 150,000 cases of AIDS were reported in the United States from June 1981 through September 1990, with more than 92,000 deaths. The Public Health Service estimates that as many as 480,000 cases will have been diagnosed by the end of 1992. According to other estimates, as of 1989, between 1 million and 1.5 million people in the United States had been infected with HIV (Human Immunodeficiency Virus), the cause of AIDS. Although there are several high risk groups associated with AIDS, intravenous drug use is implicated in 26 percent of reported cases.

HIV progressively destroys the immune system of the body, resulting in increased susceptibility to a wide variety of infections and several rare cancers, all of which can be fatal. As AIDS develops, it's also accompanied by severe mental deterioration and widespread wasting of the body. First identified in Africa as Slim Disease, AIDS began to be seen in the United States in 1981.

HIV: THE HUMAN IMMUNODEFICIENCY VIRUS

AIDS is caused by the human immunodeficiency virus (HIV), one of the lentiviruses in the retrovirus group. The HIV contains RNA (ribonucleic acid), the messenger of genetic information from DNA (deoxyribonucleic acid) to the protein-forming system of the cells.

As a retrovirus, HIV has a special enzyme (reverse transcriptase) that allows it to reverse the normal flow of genetic information from DNA to RNA to protein molecules. Thus HIV's own genes are incorporated into the genetic makeup of normal cells. The viral DNA

TABLE 17.1
Cases of Adult/Adolescent AIDS
by Exposure Categories Through September 1990

Single Mode of Exposure	Number of Cases	Percentage of Overall Cases
Male homosexual/bisexual contact	85,613	57
Intravenous (IV) drug use	27,662	19
Hemophilia/coagulation disorder	814	1
Heterosexual Contact	7,414	5
Recipient of Transfusion	3,512	2
Other/Undetermined	5,408	3
Multiple Modes of Exposure Related to IV Drug Use	10,279	7
Other	8,796	6

Source: HIV/AIDS Surveillance Centers for Disease Control, U.S. Department of Health and Human Services, Atlanta, October 1990.

then merges with the person's gene pool and remains latent until activated to make new virus particles.

Up to 1983, the HIV group hadn't been identified as a cause of disease in humans. That has led some investigators to speculate that the virus had evolved from SIV, simian immunodeficiency virus, a retrovirus that causes fatal infection in monkeys and apes.

The HIV comprises two types. HIV-1, responsible for AIDS, since its isolation in 1983 has been identified in the United States and throughout the world. HIV-2, first isolated in 1985, has been detected primarily in West Africa and in some AIDS patients in both Central Africa and Europe. The illness associated with Type 2 is often indistinguishable from that of Type 1. Even though HIV-2 is uncommon in the United States, those who appear ill with AIDS but test negative for the HIV Type 1 antibody should also be tested for HIV-2 infection.

HIV has been isolated from many body secretions in both men and women: blood, urine, semen, saliva, tears, breast milk, amniotic fluid, and genital secretions of women. HIV has been detected in those clinically ill with AIDS, as well as in those who have been exposed to the virus but show no symptoms.

Infection of the immune system by HIV results in destruction of white blood cells (T lymphocytes), which usually play a major role in stimulating the immune system. T lymphocytes consist of helper cells (T4) and suppressor cells (T8). Both groups of cells actively fight infection, and each group has a role in controlling the other group's function. As HIV infections develop, and clinical signs of early AIDS appear, many of the helper cells die, thus creating an inverse ratio between helper and suppressor cells. The remaining helper cells often function defectively, leaving the body susceptible to infections.

Some of the infections contracted by HIV-infected people are called opportunistic because they rarely occur in those with normal immune systems. The most common is pneumocystis carinii (PCC), a severe pneumonia, which until the late 1980s was almost uniformly fatal.

People with AIDS are susceptible to a whole range of severe bacterial, fungal, and viral infections. These include various pneumonias and infections of heart valves, membranes surrounding the brain and spinal cord, the skin, and the gastrointestinal tract. The most common cancer in AIDS patients is Kaposi's sarcoma, but tumors of the lymphatic system are also common. Mental deterioration (AIDS dementia), consisting of memory loss and decreased ability to concentrate, also can occur. Decreased strength in leg muscles and difficulty walking are other manifestations of the disease.

HIV Testing.   HIV antibodies in the bloodstream can be readily detected. A positive result on initial screening (ELISA), confirmed by a more specific method (Western Blot), provides a highly reliable indication of HIV infection. But false positives occur, especially when large numbers of people in low-risk groups are tested. The incidence of false positives in such groups may be as high as 175 per 100,000. A review of these screening tests by the Centers for Disease Control in 1989 found the accuracy rate to be 98.5 percent for ELISA and 91.6 percent for Western Blot.

In a high-risk group, however, a negative test doesn't eliminate the possibility of HIV infection. False negatives can occur if:

- an individual hasn't yet developed antibodies to HIV
- loss of antibodies occurs subsequent to infection while the virus remains (quite rare)
- antibody formation is delayed because of failure of the HIV to trigger the immune system
- the very rare HIV-2 infection is present

As more experience is gained in testing, and as more sensitive techniques are developed, accuracy in detection of HIV-1 may improve. Note that a positive test documents exposure to HIV, not the presence of AIDS. But it does indicate that the person is capable of transmitting the virus to others.

Testing for the HIV in intravenous drug users (IVDUs) is critical in helping to prevent transmission of the virus. Unfortunately, many of these people object to testing, believing they're already HIV-positive and will develop AIDS at some point no matter what they do. But even in areas of high HIV infection, 50 percent of IVDUs may be HIV-negative. By eliminating needle sharing and avoiding high-risk sexual behavior, they might never become infected. One study in a maintenance program found that all of those who remained negative on testing for HIV had stopped sharing needles.

An HIV Imitator: the Human T Lymphotropic Virus. The human T lymphotropic viruses, Type I (HTLV-I) and Type II (HTLV-II), are also retroviruses. Neither HTLV-I nor -II is related to HIV or to development of AIDS, and they usually aren't associated with suppression of the immune system. But HTLV-I has been identified in several groups at high risk for the HIV infection, including intravenous drug users and, to a lesser extent, those who have received multiple blood transfusions. HTLV-I is unusual in homosexuals, hemophiliacs, and sexually promiscuous heterosexuals.

Although not associated with AIDS, HTLV-I is connected with a rare form of cancer affecting the blood and lymph nodes, and with unusual degenerative neurologic diseases. Whether there is an exact cause-and-effect relationship remains to be determined. Screening tests for HTLV-I have been approved by the Food and Drug Administration. It's important to remember the difference between HTLV-I and HIV, which can exist independently of each other.

HIV Transmission: The Role of Intravenous Drug Use. HIV is transmitted through several routes, with a number of groups identified at high risk for HIV infection (Table 17.2). Sexual contact is a major path, with a positive relationship reported between infection and number of sexual partners. Anal-receptive intercourse appears to play a major role in transmission among both homosexuals and heterosexuals. But anal intercourse isn't essential for transmission. Sexual activity of any kind with an HIV-infected partner and without appropriate precautions can place one at risk.

The risk becomes greater as the number of sexual partners increases mainly because the chances for contact with an HIV-positive person increase. Among other risk-increasing factors are existence of a sexually transmitted disease and failure to use condoms. Condoms are particularly important; they decrease—but don't eliminate—risk of transmitting HIV and several other sexually transmitted diseases.

The proportion of nonintravenous drug-using heterosexuals who develop AIDS each year has remained relatively stable, approximately 4 percent of reported cases. But the actual number in this category has increased considerably, with almost all cases occurring in persons whose sexual partners are known to be at risk; 72 percent of such partners are intravenous drug users. Getting the virus through contaminated needles is, of course, a more common means of transmission.

Transfused blood contaminated with the virus is responsible for a high incidence of HIV in hemophiliacs. Blood, cellular components

---

TABLE 17.2
Groups at High Risk for HIV Infection

Gay and bisexual men

Intravenous drug users

Hemophiliacs

Heterosexual partners of HIV-infected
or recognized at-risk persons

Prostitutes

Children of HIV-infected mothers

---

of blood, and plasma clotting factors have all been means of transmitting HIV. This route has also been responsible for the development of AIDS in those who received blood transfusions before HIV was recognized and blood was regularly screened.

Prevalence of HIV intravenous drug users varies greatly between different geographic areas. In New York City, up to 61 percent of samples obtained in 1986 were positive, compared with 5 percent in Colorado, 2 percent in Texas, and 10 percent in Southern California.

Needle sharing among IVDUs is common practice everywhere. From 70 to 90 percent of such individuals share in up to half of injection episodes, making rapid spread of HIV possible. In part this is due to the fact that distributing sterile needles to IVDUs is illegal; in part it may be due to the desire to have a shared or common experience when shooting up. HIV infection among IVDUs is facilitated not just by needle sharing. The tendency for this group to engage in high-risk behavior either as a means of obtaining money to purchase drugs or as a result of impaired judgment when high also raises the risk of HIV infection.

Women and HIV Infection.   Studies reveal that 30 to 50 percent of female IVDUs have engaged in prostitution. So if these women are HIV carriers, they represent a large and significant pool capable of spreading the infection throughout the heterosexual community.

Even women who aren't IVDUs are at particular risk for HIV

infection. Active protection through the use of condoms is more often male- than female-controlled. And the increasing number of women who exchange sex for crack in crack houses are at great risk.

According to the Centers for Disease Control, the number of women with AIDS represents approximately 11 percent of reported cases. However, if one looks at the proportion of AIDS cases in women who developed AIDS from heterosexual contact with persons known to be infected with HIV or at risk of being infected, this figure increases from 13 percent in 1983 to 28 percent in 1988. The proportion is even higher in cities, particularly in low-income areas where HIV infection is endemic. Worse yet, the population of infected but not yet diagnosed women surely represents sizable numbers. And since not all physicians are yet attuned to early symptoms of HIV infection in women, diagnosis and early intervention may be delayed.

Children and HIV Infection. HIV-infected women obviously play a significant role in terms of HIV-infected newborns. Projections put the number of children who will be diagnosed with AIDS by 1991 at 3,000 to 10,000. Except for the 20 percent who are hemophiliacs infected through blood transfusions, the overwhelming majority (virtually 80 percent) of infants with AIDS are born to mothers who have had IVDUs as sexual partners or who are themselves IVDUs.

The prevalence of HIV infection among childbearing women varies greatly, from 0.21 percent in Massachusetts to 2 percent in areas of New York City. In a study in New York State, 141,000 anonymous blood specimens were taken from men and pregnant women, and 133,781 from babies born over a six-month period. The incidence of HIV infections was startling. Depending on the geographic area, up to one in 22 women tested positive. Infection was twice as high in mothers in their twenties and thirties as in those in their teens and forties.

In a subsequent study of 276,609 newborns in New York State, 0.66 percent tested positive for HIV, with a prevalence of 1.25 percent in New York City (with rates highest in areas where intravenous drug use is also high).

In New York City, black mothers were many times more likely to have HIV infections than white mothers. The rates were 2.07 percent for black mothers, 1.66 percent for Hispanic mothers, and 0.4 percent for white mothers. And when racial and geographic data were pooled, the chances of a New York City black mother and her baby being infected were 41 times higher than for a white woman and her baby living outside the city.

The actual number of HIV-infected newborns who will develop AIDS can't be predicted with certainty. One study followed 117 infants born to HIV-positive mothers for about 18 months after birth. By the end of this period, 27 percent of the children were seropositive for HIV or had died of AIDS. Of the 32 seropositives, only two remained asymptomatic. Another nine children didn't test positive for HIV but had clinical symptoms of HIV infection.

In a second study of 172 children infected with HIV perinatally, the statistics were even more ominous: half developed symptoms within the first 12 weeks; 78 percent within the first two years. Seventeen percent died in their first year; median survival time was 38 months.

Extrapolating these findings to the general population suggests that about one-third of the children born to HIV-positive women will develop evidence of HIV infection or AIDS by age 18 months, with 20 percent of them having died. AIDS is now the ninth leading cause of death among children under age 13. Data from the Centers for Disease Control reveal that AIDS cases among newborns increased 17 percent from 1988 to 1989.

Adolescents and HIV Infection. Spread of HIV infection in adolescents is increasing. Whether it's related to drug use or increased sexual activity—along with or independent of drugs—is unclear. But intravenous drug use doesn't appear to be the primary route of infection.

Screening of young recruits by the military revealed the prevalence of HIV infection to be greater than 1 percent in some cities, with an increasing proportion of women infected.

The number of teenagers with AIDS is relatively small—representing less than 0.4 percent of total reported AIDS cases. But the seven-plus years of latency between infection with HIV and development of illness may increase that number. A study of 1,500 homeless and runaway teenagers in New York City revealed 7 percent to be HIV-positive, with 16 percent of those between the ages of 18 and 20 testing positive. Between July 1989 and June 1990, the Centers for Disease Control reported an increase of 38 percent in the number of AIDS cases among teenagers.

Epidemiologic surveys suggest that the education provided to adolescents about AIDS is ineffective. From 50 to 75 percent did know that HIV could be transmitted through the blood, but up to 64 percent said it could be transmitted through public toilets. And among a subset of sexually active juvenile offenders, 35 percent had never used condoms.

AIDS AND INTRAVENOUS DRUG USE

From HIV Infection to AIDS. The period between exposure to HIV and development of AIDS varies considerably. The mean incubation period was first thought to be 30 months; evidence now suggests it might be more than seven years: one study of gay and bisexual men in San Francisco found that only 20 percent remained asymptomatic after 88 months of infection with HIV.

Also in the early stages of HIV-infection awareness, the rapidity of death once a diagnosis was made was striking—80 percent of those diagnosed before 1985 died by 1987. Of great importance, however, is that there's no conclusive evidence that everyone who is HIV-positive will develop AIDS. Accumulating evidence suggests that treatment of those who are HIV-positive, but clinically well, can at the very least delay the onset of clinical symptoms.

Intravenous Drug Use As an Increasing Risk Factor. When AIDS was first diagnosed in 1981, approximately 95 percent of cases were among gay and bisexual men. By September 1990 the proportion of IVDUs among total AIDS cases reported was 22 percent. However, when intravenous drug use as an associated risk factor is surveyed, the proportion of IVDUs increased to 33 percent (Table 17.3).

TABLE 17.3
AIDS Cases Among Intravenous Drug Users (IVDUs), 1989

Group	Number of Reported Cases*	Percentage of Cases
Males		
Heterosexual	7,647	54
Bisexual/Gay	2,387	17
Heterosexual partners of IVDUs	448	3
Females		
Heterosexual	2,273	16
Heterosexual partners of IVDUs	1,010	7
Children		
Mothers are IVDUs	306	2
Mother's sex partners are IVDUs	145	1
TOTAL	14,216	100

*This number represents 33% of 43,346 AIDS cases reported in the United States and its territories between October 1989 through September 1990.
Source: HIV/AIDS Surveillance Centers for Disease Control, U.S. Department of Health and Human Services, Atlanta, October 1990.

By 1988 the proportion of AIDS cases in heterosexual IVDUs in Connecticut, New Jersey, New York, and Puerto Rico exceeded that of gay and bisexual men (Table 17.4). In Newark the proportion of reported AIDS cases increased 65 percent between June 1988 and June 1989, with almost 75 percent of cases being associated with intravenous drug use.

In New York City the number of AIDS cases is approximately 22 percent of all cases reported nationwide. Approximately 38 percent are in some way associated with intravenous drug use. By 1991 it is estimated that New York City will have more than 40,000 cumulative AIDS cases. Close to 30,000 deaths are predicted, making AIDS the leading cause of death in men between the ages of 25 and 44, and in women between 25 and 29. From 30 to 60 percent of the estimated

250,000 IVDUs in that city are probably infected with HIV. And more than 90 percent of the infected women will have had sexual contact with male IVDUs.

Since 1985, deaths among IVDUs in New York City have increased dramatically. The deaths resulted primarily from such infections as tuberculosis, pneumonia, and endocarditis (infection of the heart valves). The number of deaths from drug overdose, however, has remained relatively constant, suggesting that the HIV infection, with accompanying immunosuppression, accounted for the overall increase.

Effects of Treatment of IVDUs on HIV Transmission. Many attempts have been made to reduce transmission of HIV through intravenous drug use. They include massive educational campaigns, distribution of bleach to disinfect needles, distribution of sterile needles, and expansion of available treatment programs. Treatment programs are obviously the preferred method for preventing the spread of HIV infection among intravenous drug users. They may either be drug free or methadone maintenance. (Chapter 5, Chapter 11).

Methadone maintenance programs. Heroin addicts appear most likely to accept methadone maintenance, so it is essential that enough treatment slots are available. Entry into maintenance programs is usually accompanied by decreased heroin use, but many addicts still inject cocaine, continuing to put themselves at risk. And since cocaine is injected more frequently than heroin, the risk rises accordingly. Continued injection of heroin by some on methadone maintenance has led critics to question the efficiency of maintenance. As noted in Chapter 11, however, failures in maintenance to prevent heroin use primarily are related to the quality of the specific program and specific methadone dose administered.

In 1984 a study of patients in New York who had been on methadone maintenance continuously prior to 1978 found only 10 percent were HIV positive. The percentage rose to 47 percent for those not on continuous treatment.

Methadone on demand. This approach has been suggested as a way to increase availability of treatment for IVDUs who are denied

TABLE 17.4
AIDS Among IVDUs by City, 1988

City*	Number of Reported Cases	Percentage of Cases in City	Percent Increase Over 1987
Atlanta	1,614	16	56
Austin	5,462	14	75
Boston	1,803	20	60
Chicago	2,247	15	71
Los Angeles	5,700	12	72
Miami	1,800	21	37
New York	17,090	38	45
Philadelphia	1,066	18	52
San Diego	1,114	13	68
San Francisco	5,558	—	39

*Reporting over 11,000 cumulative AIDS cases
Source: Adapted from "Community Epidemiology Work Group, December 1988
Epidemiologic Trends in Drug Abuse," National Institute on Drug Abuse, U.S.
Department of Health and Human Services, Public Health Service, Alcohol, Drug
Abuse and Mental Health Administration, Rockville, Md., 1989.

access to maintenance programs because of overcrowding. Its relatively low cost gives it immediate appeal, but evidence suggests that it could prove counterproductive.

A major problem is that addicts in maintenance programs where insufficient counseling is provided continue to inject cocaine. What's more, on-demand methadone has been sold on the street. An inexpensive and quick solution still awaits development.

Good methadone maintenance programs are effective in decreasing needle use. So are therapeutic communities and ambulatory day programs. Maintenance programs, however, are more successful in

TABLE 17.5
Relationship Between Heroin Use and AIDS

Facilitation of high-risk behavior, thus increasing chances for HIV infection

Transmission of HIV through needle sharing

Injection of infectious agents through contaminated drugs and unsterile needles, worsening condition of those with AIDS

Exchange of sexual favors for drugs with HIV-infected persons

Depression of immune system, with increased susceptibility to infections in those with AIDS

---

attracting and keeping IVDUs for treatment. Studies have shown that residential and outpatient programs lose 40 to 50 percent of patients in the first three months, compared with a 14 percent loss from maintenance programs. The loss rate in the latter programs can probably be lowered through appropriate staffing and closer adjustments in individual dosages.

Reduction in high-risk behavior. Therapy provides addicts with information about HIV transmission and how to reduce risk through changes in sexual behavior. But purely educational efforts to change behavior in IVDUs haven't been very successful. The reasons may be the heroin addict's general self-destructive nature or feeling of helplessness stemming from the belief that infection has already taken place. Those feelings of futility and inevitability must be overcome, because less than 50 percent of IVDUs are infected. Appropriate behavior modification may protect these people from HIV infection.

AIDS research findings have documented a deliberate reduction in high-risk behaviors once the specific risk factors are made meaningful to the drug user. Risk varies depending on total number of injections per month, percentage of injections with used needles, average number of cocaine injections per month, and frequency of sharing injection equipment with large numbers of other IVDUs. For reasons not entirely clear, cocaine injection appears to carry the greatest risk of HIV infection, with heroin next, and amphetamine injection markedly less risky.

According to some authorities, the ultimate effectiveness of behavioral changes has yet to be determined. But risk reduction has been associated with a relative stabilization of HIV prevalence among heavy drug users in New York City and San Francisco. That certainly suggests the importance of continuing and expanding behavioral-change efforts.

Directing appropriate resources to meet the needs of poor communities cannot be overemphasized. As with many communicable diseases associated with poverty, blacks and Hispanics are at particular risk for intravenous drug use and AIDS by a factor of two to one. This is especially true for women in these groups, for whom intravenous drug use is the primary route of HIV transmission.

Needles on demand. Dispensing needles on request to limit HIV transmission is a highly controversial practice. Opponents say easy access to needles will increase intravenous drug use. Proponents say the opportunity to decrease HIV transmission is reason enough to try such an approach, which may not increase drug use anyway.

Studies are under way to assess the effectiveness of needle distribution in reducing both shared-needle experiences and HIV transmission. Preliminary evidence in countries where needles are distributed suggests neither increases in intravenous use nor impressive decreases in high-risk behavior. Needle sharing is said to have decreased from 55 to 15 percent. Unfortunately, those countries have relatively small and homogeneous populations of IVDUs, making extrapolations of their findings to the United States difficult.

Preliminary studies in Tacoma, Washington, demonstrate a decrease in needle sharing by approximately 30 percent. But in Louisiana, where needles are also available by prescription, 65 percent of IVDUs are said to continue to share needles. More epidemiological evaluation is needed.

Disinfectants. An alternative to sterile syringes and needles is to disinfect them between uses. The ideal disinfectant acts quickly, is inexpensive, readily available, neutralizes viruses effectively, and is safe to the user. A solution of one part household bleach to 10 parts water works best. This solution can reduce viral activity sevenfold after 60 seconds of exposure. Between June 1986 and May 1987, several thousand bottles of bleach, along with instructions for use, were dispensed in San Francisco. A follow-up survey showed that two-thirds of those who received the bleach used it for the intended purpose.

RELATIONSHIP BETWEEN THE USE OF MOOD-ALTERING DRUGS AND HIV INFECTION

There are a number of ways that inappropriate use of mood-altering drugs may facilitate HIV infection, independent of intravenous use (Table 17.5).

Impaired Judgment. Use of mood-altering drugs, including alcohol, during sexual contact can blur judgment so that safe-sex techniques are ignored. Strong association exists between such behavior and the types of sexual activity implicated in HIV infection. According to one study, gay men who continue high-risk behavior are twice as likely to have used alcohol, and eight times as likely to have used other drugs, as those who stop such behavior. Whether drug use led to high-risk sexual activity, or whether those engaged in such activity were more apt to use drugs, is unclear. But alcohol and other mood-altering drugs release inhibitions, so it's reasonable to suppose that drug consumption might contribute to failure to take appropriate precautions during sex.

Cocaine As a Specific Risk Factor. The association between intravenous use of cocaine and HIV infection is well recognized. What remains to be clearly defined, however, is whether the association is related more to frequency of cocaine injection; its use in shooting galleries, where needles are freely exchanged; the need to barter sex for cocaine; the increase in sexual activity while on cocaine; the impaired mental judgment following cocaine use that leads to other high-risk behaviors; or the effect of cocaine itself on the immune system.

Effect of Drug Use on the Immune System. Considerable laboratory and clinical evidence suggests that alcohol adversely affects immunity. Alcoholics are more susceptible to infection than nonalcoholics, and alcohol is a risk factor in development of severe pneumonia and the virulent lung abscess. When alcohol liver damage (cirrhosis) is present, susceptibility to infection increases. Tuberculosis is also more prevalent in alcoholics.

Some evidence suggests that cocaine itself may have a detrimental effect on the immune system. Markers of cell-mediated immunity in association with cocaine use have been found to be altered in other types of retroviral infections. Similar associations between cocaine use and depression of T lymphocyte helper-suppressor ratios have also been described. In experiments on the excessive use of cocaine, replication of HIV in laboratory animals was markedly increased. A link between Kaposi's sarcoma and cocaine use has also been reported, although causality hasn't been demonstrated.

Heroin has long been known to adversely affect immune function. It also significantly reduces numbers and function of T cells. In laboratory animals, marijuana can suppress certain immune functions. While we can't clearly extrapolate that finding to humans, marijuana might act similarly in a person with an existing immune deficit. Whether central nervous system stimulants and barbiturates adversely affect human immune function is not known.

Volatile nitrites have been associated with changes in immune function even after relatively brief exposure. Such changes, however, haven't been consistently confirmed. Positive association between nitrite use and Kaposi's sarcoma has also been made. Combined with other chemicals, nitrites can form nitrosamines. Because nitrosamines can cause cancer, they may more easily do so in an AIDS victim with an already altered immune state. Kaposi's sarcoma has developed in habitual nitrite users, but a definite causal relationship has not been demonstrated.

Continued use of mood-altering drugs might have a bearing on accelerating development of AIDS in HIV-positive individuals. One study of IVDUs in New York found that those who abstained from or markedly cut down on intravenous drug use were less likely to show progression of clinical AIDS symptoms and manifestations than those who hadn't.

A large multicenter study, however, involving approximately 3,500 gay men, 38 percent of whom were HIV positive, did not find the use of any of the common mood-altering drugs to be associated with either the appearance of clinical symptoms or the speed with which AIDS developed. Compared with HIV-negative men, a significantly higher proportion of HIV-positive men had used each group of mood-altering substances more recently and more frequently during the study period. But AIDS wasn't diagnosed any earlier in the HIV-positives who also used mood-altering drugs. Alcohol consumption seen in 90 percent of all men was also found not to be a risk factor in the development of AIDS.

Even though use of mood-altering drugs may not increase the progression from HIV infection to AIDS, the role of mood-altering drugs in transmitting the HIV, either through contaminated needles or by promoting high-risk behavior, remains a concern.

Chapter 18

Drugs, Pregnancy, and the Newborn

Behold, thou shalt conceive, and bear a son; and now drink
no wine nor strong drink.

—Judges 13:7

During pregnancy a woman must take responsibility for her own
health as well as that of her fetus. Ideally, use of all mood-altering
substances should stop at least three months before conception, with
abstinence continuing throughout the pregnancy. Realistically, even
when pregnancy is planned, many women who use mood-altering
substances can't or don't stop.

INCIDENCE OF DRUG USE DURING PREGNANCY

Data from the National Institute on Drug Abuse suggest that many
of the 56 million women of childbearing age in the United States use
one or more of the following: alcohol, cocaine, marijuana, nicotine—with 15 percent believed to be using enough of these substances to compromise fetal safety in the event of a pregnancy. But
defining the proportion of women at risk for drug use when pregnant
isn't the same as identifying those who will continue to use drugs
when pregnant. Various surveys indicate that approximately 80 percent of pregnant women who use mood-altering drugs will continue
to use them in varying amounts when pregnant:

- Alcohol consumption, though down in recent years, is still
  widespread. At least one-third of pregnant women smoke to-

bacco; 60 to 90 percent use analgesics at some point during the pregnancy; 20 to 30 percent take sedative drugs; and a number continue illicit drug use.

- In Chicago, a 1989 random screening of 715 urines during first visits to public and private prenatal clinics found 15 percent positive for alcohol, marijuana, or cocaine.
- In Boston, a similar study of 1,000 pregnant women found 27 percent were using marijuana, 18 percent cocaine.
- In New York City, where confidential information on maternal consumption of mood-altering drugs is required on all birth certificates, maternal illicit drug use increased from 7.4 per 1,000 live births in 1980 to 29.7 in 1988. In the same period, cocaine use, alone or in combination with other drugs, increased twentyfold.
- In California, up to 30 percent of women in one of the state's largest health maintenance programs were using cocaine.
- The National Association for Perinatal Addiction, Research and Education estimates that up to 375,000 infants each year are born impaired in some way by their exposure to mood-altering drugs.

GENERAL EFFECTS OF DRUGS ON PREGNANCY OUTCOME

A fair amount of knowledge has accumulated on the effects of mood-altering drugs on reproduction, pregnancy, and the newborn. Most investigators in the field agree on certain key points:

All commonly used mood-altering drugs can freely pass through the placental barrier, so any drug used by the mother is present in the fetal circulation. In general, congenital defects are usually induced during the first trimester, with the risk greatest from 20 days to two months. The risk of birth defects decreases after that time, but the fetus is still vulnerable to growth retardation and other neurological or behavioral abnormalities, which become apparent after birth.

Many mood-altering substances affect uterine contractions, causing decreased blood flow and oxygen supply to the fetus. This can result in premature labor and/or spontaneous abortion. Withdrawal from narcotics or drugs in the sedative/barbiturate category also causes uterine contractions.

Dependency-producing drugs cause the newborn to go into withdrawal, necessitating treatment of the symptoms (Table 18.1). And, of course, the association of HIV and AIDS has placed infants born to intravenous drug-using women at deadly risk (Chapter 17).

Data from the New York City Board of Health reveal that the risk of giving birth to an infant of low birth weight in the presence of excessive maternal drug use is 3.8 times greater than with women who don't use drugs. The risk of infant death among drug-using women is 2.6 times greater.

A safe assumption is that any mood-altering substance used in excess during pregnancy will have a detrimental effect on the fetus. But whether minimal or even moderate use of specific substances will cause bad effects is sometimes hard to determine. One reason for difficulty in identifying effects of a specific substance is that multiple drug use is very common. Alcohol and cigarettes are used in combination with such substances as heroin, methadone, cocaine, and sedatives. Moreover, many women who use these drugs excessively are poorly nourished and don't seek adequate prenatal care and counseling.

So information often has to be obtained retrospectively, by reviewing medical charts, notoriously inaccurate when it comes to drug use. Even when women themselves provide information, drug use—particularly illicit drug use—isn't always reported.

Isolating specific drug effects in terms of future infant development has similar problems. Infants treated for withdrawal symptoms are usually given other drugs for days or weeks to alleviate symptoms. The long-term effects of these prescribed drugs aren't always measured. In addition, women with chemical dependency problems are often unable to provide adequate child care. As a result, the effect of these environmental factors on child rearing and future developmental abornmalities can't be accurately assessed.

Nevertheless, the physiologic effects of specific mood-altering substances on pregnancy, fetal development, and outcome are identifiable. Before we discuss these effects for each major drug type, it

TABLE 18.1

Adverse Effects of Mood-Altering Drugs on Pregnancy and the Newborn

Drug	Spontaneous Abortion	Premature Delivery	Perinatal Mortality	Neonatal Withdrawal	Fetal Distress	Congenital Abnormality
Alcohol	+				+	+
Amphetamines		+	+			
Barbiturates, sedatives, tranquilizers				+	+	
Cannabis					+/−	
Cocaine	+	+	+		+	+
Heroin	+	+	+	+	+	+
Marijuana						+/−
Methadone				+		
Nicotine	+				+	
Phencyclidine		+		+/−	+	

+ Adverse effects
+/− Effects not consistently documented
* Used appropriately under medical supervision

should be noted that even in the "normal" course of events, without any specific identifiable risk factors, only about half of all fertilized eggs progress through a successful pregnancy and delivery. Up to half of those lost through spontaneous abortion or miscarriage are considered structurally abnormal. As many as 3 percent of newborns have one or more congenital malformations at birth; another 3 percent are diagnosed with some developmental abnormality by the end of the first year. Subtler abnormalities may not become apparent until early childhood. Because of the existence of these general patterns, we cannot simply assume that any health problems in a child born to a pregnant woman who takes drugs must be related to specific drug effects.

Alcohol.   Alcohol's adverse effects on pregnancy have been observed for centuries. One of the first studies on the subject was published in the late 1800s by a doctor from Liverpool reporting the outcome of 600 children born to 100 alcoholic women.

Fetal alcohol syndrome.   A constellation of features called the fetal alcohol syndrome (FAS) was described in 1973. FAS, found in many infants born to women who ingested substantial amounts of alcohol during their pregnancies, consists of abnormal facial characteristics, mental retardation, hyperactivity, aggressive behavior, sleep disorders, and continuing behavioral problems (Table 18.2).

Associated abnormalities may include defects in the heart, genitals, kidneys, and muscles, as well as disturbances in vision. Alcohol is one of the few known mood-altering drugs definitively linked to congenital abnormalities and to pre- and postnatal growth retardation. Risk of spontaneous abortion accompanying excessive alcohol consumption is also real.

The surgeon general issued an advisory warning in 1981 suggesting that alcoholic beverages be avoided by pregnant women, and that they be informed of the alcoholic content of food and medications.

Concern over drinking and pregnancy resulted in the Alcoholic Beverage Labeling Act being incorporated into the Omnibus Drug Bill of 1988. It requires warnings about the potential adverse health effects of alcohol to be placed on labels for alcoholic beverages. Several states have also enacted a "point of purchase" clause, re-

TABLE 18.2
Fetal Alcohol Syndrome

Behavioral changes
Hyperactivity, irritability

Facial changes
Shortened opening between the eyelids
Depressed space between nose and mouth
Flat nose
Small head circumference
Thin upper lip

Growth retardation

quiring information on the hazards of alcohol during pregnancy to be prominently displayed wherever alcohol is sold.

The need for abstinence during pregnancy has been questioned. Critics point out that many women drink varying amounts of alcohol during pregnancy, but that the incidence of FAS is far lower than the number of pregnant drinkers. Nearly 4 million live births occur in the United States each year, and 70 to 80 percent of women of childbearing age drink sometimes during pregnancy.

Estimates put at approximately 36,000 the number of pregnancies adversely affected by alcohol, with 2,000 to 2,400 infants born with FAS. If we use a liberal estimate of 40,000 pregnancies adversely affected by alcohol, the risk to any given pregnant woman who drinks is 1 in 100. But the risk of having an infant with FAS is 1 in 1,300. Both those risk ratios are lower than the risk of a congenital abnormality in the absence of any alcohol or drug use.

Some argue that social drinking at a minimal level has never been associated with any adverse effects.

Excessive alcohol use during pregnancy is often accompanied by use of other mood-altering drugs. The role of multiple drug use in FAS is not yet clear. One study, for example, found maternal use of marijuana to be the single best predictor of FAS—an even better forecaster than alcohol use.

Some women, of course, experience needless concern and anxiety throughout their pregnancy if they drank alcohol before knowing they were pregnant. That can and does happen fairly often, since several weeks typically pass between conception and confirmation of pregnancy. By suggesting that minimal alcohol consumption always leads to impaired infants, one places drinking in the same category as those drugs that are consistently associated with risks to the pregnancy, such as heavy cigarette smoking, excessive use of alcohol, and use of illicit narcotics, cocaine, and other street drugs. Minimal drinking during pregnancy should be discouraged, but it doesn't invariably increase chances of having an impaired child. Having such a misconception might even inadvertently prompt a person to use more dangerous drugs.

Unfortunately, what constitutes a safe level of alcohol consumption has not been determined. Several studies have demonstrated that spontaneous abortion and low birth weight can occur even with "social" drinking. In a study of almost 500 pregnant women, researchers at the University of Washington found that moderate drinking (defined as one drink a day) was associated with a variety of symptoms in newborns, including weaknesses in heart and lung function and irritability. At age four, some of these children had attention deficiencies and slight decreases in intelligence.

The same investigators documented the adverse effect of alcohol on breast-feeding infants of mothers who continue to drink. Compared with a control group, infants regularly exposed to alcohol in breast milk had slightly but significantly impaired motor control.

A survey of 1,000 pregnant women suggests that education on the effects of drugs during pregnancy is working. Of those women, 70 percent decreased alcohol consumption once they became pregnant. By comparison, only 14 percent stopped smoking during pregnancy.

Amphetamines.   The specific effects of amphetamines are difficult to isolate because they're often used in conjunction with other mood-altering drugs. Studies have suggested that taking amphetamines, even for weight control, can be associated with low birth weight. Dependence on amphetamines has been linked to premature delivery and sometimes to prenatal mortality. In addition, emotional disturbances have been reported in children whose mothers were dependent on amphetamines during pregnancy. When the drug is injected, both woman and fetus are exposed to all the associated medical complications.

Caffeine.   Both pregnant and nonpregnant women consume large quantities of caffeine in coffee, tea, and cola beverages. The metabolism of caffeine, which freely crosses the placental barrier, is decreased during pregnancy. And since the fetus has no enzymes for its metabolism, caffeine may accumulate in the newborn for several days after birth.

Effects of caffeine on pregnancy are controversial, although some investigators have reported both decreased ability to conceive and increased risk of low birth-weight infants. One of the problems in singling out the effects of caffeine is that coffee, alcohol, and cigarette smoking frequently go together—and cigarette smoking is a known independent risk factor in low birth-weight infants.

A large study of 3,891 pregnant women at Yale-New Haven Hospital revealed a definite relationship between maternal coffee consumption and birth weight. Only 25 percent of the women had no caffeine intake; another 8 percent consumed the equivalent of three-plus cups of coffee per day. The latter were the only ones at significant risk for having low birth-weight infants (7.3 versus 4.1 percent among noncaffeine drinkers).

Caffeine consumption correlated positively with cigarette smoking, marijuana smoking, and alcohol drinking. Yet when those variables were accounted for, the increased risk among heavy coffee drinkers remained. The clinical importance of that finding remains to be determined. But it's probably best for women to moderate their consumption of caffeine, including coffee, teas, and cola drinks, during pregnancy.

Central Nervous System Depressants.   Many studies have shown that chronic maternal use of barbiturates and other central nervous system depressants can be associated with an accumulation of the drugs in fetal tissues. Infants born to mothers dependent on such drugs undergo withdrawal not unlike narcotic withdrawal. Depending on the specific drug, symptoms may not appear until several days after birth because of the prolonged half-life in the infant's blood. Acute, intermittent use during pregnancy can also be associated with adverse fetal effects. High doses prior to delivery can result in respiratory depression, failure to nurse, and lethargy at birth.

Cigarettes. The adverse effects of smoking on the reproductive system and pregnancy are well known. Less well known is whether they're related to nicotine or to the numerous constituents in cigarette smoke, including such toxins as lead, cadmium, and cyanide.

Smoking has been shown to decrease fertility and to increase risk of spontaneous abortion and placental problems. These include rupture of the placenta and premature rupture of the placental membranes at birth.

Smoking can also cause growth retardation, resulting in low birth weight, and has been associated with subsequent deficits in intellectual and emotional development. Conversely, smoking has been associated with decrease incidence of maternal preeclampsia and toxemia, conditions characterized by a sudden rise in blood pressure, excessive weight gain, generalized edema, and other toxic disturbances. But when those conditions do occur in smokers, the result is increased risk of infant mortality.

The effects of passive smoking on adults are relatively well known (Chapter 14), but the effects on the fetus when a pregnant woman is exposed to cigarette smoke are not well known. For example, increased levels of thiocyanate, a byproduct of tobacco smoke, have been identified in fetal tissues, but its actual effects have not been studied.

Cocaine. One nationwide survey of 36 hospitals found that 11 percent of women who delivered had exposed their fetuses to illegal drugs. Some of the hospitals reported an incidence of 27 percent. The most common drug was cocaine.

The risks to a woman and her fetus from cocaine are even greater than those from heroin (Table 18.3). The risks occur whether the drug is snorted, smoked as crack, or taken intravenously—although intravenous use introduces a new set of complications. The stimulant effects and pharmacological properties are such that even a single use can result in adverse consequences.

Cocaine rapidly crosses the placental barrier. The overall effect on the placenta is to decrease blood flow to the fetus. That can result in impairment in fetal growth, an increased growth of malformations, and often excessive bleeding and fetal death. Premature labor and decreased birth weight are common. In New York City, the risk of having a low birth-weight baby is four times greater in cocaine users than in women who don't take drugs. Rapid increases in maternal and fetal blood pressure may result in stroke or convulsion.

Mortality of infants born to women using cocaine in New York City has been three to six times greater than that of nondrug-using women. Cocaine is eliminated from an adult's body within 48 hours, but the low levels of enzymes in the fetus make metabolization there much slower. Thus cocaine may remain in fetal tissues for several days. Norcocaine, one of cocaine's breakdown products, is equally toxic and is recirculated throughout the amniotic fluid.

At birth, newborns whose mothers have used cocaine are hypersensitive and irritable, crying at the least stimulation. Conversely, they may appear oversedated. The incidence of sudden infant death syndrome (SIDS) also increases. Maternal cocaine use can interfere with parent-child bonding, and neurological impairment can persist into early childhood. Subsequent psychological and social development may also be impaired. Children who have inhaled crack or cocaine smoke in their homes become drowsy, unable to stand, or even suffer seizures. Such passive exposure results in considerable blood levels of cocaine with potentially serious effects on the brain and heart.

A Chicago study found that adverse outcomes were most severe in women who used cocaine throughout their pregnancy, as compared with those who used it only during the first several months. Effects after birth, including impairment in orientation and motor behavior, were documented in both groups.

Heroin. Illicit heroin use can expose the woman and her fetus to withdrawal and overdose. Both phenomena carry great risk for the fetus (Table 18.4). Consequently, heroin users who become pregnant are apt to experience an increased incidence of spontaneous

---

TABLE 18.3
Effects of Cocaine on Pregnant Women and Newborns

Women
Increased risk of:
    Spontaneous miscarriage (abortion)
    Decreased growth of fetus
    Premature birth
    Premature separation of placenta (abruptio placenta)
    Decreased uterine blood flow

Newborns
Low birth weight
Irritability
Tremors
Neurological abnormalities
Stroke
Damage to small intestines
Possible congenital heart and kidney deformities
Sudden infant crib death (SIDS)
More complicated and prolonged hospitalizations

---

abortion and stillbirth. Other complications include fetal distress during labor, narcotic withdrawal and low birth weight, and decreased growth rates when the infant is three to six months old.

Methadone maintenance. The best solution for a pregnant woman addicted to heroin is gradual detoxification and subsequent abstinence. In practice, however, that's often unrealistic. Clinical experience repeatedly shows that up to 70 percent of pregnant women who are detoxified from heroin resume their habits by the time they reach the third trimester. So to prevent heroin use (and clearly as a second choice), low doses of methadone have been used in maintenance therapy.

Numerous studies have tried to define the effects of methadone on the fetus, the newborn, and the developing infant. Methadone, like all narcotics, crosses the placental barrier, is found in fetal tissues,

---

TABLE 18.4
Complications of Heroin Use in Pregnant Women

Abortion

Breech presentation

Infection of amniotic fluid

Intrauterine death

Placenta insufficiency

Premature labor

Premature rupture of membranes

Toxemia

---

and results in newborn withdrawal 100 percent of the time. Pharmacologic treatment is warranted in 60 to 80 percent of such cases. Withdrawal is sufficiently mild in the rest for them to be treated without narcotic drugs.

Mothers maintained on methadone—and who don't use other drugs and are appropriately followed throughout the pregnancy—can deliver infants without significant problems. The babies may have slightly decreased birth weight, but their neonatal complication rate is the same as that of babies born to nondependent women.

Follow-up studies indicate that children born to women on methadone may exhibit a higher incidence of minor neurologic abnormalities, and somewhat lower scores on developmental evaluations during their first three years. When compared with scores in a control group, however, those differences tend to regress toward normal.

No uniform long-term effects have been consistently found. But many women on methadone also use other mood-altering drugs, including heroin and cocaine. Maintaining a woman on methadone is not as good as abstinence, and the decision to prescribe methadone is made only after realizing how difficult—if not impossible—it is for many women to remain abstinent when pregnant. The medical use of methadone is far safer than continued heroin use.

Lysergic Acid Diethylamide (LSD).   Isolated reports have linked LSD with congential malformations, but there is no consistent evidence that it causes such abnormalities.

Marijuana.   Use of marijuana during pregnancy may affect the fetus through a number of mechanisms. Marijuana is highly fat-soluble and is absorbed by the tissues, so a single administration may remain in the placenta and fetal tissues for up to 30 days. Physiologic effects resulting in increased heart rate and blood pressure may adversely affect placental blood flow. Smoking marijuana, like smoking cigarettes, results in elevated carbon monoxide levels in the blood. These levels are higher with marijuana than those from regular cigarettes because of the practice of inhaling deeply and holding the breath. The frequent use of marijuana with other drugs can result in an additive adverse effect on the fetus.

Early studies failed to demonstrate conclusively the incidence of congenital malformations increased in infants exposed to marijuana during gestation. Deficiencies in central nervous system functioning were reported by some investigators, but not confirmed by others. More recent evidence, however, suggests a positive association between marijuana use during pregnancy and congenital malformations. In fact, marijuana is the mood-altering drug most highly predictive of such abnormalities, even more so than tobacco and alcohol. But deficits present at birth don't always appear to be problematic when children are tested up to two years later.

Much higher levels of THC are being detected in marijuana; the result may be more fetal and neonatal problems.

Phencyclidine (PCP).   Use of PCP during pregnancy has rarely been associated with malformations, but its frequent combination with other mood-altering drugs makes studying its singular effects in pregnancy difficult. Incidence of PCP use in high-risk pregnancies has been estimated at 7 to 12 percent. Premature labor, fetal distress, and low birth weight have been described in women who use PCP.

Abnormal findings in the newborn consist of increased tremors, irritability, altered nursing reflex, and poor attention span. Those symptoms are similar to the withdrawal symptoms in infants of heroin-dependent mothers. But PCP is stored in the fetal tissues, so it's possible that the irritability may be due to its release rather than representing withdrawal from the drug. Agitation and restlessness can continue for several months. Several follow-up studies observed consistent borderline abilities in fine motor development, language, and in social adjustment.

TREATMENT OF DRUG USE
AND DEPENDENCY DURING PREGNANCY

Therapy for women who use mood-altering drugs while pregnant should be essentially the same as that for nonpregnant women on drugs. However, emphasis must be placed on the adverse effects that continued drug use will have, not only on the woman, but on the fetus, the newborn, and even on the child's subsequent development. As discussed earlier in this chapter, it is best for women to abstain from all mood-altering drugs while pregnant. For those women dependent on opiates who are unable or unwilling to remain abstinent, methadone maintenance is a viable alternative.

Frustration over the inability to convince women who are pregnant to abstain from illicit drug use during their pregnancies has resulted in an increasing number of communities viewing the pregnant woman as a criminal rather than a victim of drug dependency. A number of states have initiated criminal proceedings against women who continue to use drugs during their pregnancy as well as charges of child neglect once the infant has been born. In 1989 Florida became the first state to convict a woman of "drug delivery" to her infant, sentencing her to 14 years on probation. In May of 1990, a New York State Appeals Court ruled that the presence of cocaine in an infant's system, combined with a mother's admission of drug use, was sufficient to require a hearing on child neglect.

Advocates of pursuing criminal charges against drug-dependent pregnant women maintain that the infant's rights are as important as the mother's. Not surprisingly, opponents argue vehemently for "free choice" of the pregnant woman to use or not use drugs. When faced with the possibility that criminal charges may be leveled against them, pregnant women who are drug-dependent may steer clear of adequate prenatal care programs or deny drug use to their physicians, delivering the babies without the physicians' knowledge of maternal drug use.

Treatment of the newborn dependent on mood-altering substances is important and should be administered promptly. In many cases, supportive care is all that is necessary. Depending on the drug used, the level of dependency, and the effect that the drug has had on fetal development, much more may be required. Infants born dependent on opiates may require a slow detoxification to prevent the effects of withdrawal. Infants born to mothers who use cocaine have been found to suffer the most complications and require the most assistance, often including prolonged intensive care while in the hospital as well as supportive services and special education programs for learning disabilities as they get older.

The economic and social costs of caring for an infant born to a woman who uses mood-altering substances have been identified. Estimates put the cost of medical care for such infants at 50 to 100 times greater than for a healthy infant. A 1990 report from the Office of the Inspector General in the Department of Health and Human Services, studying approximately 9,000 babies in eight major cities born to women who used cocaine, estimated the cost of hospitalization as well as foster care during the first five years of these children's lives at a half billion dollars. In New York City, mothers who use drugs were responsible for more than a threefold rise in cases of child abuse during the period from 1980 to 1988.

Since there may be several million women of childbearing age who use or are dependent on illicit substances and who will give birth at some future date, projections of costs to care for their infants are staggering. Hence it becomes critically important to develop outreach programs to get pregnant drug users into counseling, to give these women early and proper prenatal care, to identify developmental problems in their infants as early as possible, and to establish appropriate home environments that allow for placement of these children in foster care if necessary.

Chapter 19

Drugs and Sports

Show me a good and gracious loser and I'll show you a loser.
—Knute Rockne

As a group, athletes are neither more nor less prone to take mood-altering substances for recreational use than others. Drinking, smoking, chewing tobacco, and drinking caffeine-containing beverages are common behaviors in most groups, including athletes. Drugs taken by athletes for restorative effects, such as analgesics to relieve pain, or steroids for specific medical conditions (diabetes or asthma), are the norm. There are also three types of drugs athletes use primarily to enhance performance: stimulants, anabolic steroids, synthetic growth hormone, and most recently erythropoietin.

STIMULANTS

Stimulants, such as amphetamines and cocaine, taken to increase aggressiveness, muscular coordination, and physical prowess, are at times also taken "defensively" to compete against opponents who also use stimulants. They're detrimental both to daily functioning and ironically to performance on the field.

ANABOLIC STEROIDS

Steroids are naturally occurring substances found in hormones and certain vitamins. They're divided into the female sex hormones (estrogen and progesterone); cortical hormones of the adrenal gland (cortisone and deoxycorticosterone); hormones from the middle of the adrenal gland (aldosterone); hormones synthesized by the liver and/or gallbladder (cholesterol and cholregad); anabolic steroids; and vitamin D_3 (cholecalciferol).

Anabolic steroids were first promoted during World War II, when the Germans supplied them to their troops to increase aggressiveness and fitness. These drugs (Table 19.1 and 19.2) are basically derivatives of testosterone, the male hormone. They were initially developed to increase body mass and muscle strength without causing the excessive masculine characteristics (androgenic effects) associated with natural testosterone. But all these drugs, to some degree, have varying androgenic effects, depending on extent and duration of use.

Anabolic steroids are approved for a variety of medical conditions. Since they are testosterone derivates, they can stimulate sexual development in men with diminished testicular function, stimulate production of red blood cells in bone marrow in certain anemias, and diminish symptoms of hereditary angioedema, an uncommon allergic condition.

TABLE 19.1
Oral Anabolic Steroids and Androgens

Brand Name	Generic Name
Dianabol,* Methandroid	Methandrostenolone
Mestoranum	Mesterolone
Anavar	Oxandrolone
Anadrol 50	Oxymetholone
Maxibolin, Orabolin	Ethylestrenol
Winstrol	Stanozolol
Android-F, Halotestin	Fluoxymesterone
Android, Metandren Oreton Methyl, Vigorex, Virilon, Testred	Methyltestosterone

*Discontinued in March 1982

TABLE 19.2
Injectable Anabolic Steroids and Long-Lasting Androgens

Brand Name	Generic Name
Anabolin, Androlene, Durabolin, Hybolin, Nandrobolic	Nandrolone phenpropionate
Analone, Androlone-D, Deca-Durabolin, Hybolin Decanoate, Decolone, Neo-Durabolic, Nandrobolic L.A.	Nandrolone decanoate
Everone, Andryl, Andro LA, Delatestryl, Delatest, Everone, Durathate Testostroval, Testrin PA, Testone LA	Testosterone enanthate
Andro-Cyp, Andronaqla, Andronate, Depo-Testosterone, Duratest, depAndro, Testa-C, Testadiate-Depo, Testoject LA, Testred	Testosterone cypionate
Testex	Testosterone propionate

They have very limited usefulness as additional therapy in treating demineralization of bone (osteoporosis). They have also been used in metastatic breast cancer.

Their first use by athletes was reported in 1954, and despite adverse publicity, use has increased over time. Frequent users are usually interested in improving muscle mass and body strength.

Prevalence of Use. Mounting evidence suggests that anabolic steroid use by athletes in the United States is equal to illicit drug use. Prevalence, however, varies by sport, and frequency by season. One survey of 3,400 male teenagers at Pennsylvania State University found that 7 percent had taken steroids. A National Collegiate Athletic Association (NCAA) survey found that one-third of players tested positive for steroids, with 25 percent having received the drugs through physicians' prescriptions.

Only 4 percent of all athletes admit using anabolic steroids, but epidemiologic surveys indicate that the actual figure may be four times higher. Approximately 1 million Americans are estimated to have taken steroids nontherapeutically, with up to 260,000 adolescents believed to have used or to be using these drugs. A report released in 1990 by the inspector general of the Department of Human Services estimates between 5 and 11 percent of teenage boys and up to 2.5 percent of teenage girls in grades seven through 12 may have used these agents.

Of 546 football players surveyed, 3.3 percent were positive in March and April, compared with 1 percent postseason. The National Football League estimates that 6 percent of its players have taken steroids.

Nearly half of 250 surveyed weight lifters admitted taking steroids sometime during their careers. Other surveys suggest that 80 to 100 percent of international body builders experiment with these drugs at some time.

Anabolic steroid use was first detected in Russian athletes in the mid-1950s, and in Americans shortly thereafter. But it wasn't until 1976 that the magnitude of the problem was acknowledged on an international level. At that time, the International Olympics Committee initiated routine urine testing to screen for steroids. At the 1983 Pan American Games in Venezuela, a number of athletes were disqualified for positive urine tests, and dozens of others withdrew before being screened. At the 1988 Olympic Games in Korea, the fastest man in the world was disqualified after running the 100-meter race in the record-breaking time of 9.79 seconds, when stanozolol, an anabolic steroid, was detected in his urine.

Steroid Economics. As with the production and sale of illicit drugs, steroid use has created a considerable economic enterprise to meet the demand. The U.S. government has identified Europe, South America, and Mexico as possible points of origin, plus up to 20 clandestine laboratories in the United States. Considerable profit can be realized from sales of homemade steroids: the U.S. Food and

Drug Administration estimates that black market sales may be $100 million annually. Steroids may be obtained in different ways: legitimate prescriptions or veterinary products may be diverted, or steroids may be synthesized outside the United States, packaged under recognized brand names, and smuggled back into the country.

Synthesis is relatively easy. And unlike cocaine and heroin, steroids are impossible to identify by taste or by quickly appearing postinjection effect. That makes it easy to substitute inactive (placebo) substances.

Patterns of Use. Anabolic steroids may be taken orally or by injection (Tables 19.1 and 19.2). The oral preparation methandrostenolone (Dianabol) was the most popular of these drugs at first. But in 1982, its manufacturer, Ciba-Geigy, withdrew it after its misuse as an appetite stimulant for young children in third-world countries was discovered. Generic methandrostenolone, however, is still available.

Injectable steroids are now more popular because they need to be administered less frequently and have a relatively low association with liver toxicity. Prescriptions from physicians may play a role in obtaining the drugs, but most are steroids from nonprescribed sources. They may come from pharmaceutical houses, friends in the health professions, or associates from other countries where drug purchases are less stringently regulated than in the United States.

The body produces four to 10 milligrams of naturally occurring steroids per day. Anabolic steroids, however, are usually taken in increasingly higher doses through a technique called "pyramiding." When several drugs are taken, it's called "stacking." The drugs are taken in a cyclic manner for four to 18 weeks, with subsequent drug-free periods of one to 12 months. Doses may range from 10 to 2,000 milligrams daily, which is up to 200 times the usual dose prescribed for specific medical conditions.

Supposed Benefits of Anabolic Steroids. Athletes take anabolic steroids for a variety of reasons, some of which have never been proven valid (Table 19.3). The drugs are claimed to increase muscle mass; decrease muscle recovery time; allow more frequent training

---

TABLE 19.3
Supposed Benefits of Anabolic Steroids

Enhanced physical appearance

Increased aggressiveness

Enhanced self-confidence

Increased lean-muscle mass

Decreased muscle-recovery time

Decreased muscle-injury healing time

Prolonged endurance

---

sessions; decrease healing time after injury, thus allowing earlier return to practice; and increase the hemoglobin concentration in the bloodstream, thus allowing more oxygen intake to prolong the duration of exercise. The perceived psychological effects—increased aggressiveness, for one—are believed to contribute to the competitive edge.

Studies to determine what role, if any, anabolic steroids have in improving performance have produced conflicting results. One comprehensive review of 25 published studies noted that when increases in strength occurred, the changes were accompanied by increases in body size and weight.

In one study, biopsies of abdominal muscles were taken from normal volunteers who had been given stanozolol before undergoing elective surgery. An increase was found in the size of the muscle fibers responsible for increasing strength after long-term aerobic exercise (Type I); muscle fibers thought to be responsible for increasing strength after body building (Type II) weren't affected.

The American College of Sports Medicine, after reviewing all published evidence of anabolic steroid effects on athletic performance, and noting that the evidence was far from conclusive, found that these drugs can increase muscular strength in excess of that seen with training alone and increase lean body mass in association with diet and exercise. But they cannot increase the capacity for aerobic work.

Differences between perception and reality can be only partially explained. For one thing, many of the studies used far lower doses than are taken by athletes, and no one questions that weight gains occur with higher doses. And because the doses used by athletes are far greater than FDA recommendations, many ethical questions surround those legitimate, randomized controlled studies.

A placebo effect can be seen in some who take steroids. Athletes who believe they're taking a drug to improve performance do indeed have improved performances when compared with control subjects.

Physiologically, anabolic steroids increase salt and water retention, which accounts for their ability to increase weight. And while it hasn't been consistently demonstrated that the drugs increase bone mass, thousands of athletes are convinced of their beneficial effects.

Adverse Effects of Steroids.   Although the ability of anabolic steroids to increase muscle strength and performance in sports requires more study, the adverse effects of large doses are already well defined. Taken in excess on a chronic basis, steroids can produce a number of severe and sometimes long-lasting abnormalities (Table 19.4).

Abnormal liver function can be detected in blood tests on athletes engaged in intense training, with or without steroids. Those using steroids who exhibited increased signs of liver dysfunction appeared to revert to normal when the drugs were discontinued. Oral steroid preparations are associated with a much higher incidence of liver disease. Cancer of the liver after steroid administration has also been reported.

Adverse effects on the cardiovascular system include an increase in low-density lipoprotein levels and up to a 30 percent decrease in high-density levels, increasing the statistical risk of heart attack with long-term use. Hypertension may also occur.

The adverse effects of chronic administration are difficult to assess because it's unethical to administer anabolic steroids in doses athletes ordinarily take over long periods of time. Most users, however, believe the practice is so widespread that any adverse effects would be

TABLE 19.4
Side Effects of Anabolic Steroids

General

Liver abnormalities,* rarely including liver cancer

Alters blood cholesterol levels predisposing to coronary artery disease (decreases high-density lipoproteins, increases low-density lipoproteins)

Disturbs electrolyte concentration; retaining sodium, potassium, chloride, phosphate, water, may promote hypertension

Acne

Increases blood pressure

Personality changes

Increases susceptibility to infections, notably tuberculosis, hepatitis, and AIDS

Men

Prepubertal
    Increases hair production
    Increases skin pigmentation
    Decreases height due to early closure of growth plates in bones
    Increases penis size and frequency of erections

Adult
    Inhibits testicular function with testicular atrophy
    Enlarges breasts
    Male-pattern hair loss
    Enlarges prostate
    Frequent erections

Women

Male-pattern hair loss
Menstrual irregularities
Deepens voice, may be permanent
Enlarges clitoris
During pregnancy, masculinizes fetus with possible birth defects

*Some anabolic steroids

readily seen. But such long-term effects as those associated with cardiovascular disease may not become apparent for years—particularly in people currently in excellent physical condition.

The behavioral effects of anabolic steroids are becoming better recognized, with subjective changes reported by up to 30 percent of regular users. Euphoria, increased motivation, and sense of well-being have been described as the positive effects of these drugs. But so have impaired judgment and increased aggressiveness. Psychiatric disturbances ranging from depression to paranoia have been reported in up to 22 percent of anabolic steroid users.

Some reports also suggest development of an addictive state, just as is seen with the more commonly recognized dependency-producing drugs: compulsive use; failure to stop despite awareness of adverse psychological effects; withdrawal or abstinence symptoms with craving to resume use; and once steroid-free, switching to other mood-altering substances when steroids are unavailable.

Such observations indicate that—at least for some long-term, high-dose users—stopping use is far from easy, both psychologically and physiologically.

Persistent high doses taken by young people have the potential for as yet unknown long-term adverse effects. Premature closure of the growth plates in the bones of adolescents whose bone growth may not be complete is one possibility. Another is premature suppression of sperm production, now known as a temporary complication of anabolic steroid use.

Detection of Anabolic Steroid Use. The Olympic Committee lists more than 3,000 drugs that can disqualify an athlete from competition. Urine tests routinely detect anabolic steroids, so athletes try various ruses to avoid detection.

They may consume only oral steroid preparations and quit a week or two before testing. They may use diuretics to dilute the urine. They try newer drugs, which are structurally different, hoping these can't be detected by current tests. Refinements in urine testing, however, have kept up. Current technology allows steroid detection at a concentration of one part per billion. Water-soluble steroids can be detected up to four days after use; fat-soluble drugs, up to two weeks.

Curbing Steroid Use. The Omnibus Drug Bill of 1988 prohibits distribution of anabolic steroids for any human use other than treatment of disease and requires a prescription. The penalties are up to six years in prison for distributing to those under age 18; up to three years for distributing to those over 18. Seizure and forfeiture of assets also await illegal distributors.

Many states have also introduced penalties or have classified anabolic steroids as Schedule II drugs. Penalties vary by state but may include prison sentences, and loss of license when physicians are involved. Such controls diminish diversion of these drugs by physicians, but they have little effect on illicit trade as long as people want to use them.

A campaign is under way to limit substance abuse in sports. Drug education in high schools is common, and owners of major professional teams have also expended considerable effort. In international competition, the Olympics Committee has initiated urine testing at all games. Moreover, the United States and the Soviet Union have signed a memorandum of agreement to test each other's Olympic athletes on a semiannual basis.

The National Football League has recently become the first professional sports association to ban anabolic steroid use. Players whose urine tests positive for steroids are subject to further testing at any time. A second positive test results in a month's suspension; a third in dismissal from the league.

The National Basketball Association, National Hockey League, and Major League Baseball have all to varying degrees stated their intolerance to use of mood-altering drugs. The corresponding players' associations have voiced similar concerns, emphasizing the importance of rehabilitation as well as sanctions.

GROWTH HORMONE

Synthesis of human growth hormone has opened a new door to inappropriate use in sports. Naturally secreted by the anterior pituitary gland, growth hormone has a number of physiologic effects, including stimulation of protein synthesis. As such, it is essential for achieving normal growth potential.

A deficit of growth hormone in childhood results in dwarfism. Fortunately, pituitary growth hormone can now be synthesized through biotechnology, all but eliminating that condition. Two synthetic growth hormone products—somatrem (Protropin) and somatropin (Humatrope)—are commercially available, albeit at exorbitant cost.

Use of these new hormones in athletics is not yet well known. But they do increase body growth and strength, and are difficult to detect in urine tests. That makes them logical as favored substances of inappropriate use, limited only by their considerable expense. According to reports, they are already being given to many athletes. Though the drugs are newly synthesized and not easily available, one physician of the United States Sports Academy was able to obtain a supply from two drug companies he contacted.

Excessive natural production of growth hormone causes well-known complications (Table 19.5). In childhood it results in gigantism; in adults it causes acromegaly, a condition associated with elevated blood sugars, increased cholesterol concentrations, high incidence of heart disease, impotence, and overgrowth of the bones in the forehead, jaws, hands, and feet. Since growth hormones have never been given to people with normal supplies, their adverse effects when used by athletes is still unknown. Potential adverse effects, however, have been categorized (Table 19.6).

TABLE 19.5
Effects of Increased Secretion of Growth Hormone

In children
Gigantism

In adults
Elevated blood sugar
Elevated cholesterol
Heart disease
Impotence
Increased bone growth of forehead, jaw, hands, and feet

TABLE 19.6
Potential Adverse Effects of Synthetic Growth Hormone

Development of antibodies to growth hormone

Hypothyroidism

Increased incidence of leukemia

Metabolic Effects
Impaired serum glucose levels
Increase in serum free fatty acids
Body retention of sodium, potassium, and phosphorus

ERYTHROPOIETIN

The use of intravenous infusions of red blood cells to enhance athletic performance (blood doping) has long been known although infrequently used because of the inherent risks associated with intravenous infusions. Recently, the human hormone erythropoietin, which stimulates the production of red blood cells from the bone marrow, has been synthesized through recombinant DNA techniques and marketed as Epoetin and Epogen. Epoetin is used for the treatment of severe anemias, most commonly those caused by chronic kidney failure. The availability of Epoetin, and its demonstrated ability to increase red blood cells, has resulted in reports of its use by athletes. Unlike traditional blood doping, which requires withdrawal of an athlete's own blood to be reinfused before a meet and which must be done in the presence of those trained in blood-storage techniques, Epoetin can be self-administered. Since there are a number of adverse effects due to increased red cell volume, including convulsions and increased clotting of blood in the tissues leading to pulmonary embolism, heart attacks, or strokes, the use of this drug may be quite dangerous. The American Medical Association Council on Scientific Affairs has strongly recommended against Epoetin use to enhance athletic performance.

Chapter 20

Why Has the War Against Drugs Failed?

Over the last two decades, the United States has spent billions of dollars trying to curtail illicit drug manufacture, sale, and use, with almost $10 billion projected to be spent by the federal government in 1990 for its drug control and treatment programs. Between 1985 and 1988 expenditures by states have increased remarkably—in some states by more than 800 percent—to a total of over $5 billion. Federal seizures of illicit drugs continue at an unparalleled rate, as have arrests of drug dealers and seizures of their assets. Yet despite all our efforts to address the issue, none of our approaches have been successful. The worldwide production of opium, cocaine, and marijuana in 1989 increased greatly over previous years, as did worldwide consumption of drugs.

Federal and state government, politicians, religious leaders, public health authorities, and many other groups and individuals have come up with strategies to prevent, reduce, or even eliminate the always controversial use of illicit mood-altering drugs. The strategies, often conflicting and always controversial, can be grouped into several categories: reducing the supply, reducing demand, eliminating the illegality of the act, and promoting treatment and rehabilitation (see Table 20.1). Although reason would suggest that only by emphasizing the reduction in demand and increasing the availability of treatment could use of drugs in the United States be markedly diminished, we continue to focus most of our energies and financial resources on the first strategy, with little evidence of success.

TABLE 20.1
Current Responses to Illicit Drug Use

Reduce supply
  At source: reduce crops, substitute other crops, spray crops with
  herbicides; provide aid to local law enforcement agencies in
  other countries; withholding aid from those countries not
  taking an active role in preventing illicit production and
  distribution

  Prevent drugs from entering United States

  Prevent chemicals needed to manufacture other illicit drugs from
  entering United States

  Prevent distribution and sales within United States

  Maximize criminal penalties

Reduce demand
  Deter use: increase penalties associated with use so as to
  diminish desire to take drug; criminal versus social

  Educate as to adverse effects of use: effective prevention
  programs

Allow "responsible use": decriminalization and/or legalization

Support treatment and rehabilitation efforts

REDUCING THE SUPPLY

Attacking the Source: Diminishing Foreign Production.   In the
early 1970s, the United States made a major commitment to eliminating illicit drug supplies. The State Department contacted representatives of the largest producer countries and asked their leaders
to take the initiative in reducing crops and preventing drug transport.
The State Department offered incentives, including financial aid to
farmers who substituted other crops and assistance from our law

enforcement agencies. In 1986 Congress passed a law allowing the president to impose economic sanctions on twenty-five countries known to be major production and distribution centers. At the top of the list were Peru, Bolivia, Colombia, and Ecuador for cocaine; Afghanistan, Guatemala, Laos, Myanmar (formerly Burma), Iran, and Thailand for opium; and Belize, Colombia, Jamaica, and Mexico for marijuana. The United States also plays a prominent role in harvesting marijuana.

U.S. foreign aid to some of these countries has been significant, and the government expected cooperation in return. But that has not happened, and the reason is obvious: drugs are highly profitable. In Colombia, the income a farmer receives from cocaine is 10 to 15 times that of his best licit cash crop. In Peru, cultivation of coca provides a profit eight times greater than that realized with other crops. In the Andes, the cocaine industry employs about 1.5 million people. The only success—and a limited one at that—has been in Turkey. Turkey, a prominent supplier of opium, decreased cultivation—but other countries soon increased theirs. Not only has every country except for Turkey and Thailand (another major producer of opium) maintained or increased production, in Guatemala and Afghanistan, two relatively minor players, production has increased dramatically. In 1988, Guatemala produced enough opium to satisfy 60 percent of U.S. needs. When the Russians withdrew from Afghanistan, the annual opium crop increased 100 percent.

This phenomenon holds for other illicit drugs. When Mexican marijuana fields were sprayed with chemicals that killed the crop, cultivation dropped; other areas quickly picked up the slack, including some regions in the United States. (The number of U.S. marijuana cultivation sites increased 100 percent between 1987 to 1988.) Spraying alone is not a long-term solution, since crops are simply relocated to more remote areas that are less accessible to authorities. Such land is abundant.

Many governments hesitate to take an active role in crop reduction and enforcement. The enormous profit—estimated at $100 billion—generated by drugs is a corrupting influence on local and even national leaders. Trafficking in Colombian cocaine grosses more than $4.5 billion per year, as compared with the $1.5 billion in profits reported in 1988 from coffee sales. One dealer in Bolivia allegedly offered to pay his country's $3.8 billion foreign debt if the government would stop enforcing narcotic laws. When bribes are rejected, violence often becomes a most effective deterrent to enforcement. Over the last several years, 22 Colombian judges and the country's attorney general were murdered for their opposition to drug cartels, despite the fact that only an estimated 14 percent of drug-related cases reach the stage when the justice system issues a verdict.

Committed governments acting alone in a military state or in concert with public commitment in a democracy can of course reduce production—but only at a price. Chile, which predated Colombia as a cocaine processing center, essentially went out of the cocaine business when the totalitarian regime of General Augusto Pinochet took power in 1973; Colombia increased its production. Growth does not occur without considerable public involvement. More than 500,000 Colombians are alleged to be involved in cocaine processing and transportation, with even greater numbers at all levels of society benefiting indirectly from the industry. In fact, if a plebiscite were taken, it is questionable whether Colombians would vote to remove cocaine from their economy, particularly if they would experience a comparable loss of income. Indeed, most Colombians oppose extradition of traffickers to the United States. In spite of the best efforts of the beleaguered and greatly endangered few in the Colombian government who attempt to eliminate the dealers, popular support for enforcement appears only transiently as an immediate response to isolated violence, but subsides as the violence escalates. Many people direct their resentment against the violence not back to the traffickers but toward those in government trying to enforce the law, and toward the United States as well.

Not surprisingly, many Colombians express anger toward the United States. By creating a booming market for cocaine, that nation is viewed as the basic cause of the Colombian problem. In addition, many of the chemicals used to process cocaine from coca originate in the United States.

The inability to conclude an international agreement over coffee prices, in large part due to U.S. objections to certain proposed regulations, resulted in a marked fall in the price of coffee—Colombia's leading export. The income from cocaine in 1989 was felt to be threefold the $1.2 billion expected from coffee sales. Both public and private efforts in the United States to protect the domestic flower industry at the expense of Colombia's flower trade—its fourth largest export—result in an annual loss to the Colombian economy of hundreds of millions of dollars. All these factors do little to convince Colombians of U.S. sincerity about providing viable alternatives to cocaine production and sales.

Still another factor inhibits U.S. efforts to reduce production: political alliance between the United States and many countries where illicit substances are produced. Members of the State Department have viewed economic sanctions against these countries as incompatible with the department's foreign-policy goals. For example, the United States has known of the Panamanian government's involvement with drug dealing since the 1970s but has only recently taken action. Mexico, Colombia, Peru, Bolivia, Paraguay, and the Bahamas have all been implicated in the drug trades yet have never been sanctioned. Myanmar (formerly Burma) remains one of the world's leading producers of opium, yet U.S. support for its government remains undaunted. The United States has not, in fact, applied economic sanctions against any nation it considers an ally. And even when action is taken, profits from the drug trade offset the loss of financial support. For example, when the United States suspended aid (approximately $100 million) to Bolivia in 1980 because of its indifference to restricting drug trade, it was alleged that various Bolivian government offices netted an estimated $1.5 billion annually from narcotic traffic. Although U.S. aid to Bolivia was resumed in 1988, by the end of 1989 it was estimated that only 3,200 acres, out of 123,000 acres where coca is grown, had been eradicated.

Conversely, the United States often has no relationship with countries where production occurs. Thus Syria and Afghanistan were the first two countries eliminated as potential foreign-aid recipients, but they receive no military or economic assistance from the United States in the first place. Although Laos and Myanmar are also involved in the drug trade, U.S. ability to influence their governments' policies is minimal.

Stopping Drugs at the Border.   It has proved next to impossible to prevent illicit drugs from entering the United States once they have been harvested or refined in other countries.

Each year more than 27,000 freighters and 220,000 smaller ships sail into U.S. waters; 355 million people enter and leave the country on 635,000 planes; 89 million cars and trucks cross the borders; and over 100 million pieces of mail are delivered. A single cargo ship can carry a year's worth of cocaine. Despite intensive efforts, the U.S. Coast Guard finds drugs on only 4 percent of the vessels it boards. Even when operating with informants—some of whom are planted by dealers to mislead—only 12 percent of the Coast Guard boardings result in drug seizures.

It is equally difficult to intercept aircraft. A plane, unlike a ship, is subject to interdiction only for short periods of time. Running the Mexican border, a plane flies in U.S. airspace for less than 30 minutes; it can land on a makeshift field, unload, and take off before any intervention is possible. Customs officers cannot easily identify travelers who smuggle drugs, although the Customs Service has developed a profile of the potential drug smuggler and uses dogs to sniff out illicit substances. Customs seizures of large quantities of drugs, even recent record-high seizures, do little to reduce the overall supply.

Frustration with current efforts has led some authorities to suggest that the military become actively involved in interdiction efforts. This possibility has caused a great deal of concern, much of it from the commanders of the armed forces. Critics question both the appropriateness and the effectiveness of direct military action. Nevertheless, the military has already increased its involvement in border interdiction; their expenditures for these activities were up to $165 million in 1987 with projections of $1.2 billion to be spent in 1990. The National Guard has also been mobilized toward these efforts, especially in the border states.

Interdiction and the Cost of Dealing.   Seizures of illicit drugs and arrests by federal, state, and local agencies for dealing and possession increase each year. In 1989, for example, authorities seized approximately 1,700 pounds of opium, 181,000 pounds of cocaine, and more than 739,000 pounds of marijuana, and arrested many important narcotics dealers, seizing assets of $1 billion. Despite these efforts, cocaine imports rose by 150 percent in 1988. Up to 750 metric tons of cocaine may have been produced in 1989—more than 85 times the amount seized and probably three times the amount consumed. Similarly, in 1987, 3,000 tons of heroin were produced, with only 70 needed to supply demands in the United States.

Attempts to discourage trafficking by aggressive interdiction have proven unsuccessful because the profits to be made encourage risk taking. Yet the greatest profits are not made outside the United States. They occur once the drug enters the country and is cut for distribution and sale (see Table 20.2). One kilogram of opium, for which a buyer pays the grower about $30 to $50, sells for $4,000 to $8,000 after losing one-tenth of its volume while being refined into heroin. After arriving in the United States, it commands a price up to $200,000. When sold on the street, it yields between $1.2 million and $2.5 million in profit. Cocaine profits may be even higher because so many more people use this drug. A kilogram of Colombian cocaine that costs a distributor $5,000 may ultimately be worth more than $500,000 on the street. Yet of the $5 one pays on the street for a piece of crack, only 10 percent represents the cost of growing, producing, and getting the drug into the United States. Profits from marijuana may increase 90 times between a producer country and the United States.

Gross revenues from all drug sales in the United States approximate $120 billion per year, with an enormous profit margin of over $100 billion. After laundering drug money in banks, usually located outside the country, drug traffickers reinvest a large proportion of it in legitimate businesses. The dealer's economic risk from interdiction or confiscation is therefore minimal: a shipment of cocaine worth $200,000 on arrival in the United States costs the dealer less than $5,000. More successful interdiction, resulting in even greater seizures, would have little effect on the drug's cost or the dealer's financial risk. A Rand Corporation study found that if total seizures rose by 58 percent, there would be only a 4 percent increase in cost of delivery to the street.

The dealer risks little personally, as well; the chances of him or

TABLE 20.2
Estimated Values (per Kg) at Different Levels of Distribution

	Cocaine	Heroin	Marijuana
Refiner	$ 5,000	$ 4,000	
Exporter	$ 20,000	$ 90,000	$ 125
Distributor	$100,000	$ 200,000	$ 750
Retailer	$625,000	$1,200,000	$1,700

her actually going to prison are relatively small. In 1987 those arrested in New York City for drug-related offenses had a 50 percent chance of indictment, a 38 percent chance of conviction, and a 15 percent chance of serving time. In Washington, D.C., between 1983 and 1987 arrests for drug-related crimes increased by 45 percent, prosecutions by 500 percent, and convictions by 700 percent. Yet only 7 percent of those arrested and 20 percent of those convicted went to jail. Washington officials paid increasing attention to sentencing in 1987, and the incarceration rate doubled: a dealer stood a 50 percent chance of serving time. But the chance of a dealer serving a full sentence is remote. A recent U.S. General Accounting Office report stated that drug traffickers serve less than 40 percent of their sentences. As is well established, prisons are overcrowded and the parole system severely understaffed; early releases are common, as is inadequate supervision when on parole.

Local pressure has generated a series of counterattacks intended to further increase the risk of dealing. Some communities have authorized seizing the assets of suspected dealers. Others evacuate residents from houses and apartments where drugs are sold—some communities even destroy houses and empty whole sections of housing projects. Some local officials have imposed strict enforcement of antiloitering laws and curfews, going so far as to cordon off streets and institute random searches. In some areas membership in gangs, which are often associated with drug sales, is considered a felony. The Drug Enforcement Agency has instituted investigations of customer lists of plant supply houses in order to identify those people who purchase equipment (for whatever reason) capable of cultivating marijuana.

All these efforts illustrate the public's frustration with and fear of illicit drugs, especially in low-income areas where cocaine sales and use are sometimes highest and most destructive. But penalizing people before establishing their guilt comes at the cost of infringement on constitutional rights.

Moreover, despite stiffer sentences, seizure of assets, and even imposition of the death penalty for murder occurring during a drug operation, in reality the risk to the mid- or low-level dealer is slight, particularly when balanced against potential profits. The real risk comes not from law enforcement, but from competitors who use murder to eliminate competition and control markets. This puts the public at risk as well; bystanders may be victims as well as the intended targets.

It is obvious that reducing supply has not worked well.

REDUCING DEMAND

Demand is reduced by various means, including deterrence, education, and provision of alternatives to drug use. Pragmatically, these can be grouped as either the "carrot" or the "stick" approach.

Deterrence. Many people advocate deterrence to reduce demand for drugs. The rationale is that a sufficiently great risk will discourage use, regardless of the pleasure obtained from the drug or the discomfort experienced if the drug is unavailable. At its most basic level, deterrence links illicit drug use with civil or criminal sanctions similar to—though perhaps not so severe as—those imposed for dealing. Two good examples of deterrence are from California and New York.

In 1968 increased concern over marijuana use in California led state legislators to rewrite criminal definitions. Possession of marijuana was considered a felony and carried a penalty of one to 10 years in prison for the first offense and life imprisonment for the third offense. This law remained on the books until 1976 when, largely through the efforts of State Senator George Moscone, possession of one ounce or less of marijuana was reduced to a misdemeanor carrying no prison term and a maximum fine of $100. Although a number of people were convicted under the harsher law, there was no appreciable increase or decrease in marijuana use. Since 1976, however, California has saved over $1 billion previously spent on arrest, court, prison—and without any marked increase in marijuana use. Indeed, 40 percent of users report that they have decreased use.

In 1973 New York State passed a law imposing stiff, mandatory minimum sentences for drug-related offenses with no possibility of plea bargaining, even for possession of relatively small amounts. A study by the New York City Bar Association found heroin use just as widespread in 1976 (the same was true for marijuana and cocaine use). Use was so widespread, in fact, that any substantial punitive action would paralyze the state's judicial system.

In 1988 approximately 800,000 people were arrested for illicit drug use in the United States. From an enforcement perspective that may seem positive, until we realize that 28 million were thought to use drugs. On a purely pragmatic basis, deterrence through increased arrests and convictions for personal use does not work.

Other deterrents may or may not be more effective. Urine testing in the workplace, either for suspected drug use or as part of routine screening, may or may not deter use—no one knows. Still, Congress has passed new and more severe antidrug legislation according to which drug users lose federal student loans, the right to occupy federally financed housing, and the right to federal mortgage guarantees; plus they incur fines of up to $10,000 for possession of even small amounts of illicit drugs. We do not know whether the system has the resources to prosecute such cases or whether the laws are constitutional.

Prevention, Education, and Rehabilitation.   One key to reducing demand lies in honestly educating the public about the effects of illicit drugs. In this regard, the slogan "just say no" is inadequate. Most Americans drink alcohol, and many smoke tobacco. Many therefore use a potent mood-altering drug of some sort. To date,

America's "war" on drugs has not told anyone to say no to alcohol or tobacco with equal vehemence.

Just as any public health campaign should be directed toward those people most at risk, so should educational efforts aimed at reducing the use of mood-altering drugs (licit or illicit).

Finally, legislators and communities must address the problem of treatment. Hospitals regularly set aside beds in the winter in anticipation of the flu season, and counties periodically review and upgrade their emergency services in preparation for large-scale catastrophe. Similarly, resources for a sufficient number of effective treatment programs should be available so that any substance user wanting help can quickly be placed. In New York City heroin addicts sometimes must wait two years or more for treatment.

DECRIMINALIZATION AND LEGALIZATION

Political debate about how to end illicit drug use generally focuses on supply and demand. The issues of decriminalization and legalization, last seriously considered in the United States two decades ago for marijuana, have resurfaced as failure to curb the flourishing drug trade or decrease the number of dependent people becomes more and more obvious. The two concepts are often confused or blurred. Decriminalization would remove (or significantly reduce) criminal penalties for possession of small amounts of illicit substances intended for personal use; legalization would remove criminal penalties for possession and sale of some (or all) currently illicit substances and also subject drug sales and use to government regulation and taxation, much the same way alcohol and tobacco are controlled.

Decriminalization and legalization have significant numbers of articulate spokespersons, but many people consider these concepts unacceptable. Nationally, advocacy of either is tantamount to political suicide, although certain states have experimented with reformed drug laws. The concepts arouse emotions and heated moral and pragmatic arguments on both sides.

A compelling argument for decriminalization or legalization is that much of the billions currently spent on enforcement of the drug laws could be redirected toward education, prevention, and treatment.

Under legalization plans, sales taxes would enhance government revenues. Critics of decriminalization and legalization fear that if illicit drugs—especially cocaine—were more readily available, drug use would escalate dramatically and adverse effects would equal or exceed those of alcohol and tobacco. This is no small concern: estimates of deaths related to alcohol and tobacco range from 200,000 to 350,000 a year, as compared with deaths from illicit drug use, which are believed to be under 4,000. Many critics argue vehemently that legalization and decriminalization "send the wrong message"—that drug use is acceptable to society—or at the least dilute efforts to raise awareness about their potential adverse effects.

Decriminalization and legalization are extraordinarily complex issues that defy generalization. The arguments of proponents usually focus on the following points:

- People have used and will always use mood-altering drugs.
- People have the right to pursue behavior as long as it does not harm others.
- As noted, production, sale, and distribution of illicit drugs continue, despite enormous investments of money and personnel. Funds currently used for this enforcement could be diverted to prevention, education, and treatment.
- Current policy has little impact on criminal activities, and slight deterrent effect on the millions who use illicit drugs.
- The failure of Prohibition can serve as a model; repealing prohibitionary measures against illicit drugs carries about the same benefits and risks as did repeal of Prohibition.
- Workable models exist in other countries that permit drug use.

The counterarguments are generally equally vehement:

- Enforcement efforts have not been pursued forcefully enough and therefore cannot be dismissed as a failure. There is no guarantee that money would be saved or that any saved money would go where it is needed.
- As noted, allowing drug use in all or certain circumstances sends the wrong message. Drug use—and costs to society—would rise dramatically if sanctions were lifted.

- Prohibition may in fact have reduced alcohol-related problems; many illicit drugs have far greater potential for addiction problems than alcohol if used widely.
- Use of drugs in the privacy of one's own home does imply health and social costs to society, just as the problems related to drinking do.
- Most of society believes that use of mood-altering drugs is morally wrong, and the majority does have the right to create legal sanctions that reflect moral values.

One of the major obstacles to establishing a rational drug policy is the moral stigma surrounding drug use. Even when that stigma is removed, an absence of hard evidence makes the predictions of either side about what would happen if certain changes were made in the current laws little more than speculation.

Models of Success and Failure.   In an attempt to draw lessons from history, both advocates and critics of drug law reform have turned to past and present models.

China and the Opium Wars.   The practice of smoking opium reached China in the seventeenth century, but at first it was not widespread and only marginally concerned authorities. In the eighteenth century, however, British influence ascended in India, a center of opium production. Opium became an important commodity in the Indian tax base. To build revenues, Britain forced the exportation of the drug throughout Asia, including China.

In response to the dramatic increase in use caused by this influx, the Chinese government prohibited opium smoking in 1729 and, since the prohibition had little effect over the course of the years, banned the importation of opium in 1800. Nevertheless, imports continued unabated, averaging 340 tons a year between 1811 and 1821. The British met the emperor of China's further attempts to curtail the opium trade with opposition, and the Opium War of 1839–1842 resulted. China suffered a devastating loss. Widespread opium use continued. The need for opium led to an increase in opium production by the Chinese.

After losing a second war in 1856, the Chinese government recognized that it was unable to control opium trade or use and dropped efforts at control. British promotion of the export of opium throughout Asia continued. By 1880, Indian imports into China reached 6,500 tons. At the end of the nineteenth century, the Royal British Commission on Opium actually concluded in its report that since China was too weak to suppress opium and the profits were too great, little needed to be done.

In the early 1900s the Chinese government again attempted to suppress opium use, but allegations abounded about the involvement of political powers in the profits from opiate trade (heroin had recently been introduced to the country). The stated position of the government against opiates, accompanied by harsh penalties for use, did not measurably affect trade. When the Communists attained power, their government was determined to eliminate opiate use and did so ruthlessly and effectively. To the present time, opium and heroin are of little concern to Chinese authorities, although use certainly continues and the government probably understates the extent of the problem.

Advocates of drug law reform point out that until the Communist regime instituted draconian measures far in excess of what a democratic society would tolerate, opiate production and use flourished despite government intervention. Critics counter that as a result of widespread legal use, China twice went to war against insurmountable odds. They note the effectiveness of a forcefully committed government in suppressing use, as opposed to the ineffectiveness of a government associated with the opium trade.

The Iranian experience. Between 1968 and 1979, partly because of its inability to control the flow of opiates from Afghanistan and Pakistan into Iran and partly in an attempt to move away from a purely punitive approach to control, the Iranian government began to make opium available to users who were judged intractable to treatment and rehabilitation. Those included medically ill opium addicts and addicts 60 years of age or older. The government set up distribution centers and issued coupons that enabled duly registered people to obtain opium at a much reduced price. By 1976, the number of registered addicts had increased from about 20,000 to 200,000, with the number of people actually purchasing opium believed to be about 400,000. Corruption pervaded the system. Younger addicts, who were ineligible for the program, received their "illicit" supplies mainly by purchasing "licit" opium from those who were registered.

Advocates of decriminalization and legalization point out that the Iranian experience is irrelevant; the programs were poorly run, and illicit use, although initially curtailed, continued and increased in Iran just as use increased throughout Southeast Asia during that period. Critics note that there is every reason to expect similar problems to arise in the United States, pointing to the current diversion of methadone from the clinics into the illicit drug market as an example. They also note that the institution of a fundamentalist government in Iran willing to execute people for possession and dealing markedly decreased use. Such measures may have driven opium use underground. However, despite its stand on the use of opium by its citizens, Iran still plays a major role in the international opium scene.

The English "system". Perhaps the most remarkable and least understood feature of the British system of drug control is that it is not a system at all. It is a simple understanding, under which the government licenses qualified physicians working in narcotic treatment centers to prescribe heroin, morphine, or methadone as they see fit. The narcotic used, the method of rehabilitation, and the support services offered those who are heroin-dependent vary from clinic to clinic. The only unifying philosophy is that morphine and heroin dependency are manifestations of an illness. In Great Britain, just as treatment of a bacterial infection calls for an antibiotic, use of narcotics is justified when treating a dependent person.

But problems exist with that system, too. Although heroin and sterile needles are readily available, Great Britain has an expanding illicit narcotics market and many heroin-dependent people share unsterile needles. A significant amount of narcotics from prescriptions is diverted to the underground market; an increasing number of addicts take narcotics orally to avoid detection, making treatment more difficult. The number of heroin addicts in England had increased steadily, from about 500 in 1965 to 3,000 in 1972 to 12,000 currently. Nevertheless, this represents less than 3 percent of the heroin-dependent people in New York City and a rate of growth consistent with increased use throughout the world. The British are more and more concerned about the "heroin problem," particularly with traffic in drugs outside the system.

The Netherlands. In the Netherlands most mood-altering drugs are effectively decriminalized. Possession of small quantities is still illegal, a misdemeanor, but the government chooses not to enforce the law. People who deal in large quantities or engage in violent activities are prosecuted. Cafes can obtain permits to sell marijuana. Addicts are regarded as people with a health problem. Physicians can provide morphine and methadone as needed, and effective educational programs document the adverse effects of mood-altering drugs.

The system appears to work in all aspects. Granted, the Netherlands is not the United States. Its social programs are infinitely better, and the number of homeless and poor minimal by comparison.

U.S. reforms at the state level. Although not heavily publicized, some states now have decriminalization laws on their books. As noted, California liberalized its laws in 1976 and saved over $1 billion in a decade. Marijuana use actually decreased. Following a state Court of Appeals ruling in 1975 in Alaska, small amounts of marijuana, kept at home for personal use, were legal until a referendum to make marijuana illegal was approved by the electorate in 1990.

Some other states are considering reforms. Under the Oregon Marijuana Initiative, that state would generate funds for drug treatment by selling personal-use certificates. These certificates would permit a holder to grow a limited amount of marijuana for personal use only. Advocates are trying to obtain signatures to bring the initiative to referendum at the ballot.

Public Concerns. Ultimately, public opinion may determine the feasibility of decriminalization or legalization. Public concern over illicit drug use is at an all-time high. In a 1989 poll taken by the *New York Times*-CBS News Service, 64 percent of those surveyed believed that drugs are the biggest problem in the United States (a similar poll taken in 1985 reported less than 1 percent of those interviewed believing drugs were the most important problem). Despite evidence that illicit drug use is down, the public perceives that Americans are losing the war and wants "something done about it."

Public concern about illicit drugs seems centered on the accompanying violence and social corrosion. Frequently, people with middle and upper incomes, whose communities feel these problems less severely, advocate decriminalization or legalization. The less affluent or those whose daily lives are most affected by cocaine and other illegal drugs are less likely to stand behind reform of the current laws. Some of their concerns may be that if more people among them were to have legal access to drugs, it might further destroy the ability of these people to function productively.

Legalizing cocaine sales to adults exclusively is meaningless in neighborhoods where people are trapped by poverty and despair. As long as government fails to improve living conditions and education in poor communities, the financial rewards from dealing drugs will remain a powerful temptation.

These problems are rarely acknowledged by advocates of legalization, whose arguments tend to focus on beneficial effects to society and on people who are dependent on heroin or even marijuana.

Many critics of legalization can agree with decriminalization's goal to eliminate punishment of the user. But this view is by no means a consensus, and when the vast majority of people want "something done," they mean stronger enforcement and harsher deterrents.

ARE WE REALLY COMMITTED?

An unpopular explanation for failure of the war on drugs, and one rarely mentioned by those in the establishment, is that the U.S. government's commitment to diminish drug use is debatable. Unfortunately, a number of factors suggest that this commitment is far from total.

In the fall of 1989, President Bush released his administration's National Drug Control Strategy under the coordination of William J. Bennett, director of the newly created White House Office of National Drug Control Policy. The plan calls for enhanced enforcement through increasing federal prison capacity, better-financed state and local law enforcement efforts, and vigorous prosecution and tougher penalties for sales and use—even casual use—of drugs. The plan also advocates increased military and economic aid to South American countries such as Bolivia, Colombia, and Peru to assist in their fight against drug producers and traffickers and new interdiction efforts to prevent chemicals used to synthesize drugs from getting into the United States. It suggests regulations to make money laundering of drug profits more difficult. It encourages international conferences to develop a coordinated effort to diminish drug use.

At home, the Drug Control Strategy calls for education, especially in schools, and communitywide drug prevention efforts. The plan wants schools, colleges, and universities to adopt a "get-tough" policy toward drug use on campuses. It suggests that the government form a Demand-Reduction Working Group to coordinate and implement all policies and strategies, including establishment of a drug-free workplace. Increased funding would go for treatment programs, and third-party carriers would be encouraged to provide insurance coverage. The plan promotes coordination and accountability among treatment programs and exploration of "civil commitment" (boot camps) as a means of expanding therapeutic alternatives. Expanded resources would allow better data collection for evaluation of treatment efficacy.

The policy appears to address the issues. But on closer scrutiny the question of commitment becomes apparent. First, the division of funds allocates 70 percent of the budget to enforcement. The 30 percent left over for programs to decrease demand represents an increase of less than 5 percent. Even with respect to the enforcement budget, which may exceed $3 billion in 1991, a significant amount will go toward increasing federal prison space, unrelated to a drug strategy. Moreover, the amount of money actually available is far less than that called for and must be taken from other programs. The social services programs, already underfunded and essential in providing effective rehabilitation, are the most vulnerable to cuts. Since the effects of drug dependency are most severe in poorer communities, insufficient funding for social programs practically guarantees failure. The administration has committed for 1991 an extra $1.13

billion to fight illicit drug use. Although in absolute dollars the amount allocated for treatment would rise by $260 million, the proportion devoted to health care programs would actually decline while the share for domestic law enforcement would increase by $5.2 billion, or 14 percent. Treatment and prevention still remain underfunded. This effort is still sorely underfunded and, when compared to the costs of rehabilitation of drug users and those children damaged by parental drug use, still inadequate.

Prosecutors cannot pursue convictions for possession of small amounts of illicit substances without becoming mired in an overburdened legal system. Further clogging of U.S. courts will allow meaningful violation of the drug laws to receive little attention. Establishing a "zero tolerance" for all drugs, including marijuana possession, and prosecuting offenses with the same vigor as cocaine and heroin trafficking will aggravate the problem.

Even the goals set by the administration appear to be rather modest. In fact, prior to the implementation of this plan, surveys of high school seniors and young adults as well as the National Household Survey on Drug Abuse revealed that the use of illicit drugs was at its lowest level in the past decade despite increased availability. Indeed, many of the Public Health Service's 1990 Health Objectives of the Nation regarding alcohol and substance abuse were already met prior to the initiation of the administration's war on drugs. This is not to suggest that there is any reason for complacency; rather, the commitment to bring about significant changes in drug use appears somewhat lacking.

Finally, it has recently been alleged that the administration has failed to satisfy its own requirement to reach agreements with other countries to identify and prevent concealment of illegal drug profits through money laundering. Under the law, any country that does not reach such an agreement with the United States could be excluded from our financial system. To avoid these sanctions, the country must agree to keep records of any large transactions made in United States dollars. These records would then be filed by banks and other financial institutions in this country. Such information can be important in tracing the flow of money from established drug dealers. Countries that have failed to reach such an agreement with the United States include some of those long suspected to be involved in money laundering, such as Panama, Colombia, and most recently Hong Kong. Although the main reason given by the administration for its decision not to enforce sanctions is that such measures will violate the country's sovereignty, this also may be viewed as a lack of total commitment.

The administration's fiscal year 1990 request of about $7.9 billion was recognized as being inadequate to accomplish its objectives. In response, Congress voted to increase funding in fiscal 1990 to $9.4 billion, to be financed by a budget cut of 0.43 percent on all domestic and military programs.

However, Congress's track record in this regard also does not lead one toward optimism. In October 1988 Congress authorized $3.8 billion to fight this "war," yet agreed to spend only $961 million, less than the cost of one Trident submarine. Although the Congressional Comprehensive Antidrug Bill contained a number of important provisions, including direction of more funds to treatment and accepting the principle of treatment on demand, implementation of this act remains to be seen.

REDRAWING THE BATTLE LINES

In our enthusiasm for joining the "war on drugs," we often forget that the reason for preventing use is related not to morality but to the adverse effects, both physical and psychological. The "war"—if one insists on using the term—is therefore primarily against the use of these substances, not against the user. More than 30 million Americans use illicit drugs; tens of millions more regularly drink alcohol or smoke tobacco. Perhaps it is the confusion over who or what is to blame—the drugs, the user, or the use—and what should be done that has led to oppressive and at times unworkable antidrug legislation and extreme attitudes that equate addiction with moral perversity.

Success therefore has been limited for a variety of reasons. Rather than blindly forging ahead, perhaps it is time to reexamine how and why we are fighting drugs. Whose war is it, and who is the enemy? What are we trying to win? It is entirely possible that we may never be able to "win" if winning is synonymous with ending all use of mood-altering drugs. No matter what the obstacles, people have always used mood-altering substances. In order to minimize the damage, we should consider and reconsider the full range of options available to us—how the laws are written, how we enforce the laws, how we deter use, and availability of treatment.

Appendix A:
Drug Use Reporting Sources

- Community Epidemiology Work Group (CEWG), Epidemiologic Trends in Drug Abuse, December 1988
  Combines data from a variety of sources, to develop current trends in and patterns of drug use. Sponsored by the National Institute on Drug Abuse.

- Drug Use, Drinking and Smoking: National Survey Results From High School, College, and Young Adult Populations, 1975–1990
  Conducted annually by Lloyd Johnston, M.D., and colleagues at the University of Michigan. Uses representative samples of approximately 17,000 seniors, 135 public and private high schools nationwide, as well as 1,200 college students and 11,000 young adults up to 11 years after high school. Sponsored by the National Institute on Drug Abuse.

- Food and Drug Administration (FDA) Annual Review of National Drug Use
  The FDA collects data on the use of prescription drugs by indication, classification of drugs, and characteristics of prescribing physician.

- National Household Survey on Drug Abuse
  Conducted every several years since 1971. It is a general population survey of more than 25,000 households, with household members age 12 and above. Sponsored by the National Institute on Drug Abuse.

- Drug Abuse Warning Network (DAWN)
  Reports from selected emergency rooms and medical examiners

offices throughout the United States. Sponsored by the National Institute on Drug Abuse.

- Client Oriented Data Acquisition Process (CODAP)
  Collects demographic data on drug-free and on-maintenance persons entering treatment programs throughout the United States. Sponsored by the National Institute on Drug Abuse.

- National Drug and Alcoholism Treatment Unit Survey (NDATUS): 1987
  Census (as of October 30, 1987) of all drug abuse and alcoholism treatment facilities in the United States. Sponsored by the National Institute on Drug Abuse and the National Institute on Alcohol Abuse and Alcoholism.

- National Disease and Therapeutic Index (NDTI)
  Data collected quarterly from individual physicians containing drug orders for patients for 48-hour period.

- National Prescription Adult (NPA)
  Produced by the trade journal *Pharmacy Times*. Lists the top 200 drugs dispensed from retail pharmacies to patients, based on a nationwide survey of 2,000 retail pharmacies reporting on approximately 36 million prescriptions filled.

- *New York Times*-CBS News Survey
  A single survey based on telephone interviews with 824 adults in the continental United States. Phone numbers selected by computer. Results differ no more than plus or minus three percentage points from those obtained had all adults been surveyed.

Appendix B:
Drug-Testing Technology

COMMON URINE-TESTING TECHNIQUES

The most common techniques are thin-layer chromatography and immunoassay for initial screening, and gas-liquid chromatography with mass spectrometry for confirmation.

Thin-Layer Chromatography (TLC). In TLC, drugs or drug products (metabolites) in the urine are treated with solvents and then allowed to move by capillary action over a coated glass plate or plastic film. The coating contains mixtures of known drug compounds, each drug represented as a separate spot and serving as a standard. As the solvent-treated urine specimen moves across the plate, the substances separate and are identified by a spray that produces color reactions in the substances in the specimen and in the standard.

TLC can provide relatively rapid, simultaneous detection of a number of mood-altering drugs or their metabolites (Table A.1) at relatively low cost. But the test is not extraordinarily sensitive, and its accuracy may depend on the skill of the technician in distinguishing the patterns and colors of the drugs being tested from other substances in the urine.

Immunoassays. In immunoassay, a laboratory animal is injected with the drug to be tested for so that its immune system develops an antibody to that drug. Serum containing the antibody (capable of binding to the drug) is drawn from the animal and placed in a test tube with a quantity of the drug—"labeled" with an enzyme or

TABLE A.1
Detection of Drugs by Thin-Layer Chromatography (TLC)

Drugs Not Readily Detected	Drugs Detectable after Use	
	After 3 to 12 Hours	After 24 or More Hours
Cannabinoids	Cocaine	Amphetamines
(marijuana)	Opiates	Benzodiazepines
Phencyclidine	Pentazocine	(Librium, Valium,
(PCP)	(Talwin)	Dalmane, etc.)
Hallucinogens		Propoxyphene (Darvon)
		Nicotine
		Tricyclic
		antidepressants

radioactive isotope. The urine specimen is added, and the mixture incubated. During this time the labeled and unlabeled drug compete for sites on the antibody, and a precipitate consisting of the antibody-drug combination is formed.

The amount of the unattached labeled drug remaining, or the amount of labeled drug attached to the precipitate, indicates the extent of drug use. Depending on the test used, the result is measured as the amount of enzyme activity remaining (EIA) or as remaining radioactivity (RIA). The fluorescence polarization immunoassay (FIA), another technique, involves the use of polarized light.

These tests are sensitive; they detect a number of substances (Tables A.2, A.3) for which there are defined minimal threshold levels. Probably the most popular test in the United States is the EIA technique called the Enzyme Multiplier Immunoassay Test (EMIT). It provides an easily measured, fairly rapid analysis of drug use.

Confirmation Tests. Both laboratory errors and substances similar in structure to drugs being tested for can produce false-positive results, so all positive results should be confirmed through more sensitive tests. Confirming tests using gas chromatography with mass spectrometry are exceptionally accurate, but expensive and complex.

TABLE A.2
Drugs Detectable by Urine Immunoassay

Alcohol	Cannabinoids (marijuana)
Amphetamines	Cocaine
	Methadone
Barbiturates	Methaqualone (Quaalude)
Benzodiazepines	Opiates (by class)
(Valium, Librium, etc.)	Phencyclidine (PCP)
	Propoxyphene (Darvon)

TABLE A.3
Timetable for Detection of Drugs by Urine Immunoassay

Drug	Days*
Amphetamines	1 to 3
Barbiturates	3 to 4
Cocaine including metabolites	2 to 3
Codeine (as morphine)	2 to 4
Heroin (as morphine)	2 to 4
Marijuana acute use	1 to 10
daily use	to 30
Phencyclidine (PCP)	2 to 7

*Variation depends on whether use is acute or chronic.

Used properly and consistently with every positive specimen, they virtually eliminate the possibility of false-positive reactions.

URINE-TESTING EFFECTIVENESS

A number of factors must be considered in evaluating the concept of widespread urine testing of those not known to be at high risk for drug abuse:

- accuracy of the testing technique
- meaning of false-positive and false-negative reactions
- limits of detection
- value of detection when employee is unimpaired at work
- value of screening to help the substance abuser
- risks to confidentiality when detected drugs were prescribed by physicians for specific medical conditions

Test Accuracy.   Despite increasing use of urine screening, the accuracy of the tests leaves something to be desired. In 1985 the Centers for Disease Control (CDC), in conjunction with the National Institute on Drug Abuse, evaluated 13 laboratories serving 262 methadone maintenance treatment programs. Error rates (false positives) on urines containing known drugs ran 11 to 94 percent for barbiturates, 19 to 100 percent for amphetamines, 0 to 33 percent for methadone, 0 to 100 percent for both cocaine and codeine, and 5 to 100 percent for morphine. For specimens not containing drugs, the error rates ran 6 percent for barbiturates, 37 percent for amphetamines, 66 percent for methadone, 6 percent for cocaine, 7 percent for codeine, and 10 percent for morphine. And in a subsequent study on 500 prospective hospital employees, 33 had initial positive results, but only 13 could be confirmed.

To rectify this high-error situation, the federal government initiated a certification program to identify laboratories believed capable of providing accurate test results in the high volume necessary. The hope is that enough laboratories with standard quality-assurance procedures can be certified to drastically cut testing errors.

Test accuracy depends on the sensitivity of the specific technique as well as on the laboratory-determined cut-off point for dividing tests into positive and negative results. Sensitivity is the point at which a particular drug can't be detected, no matter how recently it was taken.

Because the test reliability diminishes as the drug concentration in the urine decreases to the sensitivity threshold, a cut-off point is used in most laboratories (Table A.4). Concentration of a drug below that point is read as negative, even if the substance is detected. In practice, to diminish the likelihood of false positives, the cut-off point is usually set above the sensitivity of a specific test.

Certain over-the-counter preparations and other commonly used products have been known to produce false-positive readings (Table A.5).

False-negative responses are equally important. Most false-negative urine tests are the result of mechanical and logistical problems. Switching of specimens—intentionally or accidentally—obviously prevents a true reading. The newest automated analyzers can turn out 18,000 results an hour, so a mechanical switch is certainly conceivable.

Other ways of producing false-negatives include: diluting the urine to lower concentration of the drug; using diuretics, a method well known to drug users and athletes; and changing urine acidity/alkalinity (pH). Acidifying urine can increase PCP excretion fivefold. Adding large quantities of salt to urine can also interfere with detection.

Limits of Detection. Other critical factors that determine test accuracy include the amount of drug taken, frequency of use, and elapsed time between use and submission of the specimen. The role of each factor varies from drug to drug.

A positive result indicates only that the identified substance was taken sometime before the test. It doesn't indicate either past or present impairment. For example, a single marijuana cigarette can yield a positive urine test for up to three days; a chronic user may test positive for up to a month after stopping. Cocaine is rapidly eliminated from the body, but its metabolites are detectable up to

TABLE A.4
Cut-Off Levels for Drugs in Urine Immunoassay

Drug	Cut-Off Level*
Amphetamines	1,000
Cocaine metabolites	300
Marijuana (cannabinoids)	100
Opiates	300
Phencyclidine (PCP)	25

*Levels, measured in nanograms (billionths of a gram) per milliliter (ng/ml), may vary in some laboratories.

TABLE A.5
Substances Capable of Producing False-Positive Results in Urine Immunoassay

Drug Tested for	Substance Causing False-Positive Result
Amphetamines	Contac, Sudafed, diet pills, decongestants, antiasthma medications containing phenylpropanolamine and ephedrine
Opiates	Dextromethorphan cough syrups, poppy seeds*
Marijuana	Ibuprofen preparations (Advil, Haltran, Nuprin, Pamprin, Medipren, Rufen, Ifen, Trendar)**
Cocaine	Herbal teas, and as with amphetamines
Methadone	Benadryl

*Three poppy seed bagels have produced morphine levels above 2,500 ng/ml and codeine levels above 200 ng/ml.

**These substances were initially identified only with EMIT, a technique since modified to eliminate such false positives.

three days after a single dose. A single dose of amphetamine results in positive urine for one day; in a chronic user for three days.

Urines will be positive for morphine for several days after a heroin injection. But morphine is found in poppy seeds and a wide variety of drugs, so a single positive urine doesn't necessarily mean drug use.

Central nervous system depressants vary in how long they show up in urine tests. Intermediate-acting barbiturates can be detected for up to three days; some benzodiazepines for up to a month following chronic use.

Phencyclidine or its metabolites can be detected for up to a week with acute use and for several weeks in chronic users.

RISKS TO CONFIDENTIALITY

Perhaps the greatest ethical dilemma arises when a positive urine test results from a physician's prescription for a medical condition.

A former heroin addict, functioning extremely well on methadone maintenance therapy, risks being dismissed following a positive urine test, even though it is legal for methadone to be prescribed and used.

Detection of marijuana (THC) prescribed for nausea caused by chemotherapy violates a person's right to be treated for a serious disease without his or her employer's knowledge. Use of amphetamines for refractory depression falls within this realm as well. Under such circumstances, if performance isn't impaired, there's no justification for violating privacy.

Similar—though less important—situations arise with prescriptions for amphetaminelike drugs for weight loss or narcolepsy, cough suppressants or opiate analgesics for pain syndromes, use of cocaine as an anesthesia in dental or throat surgery, and, most common of all, use of central nervous system depressants for treatment of anxiety.

Perhaps the most important statement on urine screening was issued by the American Society of Clinical Pharmacology and Therapeutics (ASCPT) in 1988. This group of experts in testing agreed that a positive test provides only limited information on the drug dose or on whether its use was recent or chronic. Further, the pharmacological effect of the drug in the user—either at time of sampling, in the past, or in the future—cannot be determined. Concern was expressed that not all laboratories are following defined, high-quality testing standards.

The conclusion was that testing should be based on scientific or clinical evidence of behavioral changes that lead to impairment in the workplace. But the U.S. Supreme Court decision made clear that where public safety is concerned, testing even without suspicion of use is allowed. The ruling also was applied to those indirectly involved with public safety—federal employees who intercept drugs, carry firearms, or have classified material authorization.

Appendix C:
List of Common Street Names
for Drugs

Note: Street names may vary from one geographic area to another. Also, one street name can refer to two or more different drugs.

Street Name—Drug Name (Drug Group*)
Acapulco Gold—Marijuana
Acid—LSD (H)
Adam—Hallucinogen
Angel Dust—Phencyclidine (H)
Aroma—Nitrite Inhalant
Banapple Gas—Nitrite Inhalant
Bang—Nitrite Inhalant
Barbs—Barbiturate (H/S)
Barrels—LSD (H)
Bazooka—Crack Cocaine (S)
Beans—Barbiturate (H/S)
Bennies—Amphetamine (S)
Berkely Boo—Marijuana
Bhang—Ganga (M)
Big Chief—Peyote (H)
Big M—Narcotic
Bing—Heroin (N)
Biscuits—Barbiturate (H/S)
Biscutt—Methadone (N)
Black Tar—Heroin (N)
Blanco—Cocaine (S)
Blockbusters—Barbiturate (H/S)
Blotter—LSD (H)
Blow—Cocaine (S)
Blow—Inhalant
Blue Angels—Amphetamine (S)
Blue Birds—Barbiturate (H/S)
Blue Cap—LSD (H)
Blue Cheer—LSD (H)
Blue Devils—Barbiturate (H/S)
Blue Dots—LSD (H)
Blue Heaven—Barbiturate (H/S)
Blues—Barbiturate (H/S)
Blue Velvet—Narcotic/Antihistamine
Bolt—Nitrite Inhalant
Bombitas—Heroin/Amphetamine (N)
Boy Jive—Heroin (N)
Brick—Marijuana
Brown—Heroin (N)
Bullet—Nitrite Inhalant
Bullets—Barbiturate (H/S)

Street Name—Drug Name (Drug Group*)
Businessman's Special—Hallucinogen
Buttons—Peyote (H)
C—Cocaine (S)
Caballo—Heroin (N)
Cabona—Inhalant
Cactus—Peyote (H)
Caine—Cocaine (S)
California Sunshine—LSD (H)
Camel—LSD (H)
Candles—LSD (H)
Caplets—Amphetamine (S)
Charas—Ganga (M)
Cheery Top—LSD (H)
China White—Fentanyl (N)
Chivo—Heroin (N)
Chris/Christine—Amphetamine (S)
Christmas Trees—Barbiturate (H/S)
Climax—Nitrite Inhalant
Coca—Cocaine (S)
Coke—Cocaine (S)
Cola—Cocaine (S)
Crack—Crack Cocaine (S)
Crank—Amphetamine (S)
Crap—Heroin (N)
Crisscross—Amphetamine (S)
Crossroads—Amphetamine (S)
Crypt—Nitrite Inhalant
Crystal—Phencyclidine (H)
Crystal—Amphetamine (S)
Crystal—Crack Cocaine (S)
Cube—Narcotic
Cube-D—LSD (H)
Cum—Nitrite Inhalant
Cyclone—Phencyclidine (H)
Dead on Arrival—Heroin (N)
Dexies—Amphetamine (S)
Disks—Methadone (N)
DOA—Phencyclidine (H)
Dollies—Methadone (N)
Dolls—Barbiturate (H/S)
Doo Doo—Heroin (N)

*Drug groups indicated in parentheses are (H) = Hallucinogen, (M) = Marijuana, (N) = Narcotic or Opiate, (S) = Stimulant, (H/S) = Hypnotic/Sedative.

Street Name—Drug Name (Drug Group*)
Dope—Heroin (N)
Downers—Barbiturate (H/S)
Downs—Barbiturate (H/S)
Dragon—LSD (H)
Drops—Hypnotic/Sedative
Dugga—Ganga (M)
Duke—Heroin (N)
Dust—Phencyclidine (H)
Dynamite—Heroin (N)
Ecstasy—Hallucinogen
Elephant—Phencyclidine (H)
Estuffan—Heroin (N)
Eve—Hallucinogen
First Line—Narcotic
Flake—Cocaine (S)
Foolish Pleasure—Heroin (N)
Fool Pills—Barbiturate (H/S)
Footballs—Amphetamine (S)
Fours—Narcotic
French Fries—Crack Cocaine (S)
Fry Daddie—Crack Cocaine (S)
Funk—Heroin (N)
Girl—Cocaine (S)
Glory—Hallucinogen
Gold Dust—Cocaine (S)
Goma—Narcotic
Goma de Mota—Ganga (M)
Goofballs—Barbiturate (H/S)
Goon—Phencyclidine (H)
Grass—Marijuana
Green Dragons—Barbiturate (H/S)
Green Frogs—Hypnotic/Sedative
Greenies—Barbiturate (H/S)
H—Heroin (N)
Hard-on—Nitrite Inhalant
Hardware—Nitrite Inhalant
Hash—Hashish (M)
Hawaiian—Marijuana
Hay—Marijuana
Hearts—Amphetamine (S)
Heaven Dust—Cocaine (S)
Hemp—Marijuana
Herb—Marijuana
Highball—Nitrite Inhalant
Hits—Hypnotic/Sedative
Hombre—Heroin (N)
Horse—Heroin (N)
Ice—Amphetamine (S)
Iranian Heroin—Heroin (N)
Itog—Phencyclidine (H)
J—Marijuana
Jamaican—Marijuana
Jive—Marijuana
Jive—Heroin (N)
Joc—Nitrite Inhalant
Joint—Marijuana
Junk—Heroin (N)
Key—Marijuana
Kick—Nitrite Inhalant

Street Name—Drug Name (Drug Group*)
Kif—Ganga (M)
Killer Weed—Phencyclidine (H)
King Tut—LSD (H)
Kitty Kat—Amphetamine-like (S)
Knockout—Hypnotic/Sedative
Krystal—Phencyclidine (H)
La Bamba—Heroin (N)
Lady Line Muser—Cocaine (S)
LA Ice—Amphetamine (S)
Lid—Marijuana
Lip Poppers—Amphetamine (S)
Liquid Increase—Nitrite Inhalant
Loads (Setups)—Heroin (N)
Locker—Nitrite Inhalant
Locker Room—Nitrite Inhalant
Locoweed—Marijuana
Loveboat—Phencyclidine (H)
Love Drug—Hallucinogen
Love Pill—Hallucinogen
Ludes—Hypnotic/Sedative
Ludies—Amphetamine-like (S)
Machohina—Ganga (M)
Magic Mushroom—Psilocibin (H)
Man—LSD (H)
Marijuana—Marijuana
Mary Jane—Marijuana
MDEA—Hallucinogen
MDM—Hallucinogen
MDMA—Hallucinogen
Mean Greens—Hypnotic/Sedative
Mesc—Peyote (H)
Mescal—Peyote (H)
Mets—Amphetamine (S)
Mexicana—Hallucinogen
Mexican Brown—Heroin (N)
Mexican Mud—Heroin (N)
Mexican Reds—Barbiturate (H/S)
Microdot—LSD (H)
Micro Dots—Narcotic
Minibeenies—Amphetamine (S)
Mint—Phencyclidine (H)
Miss Emma—Narcotic
Mr. Natural—LSD (H)
MJ—Marijuana
Mollies—Amphetamine (S)
Monkey Dust—Phencyclidine (H)
Monkey Juice—Methadone (N)
Moonrock—Crack Cocaine (S), Heroin (N)
Morph—Narcotic
Morphine—Narcotic
Mota—Marijuana
MPPP—Narcotic
MPTP—Narcotic
Mud—Heroin (N)
Muggles—Marijuana
Mutah—Marijuana
Nose Candy—Cocaine (S)
Number 1—Heroin (N)
Number 2—Heroin (N)

Street Name—Drug Name (Drug Group*)
Number 3—Heroin (N)
Number 4—Heroin (N)
Oranges—Amphetamine (S)
Orange Sunshine—LSD (H)
Owsleys—LSD (H)
Pajao—Barbiturate (H/S)
Pape Acid—LSD (H)
Paradise—Cocaine (S)
PCP—Phencyclidine (H)
Peace—Hallucinogen
Peace—Phencyclidine (H)
Peace Pill—Phencyclidine (H)
Peaches—Amphetamine (S)
Pep Pills—Amphetamine (S)
Percolators—Narcotic
Perico—Cocaine (S)
Peruvian Flake—Cocaine (S)
Peter—Hypnotic/Sedative
Pink Ladies—Barbiturate (H/S)
Pinks—Amphetamine (S)
Pinks and Grays—Darvon
Plastivil—Hypnotic/Sedative
PMA—Hallucinogen
Pocket Rockets—Amphetamine-like (S)
Polvo—Cocaine (S)
Pop—Inhalant
Popper—Nitrite Inhalant
Pot—Marijuana
Purple Haze—LSD (H)
Purple Hearts—Barbiturate (H/S)
Quads—Hypnotic/Sedative
Quas—Hypnotic/Sedative
Rainbows—Barbiturate (H/S)
Ready Rock—Crack Cocaine (S)
Red Birds—Barbiturate (H/S)
Red Chicken—Heroin (N)
Red Devils—Barbiturate (H/S)
Reds—Barbiturate (H/S)
Reefer—Marijuana
Roach—Marijuana
Rock—Crack Cocaine (S)
Rojo—Barbiturate (H/S)
Rope—Hashish (M)
Rosas—Amphetamine (S)
Rush—Nitrite Inhalant
Satan's Scout—Nitrite Inhalant
Sativa—Marijuana
Scat—Heroin (N)
Scuffle—Phencyclidine (H)
Seccies—Barbiturate (H/S)
Serenity—Hallucinogen
Sherman—Phencyclidine (H)
Shit—Heroin (N)
Shroom—Psilocibin (H)
Silly Putty—Psilocibin (H)
Sinsemilla—Marijuana
Skag—Heroin (N)
Skunk—Marijuana

Street Name—Drug Name (Drug Group*)
Sleeping Pills—Barbiturate (H/S)
Smack—Heroin (N)
Snappers—Nitrite Inhalant
Sniff—Inhalant
Snow—Cocaine (S)
Soapers—Hypnotic/Sedative
Soaps—Hypnotic/Sedative
Soles—Hashish (M)
Space Base—Crack Cocaine (S)
Space Cadet—Crack Cocaine (S), PCP (H)
Speed—Amphetamine (S)
Speedball—Heroin/Cocaine (N)
Splash—Amphetamine (S)
Stick—Marijuana
STP—Hallucinogen
Stumblers—Barbiturate (H/S)
Sugar—Heroin (N)
Supergrass—Phencyclidine (H)
Superkool—Phencyclidine (H)
Superpot—Phencyclidine (H)
Surfer—Phencyclidine (H)
Sweet Jesus—Heroin (N)
Sweet Lucy—Hashish (M)
T—Phencyclidine (H)
Tac—Phencyclidine (H)
Tango and Cash—Narcotic
Tar—Crack Cocaine (S), Heroin (N)
Tea—Marijuana
Thrusters—Amphetamine (S)
Tocas Tea—Marijuana
Tooies—Barbiturate (H/S)
Toolies—Barbiturate (H/S)
Toot—Cocaine (S)
Tragic Magic—Crack Cocaine (S), PCP (H)
Tran Q—Phencyclidine (H)
Tranquillity—Hallucinogen
Trees—Barbiturate (H/S)
Truck Drivers—Amphetamine (S)
T's and Blues—Narcotic/Antihistamine
Tuiys—Barbiturate (H/S)
25—LSD (H)
Uppers—Amphetamine (S)
Ups—Amphetamine (S)
Vaporole—Nitrite Inhalant
Wafers—Methadone (N)
Wake-ups—Amphetamine (S)
Water—Amphetamine (S)
Wedges—LSD (H)
Weed—Marijuana
Weed—Phencyclidine (H)
White—Cocaine (S)
White Lightning—LSD (H)
Whites—Amphetamine (S)
Window Panes—LSD (H)
XTC—Hallucinogen
Yerba—Marijuana
Zigzag—LSD (H)

Selected References

Preface

Brecher, E. M. *Licit & Illicit Drugs. The Consumers Union Report on Narcotics, Stimulants, Depressants, Inhalants, Hallucinogens, and Marijuana—Including Caffeine, Nicotine, and Alcohol.* Boston: Little, Brown, 1972.

"Drugs of Abuse: Cannabis." *Drug Enforcement* 6 (1979): 34–37.

"Drugs of Abuse: Depressants." *Drug Enforcement* 6 (1979): 18–19.

"Drugs of Abuse: Hallucinogens." *Drug Enforcement* 6 (1979): 28–31.

"Drugs of Abuse: Narcotics." *Drug Enforcement* 6 (1979): 10–17.

"Drugs of Abuse: Stimulants." *Drug Enforcement* 6 (1979): 24–27.

Goodman Gilman, A., L. S. Goodman, T. W. Rall, et al., eds. *Goodman and Gilman's The Pharmacological Basis of Therapeutics.* 7th Edition, New York: Macmillan, 1985. 8th Edition, New York: Pergamon, 1990.

National Institute on Drug Abuse. *Drug Abuse and Drug Abuse Research II: The Triennial Report to Congress from the Secretary's Department of Health and Human Services.* Rockville, Md.: National Institute on Drug Abuse, 1984. DHHS Publication No. (ADM) 85-1372.

Schuckit, M. A. *Drug and Alcohol Abuse: A Clinical Guide to Diagnosis and Treatment.* New York: Plenum Medical Book Co., 1979.

Wilford, B. B. *Drug Abuse: A Guide for the Primary Care Physician.* Chicago: American Medical Association, 1981.

1. Who Uses Drugs

Alcohol and Health: Seventh Special Report to the United States Congress from the Secretary of Health and Human Services. Rockville, Md.: U.S. Dept. of Health and Human Services, 1990.

Avorn, J., P. Dreyer, K. Connelly, et al. "Use of Psychoactive Medication and the Quality of Care in Rest Homes." *New England Journal of Medicine* 320 (1989): 227–32.

Barnes, D. M. "Drugs: Running the Numbers." *Science* 240 (1988): 1729–31.

Bell, C. S., and R. Battjes. *Prevention Research: Deterring Drug Abuse Among Children and Adolescents.* NIDA Research Monograph 63. Rockville, Md.: U.S. Dept. of Health and Human Services, Public Health Service, Alcohol, Drug Abuse, and Mental Health Administration, 1985.

Berke, R. L. "Poll Finds Many in U.S. Back Bush Strategy on Drugs." *The New York Times,* September 12, 1989, A14.

Blum, R. H., and Associates. *Utopiates: The Use and Users of LSD 25.* Stanford University. Institute for the Study of Human Problems. New York: Atherton Press, 1970.

Bradley, A. M. "Capsule Review of the State of the Art: The Sixth Special Report to the U.S. Congress on Alcohol and Health." *Alcohol Health & Research World* 11 (1987): 4–9.

Brook, J. S., D. J. Lettieri, and D. W. Brook. "Alcohol and Substance Abuse in Adolescence." Special issue of *Advances in Alcohol & Substance Abuse* 4 (3/4) (1985): 1–204.

"CEOs See Drug Abuse as a Growing Problem." *American Medical News,* September 1, 1989, 20.

Community Epidemiology Work Group. *Epidemiologic Trends in Drug Abuse Proceedings.* Rockville, Md.: National Institute on Drug Abuse, 1989.

Cook, R. F. "Drug Use Among Working Adults: Prevalence Rates and Estimation Methods." In *Drugs in the Workplace.* NIDA Research Monograph 91. Rockville, Md.: U.S. Dept. of Health and Human Services, 1989.

Gunby, P. "Nation's Expenditures for Alcohol, Other Drugs, in Terms of Therapy, Prevention, Now Exceed $1.6 Billion." *Journal of the American Medical Association* 258 (1987): 2023.

Johnston, L. P., M. O'Malley, and J. G. Bachman. *Drug Use, Drinking and Smoking: National Survey Results from High School, College and Young Adult Population, 1975–1988.* Rockville, Md.: National Institute on Drug Abuse. Alcohol, Drug Abuse, and Mental Health Administration, 1989.

Jones, C. L., and R. J. Battjes. *Etiology of Drug Abuse: Implications for Prevention.* National Institute on Drug Abuse Research

Monograph 56. Rockville, Md.: U.S. Dept. of Health and Human Services, Public Health Service, Alcohol, Drug Abuse and Mental Health Administration, 1986.

Kaestner, E., B. Frank, R. Marel, et al. "Substance Use Among Females in New York State: Catching Up with the Males." *Advances in Alcohol & Substance Abuse* 5(3) (1986): 29–49.

Kozel, N. J., and E. H. Adams. "Epidemiology of Drug Abuse: An Overview." *Science* 234 (1986): 970–74.

Lewin, L. *Phantastica: Narcotic and Stimulating Drugs: Their Use and Abuse.* Translated by P. A. Wirth. London: Kegan Paul, Trench, Trubner, 1931. Republished London: Routledge and Kegan, 1964.

Lund, A. K., D. F. Preusser, R. D. Blomberg, et al. "Drug Use by Tractor-Trailer Drivers." *Journal of Forensic Sciences* 33 (1988): 648–61.

National Institute on Alcohol Abuse and Alcoholism. *Alcohol and Aging.* Rockville, Md.: U.S. Dept. of Health and Human Services, Public Health Service, Alcohol, Drug Abuse, and Mental Health Administration, 1988.

Newcomb, M. D., and P. M. Bentler. *Consequences of Adolescent Drug Use.* Newbury Park, Calif.: Sage Publications, 1988.

Overview of the 1988 National Household Survey on Drug Abuse. NIDA Capsules. Rockville, Md.: National Institute on Drug Abuse, 1989.

Ruben, D. H. "The Elderly Alcoholic: Some Current Dimensions." *Advances in Alcohol & Substance Abuse* 5(4) (1986): 59–70.

Simonsen, L. L. "Top 200 Drugs of 1987: New Prescription Volume Increases 4.2% Moving Total Rxs Up 1.4%." *Pharmacy Times* 54 (1988): 38–46.

Stanford Research Institute, National Institute on Drug Abuse, Services Research Branch. *The Aging Process and Psychoactive Drug Use.* Rockville, Md.: U.S. Dept. of Health, Education, and Welfare, Public Health Service, Alcohol, Drug Abuse, and Mental Health Administration, Services Research Branch, Division of Resource Development, National Institute on Drug Abuse; DHEW Publication No. (ADM) 79–813; Washington, D.C.: U.S. Government Printing Office, 1979.

Trimble, J., A. Padilla, and C. Bell. *Drug Abuse Among Ethnic Minorities.* DHHS Publishing No. 87-1474. Rockville, Md.: National Institute on Drug Abuse, 1987.

United States General Accounting Office. *Comprehensive Approach Needed to Help Control Prescription Drug Abuse Summary: Report to the Congress of the United States by the Comptroller General.* Washington, D.C.: U.S. General Accounting Office, 1982.

Washton, A. M., and M. S. Gold. "Recent Trends in Cocaine Abuse: A View from the National Hotline, '800-COCAINE.' " *Advances in Alcohol & Substance Abuse* 6(2) (1986): 31–47.

2. Classifying Mood-Altering Drugs

Barnett, G., and R. S. Rapaka. "Designer Drugs: An Overview." In *Cocaine, Marijuana, Designer Drugs: Chemistry, Pharmacology, and Behavior,* edited by K. K. Redda, C. A. Walker, and G. Barnett. Boca Raton: CRC Press, 1989.

Culhane, C. "Court Says No to Peyote." *The U.S. Journal,* September 1990, 10.

Nahas, G. G. "A Pharmacological Classification of Drugs of Abuse." *Bulletin on Narcotics* 33 (1981): 1–19.

Nichols, D. E. "Discovery of Novel Psychoactive Drugs: Has It Ended?" *Journal of Psychoactive Drugs* 19 (1987): 33–37.

3. Habituation, Dependency, and Addiction

Barnes, D. M. "The Biological Tangle of Drug Addiction." *Science* 241 (1988): 415–17.

Goldstein, A. "The Pharmacologic Basis of Methadone Therapy." *Proceedings of the Fourth National Conference on Methadone Treatment.* National Association on Prevention of Addiction to Narcotics, 1972, New York.

Goodwin, F. K. "Cannabinoid Receptor Gene Cloned." *Journal of the American Medical Association* 264 (1990): 1389.

Rinaldi, R. C., E. M. Steindler, B. B. Wilford, et al. "Clarification and Standardization of Substance Abuse Terminology." *Journal of the American Medical Association* 259 (1988): 555–57.

Snyder, S. *Drugs and the Brain.* New York: Scientific American Books, 1986.

Stimmel, B. *Pain, Analgesia and Addiction: The Pharmacologic Treatment of Pain.* New York: Raven Press, 1983.

————. ed. *Opiate Receptors, Neurotransmitters & Drug Dependence: Basic Science-Clinical Correlates.* New York: Haworth Press, 1981.

Stimmel, B., and S. D. Glick. "Animal-Human Correlates of Narcotic Dependence: A Brief Review." *American Journal of Psychiatry* 135 (1978): 821–25.

4. Why People Use Drugs

Bell, C. S., and R. Battjes. *Prevention Research: Deterring Drug Abuse Among Children and Adolescents.* NIDA Research Monograph 63. Rockville, Md.: U.S. Dept. of Health and Human Services, Public Health Service, Alcohol, Drug Abuse, and Mental Health Administration, 1985.

Brook, J. S., D. J. Lettieri, and D. W. Brook. "Alcohol and Substance Abuse in Adolescence." Special issue of *Advances in Alcohol & Substance Abuse* 4 (3/4) (1985): 1–204.

Charness, M. E., R. P. Simon, and D. A. Greenberg. "Ethanol and the Nervous System." *New England Journal of Medicine* 321 (1989): 442–54.

Goleman, D. "Scientists Pinpoint Brain Irregularities in Drug Addicts." *The New York Times,* June 26, 1990, C1.

Jones, C. L., and R. J. Battjes. *Etiology of Drug Abuse: Implications for Prevention.* NIDA Research Monograph 56. Rockville, Md.: U.S. Dept. of Health and Human Services, Public Health Service, Alcohol, Drug Abuse, and Mental Health Administration, 1986.

Kauffman, J. F., H. Shaffer, and M. E. Burglass. "A Strategy for the Biological Assessment of Addiction." *Advances in Alcohol & Substance Abuse* 3(1–2) (1983–84): 7–18.

Marx, J. "Marijuana Recepter Gene Cloned." *Science* 249 (1990): 624–626.

Newcomb, M. D., and P. M. Bentler. *Consequences of Adolescent Drug Use.* Newbury Park, Calif.: Sage Publications, 1988.

5. Identifying and Treating Drug Dependency

Anglin, M. D. "The Efficacy of Civil Commitment in Treating Narcotic Addiction." In *Compulsory Treatment of Drug Abuse: Research and Clinical Practice,* edited by C. G. Leukefeld and F. M. Tims. NIDA Research Monograph Series 86. Rockville, Md.: U.S. Dept. of Health and Human Services, ADAMHA-NIDA, 1986.

Ashery, R. S., ed. *Progress in the Development of Cost-Effective Treatment for Drug Abusers.* NIDA Research Monograph Series 58,

DHHS-PUB-ADM-85-1401. Rockville, Md.: National Institute on Drug Abuse, 1985.

Bullock, M. L., P. D. Culliton, and R. T. Olander. "Controlled Trial of Acupuncture for Severe Recidivist Alcoholism." *Lancet* 1 (1989): 1435–39.

"Court Rejects Some Drug Testing of U.S. Workers." *The New York Times,* November 18, 1990, A31.

Curran, W. J. "Compulsory Drug Testing: The Legal Barriers." *New England Journal of Medicine* 316 (1987): 318–21.

De Leon, G. *The Therapeutic Community: Study of Effectiveness: Social and Psychological Adjustment of 400 Dropouts and 100 Graduates from the Phoenix House Therapeutic Community.* DHHS Publication No. (ADM) 84-1286. Treatment Research Monograph Series. Rockville, Md.: U.S. Dept. of Health and Human Services, Public Health Service, Alcohol, Drug Abuse, and Mental Health Administration, National Institute on Drug Abuse, 1984.

"Eosinophilia-Myalgia Syndrome—New Mexico." *Morbidity and Mortality Weekly Report* 38 (1989): 765–67.

"Eosinophilia-Myalgia Syndrome—Canada." *Morbidity and Mortality Weekly Report* 39 (1990): 89–91.

Gerstein, D. R., and L. S. Lewin. "Treating Drug Problems." *New England Journal of Medicine* 323 (1990): 844–46.

Hansen, H. J., S. P. Caudill, and D. J. Boone. "Crisis in Drug Testing: Results of CDC Blind Study." *Journal of the American Medical Association* 253 (1985): 2382–87.

Hawks, R. L., and C. N. Chiang, eds. *Urine Testing for Drugs of Abuse.* NIDA Research Service Monograph 73. USPHS ADAMHA. Rockville, Md.: National Institute on Drug Abuse, 1986.

Hubbard, R. L., M. E. Marsden, J. Rachas, et al. *Drug Abuse Treatment: A National Study of Effectiveness.* Chapel Hill: University of North Carolina Press, 1989.

Hunt, G. H., and M. E. Odoroff. "Follow-up Study of Narcotic Drug Addicts after Hospitalization." *Public Heath Reports* 77 (1962): 41–54.

Marshall, E. "Testing Urine for Drugs." *Science* 241 (1988): 150–52.

McLellan, A. T., L. Luborsky, C. P. O'Brien, et al. "Alcohol and Drug Abuse Treatment in Three Different Populations: Is There Improvement and Is It Predictable?" *American Journal of Drug and Alcohol Abuse* 12 (1986): 101–20.

McLellan, A. T., G. E. Woody, L. Luborsky, et al. "Increased Effectiveness of Substance Abuse Treatment. A Prospective Study of Patient-Treatment 'Matching.' " *Journal of Nervous and Mental Disease* 171 (1983): 597–605.

Musto, D. F. *The American Disease: Origins of Narcotic Control.* New Haven: Yale University Press, 1973.

National Drug and Alcoholism Treatment Unit Survey (NDATUS) 1987: Final Report. Rockville, Md.: U.S. Dept. of Health and Human Services, U.S. Public Health Service, ADAMHA National Institute on Drug Abuse and National Institute on Alcohol Abuse and Alcoholism, 1988.

O'Keefe, A. M. "The Case Against Drug Testing." *Psychology Today* 21 (1987): 34–38.

Schmeck, H. M., Jr. "Drug-Testing Technology Speeds Up." *The New York Times,* November 20, 1988, E7.

Simpson, D. D., G. W. Joe, W. E. Lehman, et al. "Addiction Careers: Etiology, Treatment, and 12-Year Follow-Up Outcomes." *Journal of Drug Issues* 16 (1986): 107–22.

Smith, M. O., and I. Kahn. "An Acupuncture Programme for the Treatment of Drug-Addicted Persons." *Bulletin on Narcotics* 40 (1988): 35–41.

Tennant, F. "Clinical Diagnosis and Treatment of the Post Drug Impairment Syndrome." *Psychiatry Letter* 1982.

Westermeyer, J. "Nontreatment Factors Affecting Treatment Outcome for Substance Abuse." *American Journal of Drug and Alcohol Abuse* 15 (1989): 13–29.

Winick, C. "Some Policy Implications of the New York State Civil Commitment Program." *Journal of Drug Issues* 18 (1988): 561–74.

Wolf, C. "Judge Rejects Broad Testing for Drug Use." *The New York Times,* June 7, 1990, B1.

6. Alcohol

Alcohol and the Impaired Driver: A Manual on the Medicolegal Aspects of Chemical Tests for Intoxication. Chicago: American Medical Association, Committee on Medicolegal Problems, 1968.

"Alcohol-Related Traffic Fatalities during Holidays—United States, 1988." *Morbidity and Mortality Weekly Report* 38 (1989): 861–63.

"Alcohol Use in the United States." *Statistical Bulletin/Metropolitan Insurance Companies* 68 (1987): 20–25.

Anda, R. F., D. F. Williamson, and P. L. Remington. "Alcohol and Fatal Injuries Among U.S. Adults." *Journal of the American Medical Association* 260 (1988): 2529–32.

Annis, H. M. "Is Inpatient Rehabilitation of the Alcoholic Cost Effective? Con Position."*Advances in Alcohol & Substance Abuse* 5(1–2) (1985–1986): 175–90.

Banys, P. "The Clinical Use of Disulfiram (Antabuse): A Review." *Journal of Psychoactive Drugs* 20 (1988): 243–60.

Blum, K., E. P. Nobel, P. J. Sheridan, et al. "Allelic Association of Human Dopamine D_2 Receptor Gene in Alcoholism." *Journal of the American Medical Association* 263 (1990): 2055–60.

Bowen, O. R., and J. H. Sammons. "The Alcohol-Abusing Patient: A Challenge to the Profession." *Journal of the American Medical Association* 260 (1988): 2267–70.

Charness, M. E., R. P. Simon, and D. A. Greenberg. "Ethanol and the Nervous System." *New England Journal of Medicine* 321 (1989): 442–54.

Cloninger, C. R. "Neurogenetic Adaptive Mechanisms in Alcoholism." *Science* 236 (1987): 410–16.

Diagnostic and Statistical Manual of Mental Disorders. American Psychiatric Association, DSMIV, In preparation, Washington, D. C.

"Disulfiram Treatment of Alcoholism. American College of Physicians." *Annals of Internal Medicine* 111 (1989): 943–45.

Emrick, C. D. "Alcoholics Anonymous: Affiliation Processes and Effectiveness as Treatment."*Alcoholism* (N.Y.) 11 (1987): 416–23. [Published erratum appears in *Alcoholism* (N.Y.) 12 (1988): 29.]

Feinman, L., and C. S. Lieber. "Toxicity of Ethanol and Other Components of Alcoholic Beverages." *Alcoholism* (N.Y.) 12 (1988): 2–6.

Fell, J. C., and C. E. Nash. "The Nature of the Alcohol Problem in U.S. Fatal Crashes." *Health Education Quarterly* 16 (1989): 335–43.

Frezza, M., C. di Padova, G. Pozzato, et al. "High Blood Alcohol Levels in Women. The Role of Decreased Gastric Alcohol Dehydrogenase Activity and First-Pass Metabolism." *New*

England Journal of Medicine 322 (1990): 95–99. [Published erratum appears in *New England Journal of Medicine* 322 (1990): 1540.]

Gallant, D. M. "The Type 2 Primary Alcoholic." *Alcoholism: Clinical and Experimental Research* 14 (1990): 631.

Goodwin, D. W. *Alcoholism, the Facts.* New York: Oxford University Press, 1981.

Handa, K., J. Sasaki, K. Saku, et al. "Alcohol Consumption, Serum Lipids and Severity of Angiographically Determined Coronary Artery Disease." *American Journal of Cardiology* 65 (1990): 287–89.

Heath, A. C., R. Jardine, and N. G. Martin. "Interactive Effects of Genotype and Social Environment on Alcohol Consumption in Female Twins." *Journal of Studies on Alcohol* 50 (1989): 38–48.

Heath, A. C., and N. G. Martin. "Teenage Alcohol Use in the Australian Twin Register: Genetic and Social Determinants of Starting to Drink." *Alcoholism* (N.Y.) 12 (1988): 735–41.

Kaprio, J., M. Koskenvuo, H. Langinvainio, et al. "Genetic Influences on Use and Abuse of Alcohol: A Study of 5638 Adult Finnish Twin Brothers." *Alcoholism* (N.Y.) 11 (1987): 349–56.

Marlatt, G. A. "Alcohol, Expectancy, and Emotional States: How Drinking Patterns May Be Affected by Beliefs About Alcohol's Effects." *Alcohol Health and Research World* 11 (1987): 10–13, 80–81.

Milgram, G. G., and Consumer Reports Books. *The Facts About Drinking: Coping with Alcohol Use, Abuse and Alcoholism.* Mount Vernon, New York: Consumers Union, 1990.

Miller, W. R., and R. K. Hester. "The Effectiveness of Alcoholism Treatment: What Research Reveals." In *Treating Addictive Behaviors: Processes of Change,* edited by W. R. Miller and N. Heather. New York: Plenum Press, 1986.

Orford, J., and A. Keddie. "Abstinence or Controlled Drinking in Clinical Practice: Indications at Initial Assessment." *Addictive Behaviors* 11 (1986): 71–86.

Peele, S. "Can Alcoholism and Other Drug Addiction Problems Be Treated Away or Is the Current Treatment Binge Doing More Harm Than Good?" *Journal of Psychoactive Drugs* 20 (1988): 375–83.

Roizen, R. "The Great Controlled-Drinking Controversy." *Recent Developments in Alcoholism* 5 (1987): 245–79.

Schuckit, M. A., M. Irwin, and H. I. M. Mahler. "Tridimensional Personality Questionnaire Scores of Sons of Alcoholic and Nonalcoholic Fathers." *American Journal of Psychiatry* 147 (1990): 481–87.

Secretary of Health and Human Services. *Alcohol and Health: Seventh Special Report to the United States Congress.* PHS, ADAMHA, NIAAA. Rockville, Md.: U.S. Dept. of Health and Human Services, January 1990.

Special Report to the U.S. Congress on Alcohol and Health from the Secretary of Health and Human Services (6th). PC A08/MF A01. Rockville, Md.: Alcohol, Drug Abuse, and Mental Health Administration, 1987.

Surgeon General's Workshop on Drunk Driving: Proceedings. December 14–16, 1988, Washington, D.C. Rockville, Md.: U.S. Dept. of Health and Human Services.

Wallack, L., W. Breed, and J. Cruz. "Alcohol on Prime Time Television." *Journal of Studies on Alcohol* 48 (1987): 33–38.

7. Central Nervous System Depressants

"Benzodiazepines: Prescribing Declines Under Triplicate Program." *Epidemiology Notes,* New York State Department of Health 4 (1989): No. 12.

Gonzalez, E. R. "Methaqualone Abuse Implicated in Injuries, Deaths Nationwide." *Journal of the American Medical Association* 246 (1981): 813–15.

Greenblatt, D. J., R. I. Shader, and D. R. Abernethy. "Drug Therapy: Current Status of Benzodiazepines." *New England Journal of Medicine* 309 (1983): 410–16.

Murphy, S. M., R. T. Owen, and P. J. Tyrer. "Withdrawal Symptoms After Six Weeks' Treatment with Diazepam." Letter. *Lancet* 2 (1984): 1389.

"Prescribing of Minor Tranquilizers." *Food and Drug Administration Drug Bulletin* 10 (1980): 2–3.

Rickels, K., W. G. Case, E. E. Schweizer, et al. "Low-Dose Dependence in Chronic Benzodiazepine Users: A Preliminary Report on 119 Patients." *Psychopharmacological Bulletin* 22 (1986): 407–15.

Roy Byrne, P. P., and D. Hommer. "Benzodiazepine Withdrawal: Overview and Implications for the Treatment of Anxiety." Review. *American Journal of Medicine* 84 (1988): 1041–52.

Shader, R. I., C. L. Anglin, et al. *Emergency Room Study of Sedative-Hypnotic Overdosage: A Study of the Issues.* Rockville, Md.: U.S. Dept. of Health and Human Services, Public Health Service, Alcohol, Drug Abuse, and Mental Health Administration, National Institute on Drug Abuse; Washington, D.C.: Treatment Research Monograph Series. DHHS Publication No. (ADM) 82-1118.

8. Powerful Hallucinogens and Phencyclidine

Bergman, R. L. "Navajo Peyote Use: Its Apparent Safety." *American Journal of Psychiatry* 128 (1971): 695–99.

Clouet, D. H., ed. *Phencyclidine: An Update.* NIDA Research Monograph Series 64. DHHS Publication No. (ADM) 86-1443. Rockville, Md.: Dept. of Health and Human Services, Public Health Service, Alcohol, Drug Abuse, and Mental Health Administration, National Institute on Drug Abuse, 1986.

Grinspoon, L., and J. B. Bakalar. *Psychedelic Drugs Reconsidered.* New York: Basic Books, 1979.

Martin, W. R., and J. W. Sloan. "Pharmacology and Classification of LSD Hallucinogens." In *Drug Addictions II: Amphetamine, Psychotogen, and Marijuana Dependence,* edited by W. R. Martin. Berlin: Springer-Verlag, 1977.

Petersen, R. C., and R. C. Stillman, eds. "Phencyclidine (PCP) Abuse: An Appraisal." Based upon papers presented at a conference held Feb. 2–28, 1978, Pacific Grove, California. National Institute on Drug Abuse Research Monograph Series 21. DHEW Publication No. (ADM) 78-728. Rockville, Md.: Dept. of Health, Education, and Welfare, Public Health Service, Alcohol, Drug Abuse, and Mental Health Administration, National Institute on Drug Abuse, Division of Research, 1978.

Redda, K. K., C. A. Walker, and G. Barnett. *Cocaine, Marijuana, Designer Drugs: Chemistry, Pharmacology and Behavior.* Boca Raton: CRC Press, 1989.

Seymour, R., D. Smith, D. Inaba, et al. *The New Drugs: Look Alikes:*

Drugs of Deception and Designer Drugs. Center City: Hazelden Press, 1989.

Siegel, R. K. "Herbal Intoxication: Psychoactive Effects from Herbal Cigarettes, Tea, and Capsules." *Journal of the American Medical Association* 236 (1976): 473–76.

9. Marijuana

Astin, A. W., et al. *The American Freshman: Twenty-Year Trends, 1966–1985.* Cooperative Institutional Research Program. University of California, Higher Education Research Institute, Graduate School of Education, Los Angeles, 1987.

Cohen, S. "Marijuana. Does It Have a Possible Therapeutic Use?" *Journal of the American Medical Association* 240 (1978): 1761–63.

"Drugs of Abuse: Cannabis." *Drug Enforcement* 6 (1979): 34–37.

Dupont, R. L., A. Goldstein, and J. O'Donnell, eds. *Handbook on Drug Abuse.* Rockville, Md.: U.S. Dept. of Health, Education, and Welfare, Public Health Service, Alcohol, Drug Abuse, and Mental Health Administration, National Institute on Drug Abuse, 1979.

Gieringer, D. H. "Marijuana, Driving, and Accident Safety." *Journal of Psychoactive Drugs* 20 (1988): 93–101.

McConnell, H. "Marijuana Anonymous." *The Journal* July/August 1989. Toronto: Addiction Research Foundation.

Mikuriya, T. H., and M. R. Aldrich. "Cannabis 1988: Old Drug, New Dangers. The Potency Question." Review. *Journal of Psychoactive Drugs* 20 (1988): 47–55.

Nahas, G. "Symposium on Marijuana: Rheims, France, 22–23 July 1978." *Bulletin on Narcotics* 30 (1978): 23–32.

Plisko, V. W. and J. D. Stern, eds. *The Condition of Education: A Statistical Report.* Washington, D. C.: U.S. Government Printing Office, 1985.

Schwartz, R. H. "Marijuana: An Overview." Review. *Pediatric Clinics of North America* 34 (1987): 305–17.

"Short-Term Memory Impairment in Chronic Cannabis Abusers." *Lancet* 2 (1989): 1254–55.

Yesavage, J. A., V. O. Leirer, M. Denari, et al. "Carry-Over Effects of Marijuana Intoxication on Aircraft Pilot Performance: A Preliminary Report." *American Journal of Psychiatry* 142 (1985): 1325–29.

10. Opiates and Opioids

Cushman, P. "Propoxyphene Revisited." *American Journal of Drug and Alcohol Abuse* 6 (1979): 245–49.

Goodman Gilman, A., L. S. Goodman, T. W. Rall, et al., eds. *Goodman and Gilman's The Pharmacological Basis of Therapeutics.* 7th Edition. New York: Macmillan, 1985.

Lange, W. R., and D. R. Jasinski. "The Clinical Pharmacology of Pentazocine and Tripelennamine (T's and Blues)." *Advances in Alcohol & Substance Abuse* 5(4) (1986): 71–83.

"New Warning on Propoxyphene." *Food and Drug Administration Drug Bulletin* 9 (1979): 22–23.

Pasternak, G. W. "Multiple Morphine and Enkephalin Receptors and the Relief of Pain." Review. *Journal of the American Medical Association* 259 (1988): 1362–67.

Peachey, J. E. "Clinical Observations of Agonist-Antagonist Analgesic Dependence." Review. *Drug and Alcohol Dependence* 20 (1987): 347–65.

Showalter, C. V. "T's and Blues: Abuse of Pentazocine and Tripelennamine." *Journal of the American Medical Association* 244 (1980): 1224–25.

Smith, R. J. "Federal Government Faces Painful Decision on Darvon." *Science* 203 (1979): 857–58.

Stimmel, B. "Pain, Analgesia, and Addiction: An Approach to the Pharmacologic Management of Pain." *The Clinical Journal of Pain* 1 (1985): 14–22.

"Treatment of Dextropropoxyphene Poisoning." Editorial. *Lancet* 2 (1977): 542.

11. Heroin Addiction

Allison, M., R. L. Hubbard, J. V. Rachal. *Treatment Process in Methadone, Residential, and Outpatient Drug Free Programs.* Treatment Research Monograph Series. DHHS Publication No. (ADM) 85-1388. Rockville, Md.: U.S. Dept. of Health and Human Services, Public Health Service, Alcohol, Drug Abuse, and Mental Health Administration, National Institute on Drug Abuse, Division of Clinical Research, 1985.

Barnes, D. M. "Breaking the Cycle of Addiction." *Science* 241 (1988): 1029–30.

Cooper, J. B. "Methadone Treatment in the United States." In *Methadone in the Management of Opioid Dependence: Programs and*

Policies Around the World, edited by A. Arif and J. Wester-meyer. Minneapolis: University of Minnesota Press, 1988.

De Leon, G. "The Therapeutic Community and Behavioral Science." In *Learning Factors in Substance Abuse,* edited by B. A. Ray. NIDA Research Monograph 84. Rockville, Md.: U.S. Dept. of Health and Human Services, USPH ADAMH, 1988, 74–99.

Des Jarlais, D. C., H. Joseph, V. P. Dole, et al. "Predicting Post-Treatment Narcotic Use Among Patients Terminating from Methadone Maintenance." *Advances in Alcohol & Substance Abuse* 2(1) (1982): 57–68.

Dole, V. P. "Implications of Methadone Maintenance for Theories of Narcotic Addiction." *Journal of the American Medical Association* 260 (1988): 3025–29.

Ginzburg, H. M. "Naltrexone: Its Clinical Utility." National Institute on Drug Abuse Treatment Research Report. USPHS ADAMHA. Rockville, Md.: U.S. Dept. of Health and Human Services, 1988.

Gold, M. S., and C. A. Dackis. "New Insights and Treatments: Opiate Withdrawal and Cocaine Addiction." *Clinical Therapeutics* 7 (1984): 6–21.

Goldstein, M. S., M. Surber, and D. M. Wilner. "Outcome Evaluations in Substance Abuse: A Comparison of Alcoholism, Drug Abuse, and Other Mental Health Interventions." *International Journal of the Addictions* 19 (1984): 479–502.

Himmelsbach, C. *Clinical Studies of Morphine Addiction: Nathan B. Eddy Memorial Award Lecture.* National Institute on Drug Abuse Research Monograph Series 81 (1988): 8–18.

Narayanaswami, K. "Parameters for Determining the Origin of Illicit Heroin Samples." *Bulletin on Narcotics* 37 (1985): 49–62.

Newman, R. G. "Methadone Treatment: Defining and Evaluating Success." *New England Journal of Medicine* 317 (1987): 447–50.

Newmeyer, J. A., G. Johnson, and S. Klot. "Acupuncture as a Detoxification Modality." *Journal of Psychoactive Drugs* 16 (1984): 241–61.

Okpaku, S. O. "Psychoanalytically Oriented Psychotherapy of Substance Abuse (With Observations on the Penn-VA Study)." *Advances in Alcohol & Substance Abuse* 6(1) (1986): 17–33.

Rawson, R. A., A. M. Washton, R. B. Resnick, et al. "Clonidine Hydrochloride Detoxification from Methadone Treatment: The

Value of Naltrexone Aftercare.'' *Advances in Alcohol & Substance Abuse* 3(3) (1984): 41–49.

Roehrich, H., and M. S. Gold. "Clonidine.'' *Advances in Alcohol & Substance Abuse* 7(1) (1987): 1–16.

Shakur, M., and M. Smith. "The Use of Acupuncture to Treat Drug Addiction and the Development of an Acupuncture Training Pro-. gram." Presented at the 1977 National Drug Abuse Conference, San Francisco, California.

Simpson, D. D. and S. B. Sells. "Effectiveness of Treatment for Drug Abuse: An Overview of the DARP Research Program.'' *Advances in Alcohol & Substance Abuse* 2(1) (1982): 7–29.

Sorensen, J. L., D. A. Deitch, and A. Acampora. "Treatment Collaboration of Methadone Maintenance Programs and Therapeutic Communities.'' Review. *American Journal of Drug and Alcohol Abuse* 10 (1984): 347–59.

Stimmel, B. *Heroin Dependency: Medical, Economic and Social Aspects*. New York: Stratton Intercontinental Medical Book Corp., 1975.

"Trexan: A Pharmacologic Adjunct for the Detoxified Opioid Addict." Dupont Pharmaceuticals, 1984.

Wen, H. L., and S. Y. C. Cheung. "Treatment of Drug Addiction by Acupuncture and Electrostimulation.'' *Asian Journal of Medicine* (1973): 138–41.

Whitehead, P. C. "Acupuncture in the Treatment of Addiction: A Review and Analysis.'' *International Journal of the Addictions* 13 (1978): 1–16.

Woody, G. E., A. T. McLellan, L. Luborsky, et al. "Sociopathy and Psychotherapy Outcome.'' *Archives of General Psychiatry* 42 (1985): 1081–86.

12. Amphetamines, Amphetamine-like Drugs, and Caffeine

American Medical Association Committee on Alcoholism, Addiction and Mental Health. "Dependence on Amphetamine and Other Stimulant Drugs.'' *Journal of the American Medical Association* 197 (1966): 1023–27.

Berglund, B., and P. Hemmingsson. "Effects of Caffeine Ingestion on Exercise Performance at Low and High Altitudes in Cross-Country Skiers.'' *International Journal of Sports Medicine* 3 (1982): 234–36.

Bishop, K. "Fear Grows Over Effects of a New Smokable Drug." *The New York Times,* September 16, 1989: 1.

Cho, A. K. "Ice: A New Dosage Form of an Old Drug." *Science* 249 (1990): 631–34.

Cowart, V. S. "The Ritalin Controversy: What's Made This Drug's Opponents Hyperactive?" *Journal of the American Medical Association* 259 (1988): 2521–23.

Gilbert, R. "Caffeine: Cardiovascular Effects." *The Journal* 17 (May 1, 1988).

Gilliland, K., and W. Bullock. "Caffeine: A Potential Drug of Abuse." *Advances in Alcohol & Substance Abuse* 3(1–2) (1983–1984): 53–73.

Grinspoon, L., and P. Hedblom. *The Speed Culture: Amphetamine Use and Abuse in America.* Cambridge: Harvard University Press, 1975.

Herbel, E. S., and J. Scala. "Coffee, Tea, and Coronary Heart-Disease." *Lancet* 2 (1973): 152–53.

Morgan, J. P. "Over the Counter Medication: Availability and Issues." In *Phenylpropanolamine: Risks, Benefits and Controversies,* edited by J. P. Morgan, D. U. Kagan, and J. S. Brody. Clinical Pharmacology and Therapeutics Series, vol. 5. New York: Praeger, 1985.

Morgan, J. P., D. R. Wesson, K. S. Puder, et al. "Duplicitous Drugs: The History and Recent Status of Look-Alike Drugs." *Journal of Psychoactive Drugs* 19 (1987): 21–31.

Nencini, P., and A. M. Ahmed. "Khat Consumption: A Pharmacological Review." *Drug and Alcohol Dependence* 23 (1989): 19–29.

Rosmarin, P.C., W. B. Applegate, and G. W. Somes. "Coffee Consumption and Serum Lipids: A Randomized, Crossover Clinical Trial." *American Journal of Medicine* 88 (1990): 349–56.

Walsh, J. "Psychotoxic Drugs: Dodd Bill Passes Senate, Comes to Rest in the House; Critics Are Sharpening Their Knives." *Science* 145 (1964): 1418–20.

13. Cocaine

Belongia, E. A., C. W. Hedberg, G. J. Gleich, et al. "An Investigation of the Cause of the Eosinophilia-Myalgia Syndrome Associated with Tryptophan Use." *New England Journal of Medicine* 323 (1990): 357–65.

Byck, R., ed. *The Cocaine Papers by Sigmund Freud*. New York: Stonehill Press, 1974.

Cave, L. J. "Cocaine/Crack: The Big Lie." DHHS Publication No. (ADM) 87-1427. Rockville, Md.: U.S. Dept. of Health and Human Services, Public Health Service, Alcohol, Drug Abuse, and Mental Health Administration, 1987.

"Controlled Substances: Uses and Effects." *Drug Enforcement* 6 (1979): 20–21.

"Crack." Editorial. *Lancet* 2 (1987): 1061–62.

Culhane, C. "Dealer Stockpiling Drives Cocaine Prices Up." *The U.S. Journal*, September 1990, 10.

Estroff, T. W., and M. S. Gold. "Medical and Psychiatric Complications of Cocaine Abuse with Possible Points of Pharmacological Treatment." *Advances in Alcohol & Substance Abuse* 5(1–2) (1985–1986): 61–76.

Galanter, M. "Social Network Therapy for Cocaine Dependence." *Advances in Alcohol & Substance Abuse* 6(2) (1986): 159–75.

Gawin, F. H., and E. H. Ellinwood, Jr. "Cocaine and Other Stimulants: Actions, Abuse, and Treatment." *New England Journal of Medicine* 318 (1988): 1173–82.

Gold, M. S., C. A. Dackis, A. L. Pottash, et al. "Cocaine Update: From Bench to Bedside." *Advances in Alcohol & Substance Abuse* 5 (1/2) (1985–1986): 35–60.

Herridge, P., and M. S. Gold. "Pharmacological Adjuncts in the Treatment of Opioid and Cocaine Addicts." *Journal of Psychoactive Drugs* 20 (1988): 233–42.

Isner, J. M., and S. K. Chokshi. "Cocaine and Vasospasm." *New England Journal of Medicine* 321 (1989): 1604–06.

Lange, R. A., R. G. Cigarroa, C. W. Yancy, Jr., et al. "Cocaine-Induced Coronary-Artery Vasoconstriction." *New England Journal of Medicine* 321 (1989): 1557–62.

Levine, S. R., J. C. M. Brust, N. Futrell, et al. "Cerebrovascular Complications of the Use of the 'Crack' Form of Alkaloidal Cocaine." *New England Journal of Medicine* 323 (1990): 699–704.

Lowenstein, D. H., and S. M. Massa. "Acute Neurologic and Psychiatric Complications Associated with Cocaine Abuse." *American Journal of Medicine* 83 (1987): 841–46.

Marzuk, P. M., K. Tardiff, A. C. Leon, et al. "Prevalence of Recent Cocaine Use Among Motor Vehicle Fatalities in New York

City." *Journal of the American Medical Association* 263 (1990): 250–56.

May, C. D. "Coca-Cola Discloses an Old Secret." *The New York Times,* July 1, 1988, 25.

Musto, D. F. *The American Disease: Origins of Narcotic Control.* Expanded Edition. New York: Oxford University Press, 1987.

Shenon, P. "U.S. Says Hospital Statistics Show Use of Cocaine May Have Peaked." *The New York Times,* September 1, 1990, 9.

Siegel, R. K. "Cocaine: Recreational Use and Intoxication." In *Cocaine: 1977,* edited by R. C. Petersen and R. C. Stillman. National Institute on Drug Abuse Research Monograph 13 DHEW Publication No. (ADM) 77-741. Washington, D.C.: Supt. of Docs. U.S. Government Printing Office 1977, 119–36.

Trachtenberg, M. C., and K. Blum. "Improvement of Cocaine-Induced Neuromodulator Deficits by the Neuronutrient Tropamine." *Journal of Psychoactive Drugs* 20 (1988): 315–31.

Virmani, R., M. Robinowitz, J. E. Smialek, et al. "Cardiovascular Effects of Cocaine: An Autopsy Study of 40 Patients." *American Heart Journal* 115 (1988): 1068–76.

Washton, A. M. "Structured Treatment of Cocaine Abuse." *Advances in Alcohol & Substance Abuse* 6(2) (1986): 142–57.

Washton, A. M., and M. S. Gold. *Cocaine: A Clinician's Handbook.* New York: The Guilford Press, 1987.

———. "Recent Trends in Cocaine Abuse: A View from the National Hotline, '800-COCAINE.' " *Advances in Alcohol & Substance Abuse* 6(2) (1986): 31–47.

Weiss, R. D., S. M. Mirin, and J. L. Michael. "Psychopathology in Chronic Cocaine Abusers." *American Journal of Drug and Alcohol Abuse* 12 (1986): 17–29.

14. Nicotine

Barry, J., K. Mead, E. G. Nabel, et al. "Effect of Smoking on the Activity of Ischemic Heart Disease." *Journal of the American Medical Association* 261 (1989): 398–402.

Benowitz, N. L. "Drug Therapy. Pharmacologic Aspects of Cigarette Smoking and Nicotine Addiction." *New England Journal of Medicine* 319 (1988): 1318–30.

———. "Health and Public Policy Implications of the 'Low Yield' Cigarette." *New England Journal of Medicine* 320 (1989): 1619–21.

Brooks, J. E. *The Mighty Leaf: Tobacco through the Centuries*. London: Alvin Redman Ltd., 1953.

Bruerd, B. "Smokeless Tobacco Use Among Native American School Children." *Public Health Reports* 105 (1990): 196–201.

Byrd, J. C., R. S. Shapiro, and D. L. Schiedermayer. "Passive Smoking: A Review of Medical and Legal Issues." *American Journal of Public Health* 79 (1989): 209–15.

"Cigarette Advertising—United States, 1988." *Morbidity and Mortality Weekly Report* 39 (1990): 261–65.

Cohen, R. Y., J. Sattler, M. R. Felix, et al. "Experimentation with Smokeless Tobacco and Cigarettes by Children and Adolescents: Relationship to Beliefs, Peer Use, and Parental Use." *American Journal of Public Health* 77 (1987): 1454–56.

Cone, E. J., and J. E. Henningfield. "Premier 'Smokeless Cigarettes' Can Be Used to Deliver Crack." Letter. *Journal of the American Medical Association* 261 (1989): 41.

Davis, R. M., P. Healy, and S. A. Hawk. "Information on Tar and Nicotine Yields on Cigarette Packages." *American Journal of Public Health* 80 (1990): 551–53.

Donnan, G. A., J. J. McNeil, M. A. Adena, et al. "Smoking as a Risk Factor for Cerebral Ischaemia." *Lancet* 2 (1989): 643–47.

Fielding, J. E., and K. J. Phenow. "Health Effects of Involuntary Smoking." *New England Journal of Medicine* 319 (1988): 1452–60.

Fiore, M. C., T. E. Novotny, J. P. Pierce, et al. "Methods Used to Quit Smoking in the United States: Do Cessation Programs Help?" *Journal of the American Medical Association* 263 (1990): 2760–65.

Frye, R. E., B. S. Schwartz, and R. L. Doty. "Dose-Related Effects of Cigarette Smoking on Olfactory Function." *Journal of the American Medical Association* 263 (1990): 1233–36.

Glassman, A. H., F. Stetner, B. T. Walsh, et al. "Heavy Smokers, Smoking Cessation, and Clonidine. Results of a Double-Blind, Randomized Trial." *Journal of the American Medical Association* 259 (1988): 2863–66.

Goldsmith, M. F. "Increasing Use of Smokeless Tobacco Leads to Fears of Young Lives Being 'Snuffed Out.' " *Journal of the American Medical Association* 260 (1988): 1511–12.

Hall, R. L., and D. Dexter. "Smokeless Tobacco Use and Attitudes Toward Smokeless Tobacco Among Native Americans and

Other Adolescents in the Northwest." *American Journal of Public Health* 78 (1988): 1586–88.

"The Health Consequences of Involuntary Smoking: A Report of the Surgeon General." DHHS (CDC) 87-8398. Rockville, Md.: U.S. Dept. of Health and Human Services, Public Health Service, Centers for Disease Control, Center for Health Promotion and Education, Office on Smoking and Health, 1986.

"The Health Consequences of Smoking: Nicotine Addiction: A Report of the Surgeon General, 1988." DHHS Publication No. (CDC) 88-8406. Rockville, Md.: U.S. Dept. of Health and Human Services, Public Health Service, Centers for Disease Control, Center for Health Promotion and Education, Office on Smoking and Health, 1988.

Hermanson, B., G. S. Omenn, R. A. Kronmal, et al. "Beneficial Six-Year Outcome of Smoking Cessation in Older Men and Women with Coronary Artery Disease. Results from the CASS Registry." *New England Journal of Medicine* 319 (1988): 1365–69.

Johnston, L. M., and M. B. Glasg. "Tobacco Smoking and Nicotine." *Lancet* 3 (1942): 742.

Kozlowski, L. T., D. A. Wilkinson, W. Skinner, et al. "Comparing Tobacco Cigarette Dependence with Other Drug Dependencies." *Journal of the American Medical Association* 261 (1989): 898–901.

Layde, P. M. "Smoking and Cervical Cancer: Cause or Coincidence?" *Journal of the American Medical Association* 261 (1989): 1631–32.

Mattson, M. E., G. Boyd, D. Byar, et al. "Passive Smoking on Commercial Airline Flights." *Journal of the American Medical Association* 261 (1989): 867–72.

McGinn, P. R. "Cigarette's 'Denicotined' Advertising Hit." *American Medical News,* September 8, 1989, 3.

O'Connolly, G. N., C. T. Orleans, and M. Kogan. "Use of Smokeless Tobacco in Major-League Baseball." *New England Journal of Medicine* 318 (1988): 1281–85.

Palmer, J. R., L. Rosenberg, and S. Shapiro. " 'Low-Yield' Cigarettes and the Risk of Nonfatal Myocardial Infarction in Women." *New England Journal of Medicine* 320 (1989): 1569–73.

Pierce, J. P., M. C. Fiore, T. E. Novotny, et al. "Trends in Cigarette Smoking in the United States. Projections to the Year 2000."

Journal of the American Medical Association 261 (1989): 61–65.

"Prevalence of Oral Lesions and Smokeless Tobacco Use in Northern Plains Indians." *Morbidity and Mortality Weekly Report* 37 (1988): 608–11.

"State-Specific Estimates of Smoking-Attributable Mortality and Years of Potential Life Lost—United States, 1985." *Morbidity and Mortality Weekly Report* 37 (1988): 689–93.

The Surgeon General's 1989 Report on Reducing the Health Consequences of Smoking: 25 Years of Progress. *Morbidity and Mortality Weekly Report* 38 (1989): 1–32.

"Tobacco Lessons: Crossing Substance Abuse Boundaries." *The Journal* 17 (1988): 7.

"Tobacco Use by Adults—United States, 1987." *Morbidity and Mortality Weekly Report* 38 (1989): 685–87.

Warner, K. E. "Health and Economic Implications of a Tobacco-Free Society." *Journal of the American Medical Association* 258 (1987): 2080–86.

Willett, W. C., A. Green, M. J. Stampfer, et al. "Relative and Absolute Excess Risks of Coronary Heart Disease Among Women Who Smoke Cigarettes." *New England Journal of Medicine* 317 (1987): 1303–09.

Wolf, P. A., R. B. D'Agostino, W. B. Kannel, et al. "Cigarette Smoking as a Risk Factor for Stroke: The Framingham Study." *Journal of the American Medical Association* 259 (1988): 1025–29.

15. Volatile Solvents, Inhalants, Anesthetics

Beschner, G. M., and A. S. Friedman. *Teen Drug Use*. Lexington, Mass.: Lexington Books, 1986.

Cohen, S. "Inhalant Abuse: An Overview of the Problem." In *Review of Inhalants: Euphoria to Dysfunction*, edited by C. W. Sharp and M. L. Brehm. NIDA Research Monograph Series 15. DHEW Publications No. (ADM) 77-553.

Cohen, S. "Inhalants and Solvents." In *Youth Drug Abuse: Problems, Issues, and Treatments*, edited by G. M. Beschner and A. S. Friedman. Lexington, Mass.: Lexington Books, 1979.

Crider, R. A., and B. A. Rouse. "Epidemiology of Inhalant Abuse: An Update." NIDA Research Monograph Series 85. DHHS Publication No. (ADM) 88-1577. Rockville, Md.: National Institute on Drug Abuse, 1988.

Haverkos, H. W., and J. A. Dougherty. *Health Hazards of Nitrite Inhalants.* DHHS Publication No. (ADM) 88-1573. Research Monograph Series 83. Veteran's Administration Medical Center, Lexington, Ky. Rockville, Md.: National Institute on Drug Abuse, 1988.

Lange, W. R., C. A. Haertzen, J. E. Hickey, et al. "Nitrite Inhalants: Patterns of Abuse in Baltimore and Washington, D.C." *American Journal of Drug and Alcohol Abuse* 14 (1988): 29–39.

McHugh, M. J. "The Abuse of Volatile Substances." Review. *Pediatric Clinics of North America* 34 (1987): 333–40.

Sharp, C. W., and M. L. Brehm. *Review of Inhalants: Euphoria to Dysfunction.* DHEW Publication No. (ADM) 77-553. Research Monograph Series 15. Rockville, Md.: National Institute on Drug Abuse, 1977.

16. Multiple Drug Use

Bobo, J. K. "Nicotine Dependence and Alcoholism Epidemiology and Treatment." *Journal of Psychoactive Drugs* 21 (1989): 323–29.

De Leon, G. "Alcohol Use Among Drug Abusers. Treatment Outcomes in a Therapeutic Community." *Alcoholism: Clinical and Experimental Research* 11 (1987): 430–36.

Grant, B. F., and T. C. Harford. "Concurrent and Simultaneous Use of Alcohol with Cocaine: Results of National Survey." *Drug and Alcohol Dependence* 25 (1990): 97–104.

Hasin, D. S., B. F. Grant, J. Endicott, et al. "Cocaine and Heroin Dependence Compared in Poly-Drug Abusers." *American Journal of Public Health* 78 (1988): 567–69.

Henningfield, J. E., R. Clayton, and W. Pollin. "Involvement of Tobacco in Alcoholism and Illicit Drug Use." *British Journal of Addiction* 85 (1990): 279–91.

Hoyumpa, A. M., Jr. "Alcohol Interactions with Benzodiazepines and Cocaine." *Advances in Alcohol & Substance Abuse* 3(4) (1984): 21–34.

Kaufman, E. "The Relationship of Alcoholism and Alcohol Abuse to the Abuse of Other Drugs." *American Journal of Drug and Alcohol Abuse* 9 (1982): 1–17.

Kornblith, A. B. "Multiple Drug Abuse Involving Nonopiate, Nonalcoholic Substances. II. Physical Damage, Long-Term Psychological Effects and Treatment Approaches and Success." *International Journal of the Addictions* 16 (1981): 527–40.

Kosten, T. R., F. H. Gawin, B. J. Rounsaville, et al. "Cocaine Abuse Among Opioid Addicts: Demographic and Diagnostic Factors in Treatment." *American Journal of Drug and Alcohol Abuse* 12 (1986): 1–16.

McLellan, A. T., L. Luborsky, C. P. O'Brien, et al. "Alcohol and Drug Abuse Treatment in Three Different Populations: Is There Improvement and Is It Predictable?" *American Journal of Drug and Alcohol Abuse* 12 (1986): 101–20.

Norton, R., and J. Noble. "Combined Alcohol and Other Drug Use and Abuse." *Alcohol Health and Research World* 11 (1987): 78–80.

Yamaguchi, K., and D. B. Kandel. "Patterns of Drug Use from Adolescence to Young Adulthood: II. Sequences of Progression." *American Journal of Public Health* 74 (1984): 668–72.

17. AIDS and Drug Use

"AIDS and Human Immunodeficiency Virus Infection in the United States: 1988 Update." *Morbidity and Mortality Weekly Report* 38 Suppl 4 (1989): 1–38.

AIDS 89 Summary: A Practical Synopsis of the Vth International Conference, June 4–9, 1989. Philadelphia: Philadelphia Sciences Group, 1990.

AIDS Trends to 1990. *City Health Information (CHI)* 9(3) New York City Department of Health, May 1990.

Blanche, S., C. Rouzioux, M. L. Moscato, et al. "A Prospective Study of Infants Born to Women Seropositive for Human Immunodeficiency Virus Type 1." *New England Journal of Medicine* 320 (1989): 1643–48.

Brickner, P. W., R. A. Torres, M. Barnes, et al. "Recommendations for Control and Prevention of Human Immunodeficiency Virus (HIV) Infection in Intravenous Drug Users." *Annals of Internal Medicine* 110 (1989): 833–37.

Chaisson, R. E., P. Bacchetti, D. Osmond, et al. "Cocaine Use and HIV Infection in Intravenous Drug Users in San Francisco." *Journal of the American Medical Association* 261 (1989): 561–65.

Community Epidemiology Work Group: Epidemiologic Trends in Substance Abuse. Proceedings, June 1989, National Institute on Drug Abuse, Rockville, Md.

Cooper, J. R. "Methadone Treatment and Acquired Immunodeficiency Syndrome." *Journal of the American Medical Association* 262 (1989): 1664–68.

Curran, J. W., H. W. Jaffe, A. M. Haroy, et al. "Epidemiology of HIV Infection and AIDS in the United States." *Science* 239 (1988): 610–16.

Des Jarlais, D. C., and S. R. Friedman. "AIDS and IV Drug Use." *Science* 245 (1989): 578.

Dole, V. P. "Methadone Treatment and the Acquired Immunodeficiency Epidemic." *Journal of the American Medical Association* 262 (1989): 1681–82.

"First 100,000 Cases of Acquired Immunodeficiency Syndrome— United States." *Journal of the American Medical Association* 262 (1989): 1453–56.

Gayle, J. A., R. M. Selik, and S. Y. Chu. "Surveillance for AIDS and HIV Infection Among Black and Hispanic Children and Women of Childbearing Age, 1981–1989." *Morbidity and Mortality Weekly Report* 39 Suppl 3 (1990): 23–30.

Guinan, M. E., and A. Hardy. "Epidemiology of AIDS in Women in the United States. 1981 through 1986." *Journal of the American Medical Association* 257 (1987): 2039–42. [Published erratum appears in *Journal of the American Medical Association* 258 (1987): 206.]

Hahn, R. A., I. M. Onorato, T. S. Jones, et al. "Prevalence of HIV Infection Among Intravenous Drug Users in the United States." *Journal of the American Medical Association* 261 (1989): 2677–84.

Harris, L. S. "Problems of Drug Dependence, 1985." National Institute on Drug Abuse, Rockville, Md. Office of Science. Proceedings of the Annual Scientific Meeting (47th) of the Committee on Problems of Drug Dependence, Inc., held in Baltimore, Md., June 10–12, 1985.

Haverkos, H. W., and R. Edelman. "The Epidemiology of Acquired Immunodeficiency Syndrome Among Heterosexuals." *Journal of the American Medical Association* 260 (1988): 1922–29.

Heyward, W. L., and J. W. Curran. "The Epidemiology of AIDS in the U.S." *Scientific American* 259 (1988): 72–81.

HIV/AIDS Surveillance: U.S. AIDS Cases Reported Through September 1990. Centers for Disease Control, October 1990, Atlanta, Georgia.

Holmes, K. K., J. M. Karon, and J. Kreiss. "The Increasing Frequency of Heterosexually Acquired AIDS in the United States, 1983–88." *American Journal of Public Health* 80 (1990): 858–63.

Human Immunodeficiency Virus Infection in the United States: A Review of Current Knowledge. Review. *Morbidity and Mortality Weekly Report* 36 Suppl 6 (1987): 1–48. [Published erratum appears in *Morbidity and Mortality Weekly Report* 37 (1988): 479.]

Joseph, S. C. "Current and Future Trends in AIDS in New York City." *Advances in Alcohol & Substance Abuse* 7(2) (1987): 159–74.

Kaslow, R. A., W. C. Blackwelder, D. G. Ostrow, et al. "No Evidence for a Role of Alcohol or Other Psychoactive Drugs in Accelerating Immunodeficiency in HIV-I Positive Individuals. A Report from the Multicenter AIDS Cohort Study." *Journal of the American Medical Association* 261 (1989): 3424–29.

Lambert, B. "New AIDS Data Show the Course of Infection." *The New York Times,* July 15, 1988, B1.

Licensure of Screening Tests for Antibody to Human T-Lymphotropic Virus Type I. *Morbidity and Mortality Weekly Report* 37 (1988): 736–40, 745–47.

MacGregor, R. R. "Alcohol and Drugs As Co-Factors for AIDS." *Advances in Alcohol & Substance Abuse* 7(2) (1987): 47–71.

Novick, D. M., M. J. Kreek, D. C. Des Jarlais, et al. *Antibody to LAV, the Putative Agent of AIDS, in Parenteral Drug Abusers and Methadone Maintained Patients.* In Proceedings of the 47th Annual Scientific Meeting of the Committee on Problems of Drug Dependence, edited by L. Harris. NIDA Research Monograph Series 67 (1986): 318–320. DHHS Publication No. (ADM) 86-1448. Rockville, Md.: National Institute on Drug Abuse.

Novick, L. F., D. Berns, R. Stricof, et al. "HIV Seroprevalence in Newborns in New York State." *Journal of the American Medical Association* 261 (1989): 1745–50.

Popescu, C. B. "Answers About AIDS: A Report by the American Council on Science and Health." The Council, New York, 1988.

Schoenbaum, E. E., D. Hartel, P. A. Selwyn, et al. "Risk Factors for Human Immunodeficiency Virus Infection in Intravenous Drug Users." *New England Journal of Medicine* 321 (1989): 874-79.

Scott, G. B., C. Hutto, R. W. Makuch, et al. "Survival in Children with Perinatally Acquired Human Immunodeficiency Virus Type

1 Infection." *New England Journal of Medicine* 321 (1989): 1791–06.

Siegel, L., and M. Korcok. *AIDS: The Drug and Alcohol Connection: What Health Care Professionals Need to Know.* Center City: Hazelden Press, 1989.

Stall, R. "The Prevention of HIV Infection Associated with Drug and Alcohol Use During Sexual Activity." *Advances in Alcohol & Substance Abuse* 7(2) (1987): 73–88.

"Update: Acquired Immunodeficiency Syndrome Associated with Intravenous Drug Use—United States, 1988." *Morbidity and Mortality Weekly Report* 38 (1989): 165–70.

"Update: Acquired Immunodeficiency Syndrome—United States, 1989." *Morbidity and Mortality Weekly Report* 39 (1990): 81–86.

"Update: Reducing HIV Transmission in Intravenous Drug Users Not in Drug Treatment—United States." *Morbidity and Mortality Weekly Report* 39 (1990): 529, 535–38.

"Update: Serologic Testing for HIV-1 Antibody—United States, 1988 and 1989." *Morbidity and Mortality Weekly Report* 39 (1990): 380–83.

van den Hoek, J. A., H. J. van Haastrecht, and R. A. Coutinho. "Risk Reduction Among Intravenous Drug Users in Amsterdam Under the Influence of AIDS." *American Journal of Public Health* 79 (1989): 1355–57.

Weiss, S. H. "Links Between Cocaine and Retroviral Infection." *Journal of the American Medical Association* 261 (1989): 607–09.

Zylke, J. W. "Interest Heightens in Defining, Preventing AIDS in High-Risk Adolescent Population." *Journal of the American Medical Association* 262 (1989): 2197.

18. Drugs, Pregnancy, and the Newborn

Abel, E. L. "Smoking and Pregnancy." *Journal of Psychoactive Drugs* 16 (1984): 327–38.

Baquet, D. "New York City Neglect Hearings Upheld in Newborn Cocaine Cases." *The New York Times,* May 30, 1990, B3.

Brody, J. E. "Cocaine: Litany of Fetal Risks Grows." *The New York Times,* September 6, 1988, 19.

Chasnoff, I. J., D. R. Griffith, S. MacGregor, et al. "Temporal Patterns of Cocaine Use in Pregnancy. Perinatal Outcome." *Journal of the American Medical Association* 261 (1989): 1740–44.

Chasnoff, I. J., H. J. Landress, and M. E. Barrett. "The Prevalence of Illicit-Drug or Alcohol Use During Pregnancy and Discrepancies in Mandatory Reporting in Pinellas County, Florida." *New England Journal of Medicine* 322 (1990): 1202–06.

Chiang, C. N., and C. C. Lee, eds. *Prenatal Drug Exposure: Kinetics and Dynamics*. NIDA Research Monograph Series 60. DHHS Publication No. (ADM) 85-1413. Rockville, Md.: U.S. Dept. of Health and Human Services, Public Health Service, Alcohol, Drug Abuse, and Mental Health Administration, National Institute on Drug Abuse, 1985.

Clouet, D. H., ed. *Phencyclidine: An Update*. NIDA Research Monograph Series 64. DHHS Publication No. (ADM) 86-1443. Rockville, Md.: U.S. Dept. of Health and Human Services, Public Health Service, Alcohol, Drug Abuse, and Mental Health Administration, National Institute on Drug Abuse, 1986.

Fielding, J. E. "Smoking and Women: Tragedy of the Majority." Editorial. *New England Journal of Medicine* 317 (1987): 1343–45.

Fingerhut, L. A., J. C. Kleinman, and J. S. Kendrick. "Smoking Before, During, and After Pregnancy." *American Journal of Public Health* 80 (1990): 541–44.

Hinds, M. deCourcy. "Drug-Laced Air Called Risk to Babies." *The New York Times,* January 31, 1990, A18.

Hingson, R., J. J. Alpert, N. Day, et al. "Effects of Maternal Drinking and Marijuana Use on Fetal Growth and Development." *Pediatrics* 70 (1982): 539–46.

Hoffman, J. "Pregnant, Addicted and Guilty?" *The New York Times,* Sunday Magazine, August 19, 1990, 32.

Joesoef, M. R., V. Beral, R. T. Rolfs, et al. "Are Caffeinated Beverages Risk Factors for Delayed Conception?" *Lancet* 335 (1990): 136–37.

Little, R. E., K. W. Anderson, C. H. Ervin, et al. "Maternal Alcohol Use During Breast-Feeding and Infant Mental and Motor Development at One Year." *New England Journal of Medicine* 321 (1989): 425–30.

Martin, T. R., and M. B. Bracken. "The Association Between Low Birth Weight and Caffeine Consumption During Pregnancy." *American Journal of Epidemiology* 126 (1987): 813–21.

Maternal Drug Abuse—New York City. *City Health Information* 8(8), September 1, 1989, New York City Department of Health.

McCann, J. "Heart Defects Now Seen in Cocaine Babies." *The Journal*, March 1, 1990, 5.

"The Multiple Deficits of Prenatal Drug Abuse." *Science Focus* (New York Academy of Sciences) 3 (1988): 1, 10–11.

National Institute on Drug Abuse, Services Research Branch. "Drug Dependence in Pregnancy: Clinical Management of Mother and Child." Rockville, Md.: U.S. Department of Health, Education and Welfare, Public Health Service, Alcohol, Drug Abuse, and Mental Health Administration, National Institute on Drug Abuse, Division of Resource Development, Services Research Branch, 1979.

Neerhof, M. G., S. N. MacGregor, S. S. Retzky, et al. "Cocaine Abuse During Pregnancy: Peripartum Prevalence and Perinatal Outcome." *American Journal of Obstetrics and Gynecology* 161 (1989): 633–38.

Niebyl, J. R. *Drug Use in Pregnancy*. 2nd Edition. Philadelphia: Lea & Febiger, 1988.

"Perinatal Toxicity of Cocaine." *Medical Letter on Drugs and Therapeutics* 30 (1988): 59–60.

Pinkert, T. M. *Current Research on the Consequences of Maternal Drug Abuse*. Research Monograph Series 59. DHHS Publication No. (ADM) 85-1400. Rockville, Md.: National Institute on Drug Abuse, 1985.

Pinkney, D. S. "Costs Increase with Numbers of 'Crack Babies.' " *American Association World News*, April 6, 1990, 15.

Pinkney, D. S. "Drug-Addicted Newborns Increasing: MDs, Hospitals Face Care Dilemma." *American Medical News*, February 3, 1989, 2.

Plant, M. *Women, Drinking, and Pregnancy*. London: Tavistock Publications, 1985.

Roll, D. B., T. Smith, and E. M. Whelan. "Alcohol Use During Pregnancy: What Advice Should Be Given to the Pregnant Woman?" In *Current Controversies in Alcoholism*, edited by B. Stimmel. New York: Haworth Press, 1983.

Silverman, S. "Scope, Specifics of Maternal Drug Use, Effects on Fetus Are Beginning to Emerge from Studies." *Journal of the American Medical Association* 261 (1989): 1688–89.

"Smoking and Health, a National Status Report: A Report to Congress." DHHS Publication No. (CDC) 87-8396, Rockville, Md.: U.S. Dept. of Health and Human Services, Public Health

Service, Centers for Disease Control, Center for Health Promotion and Education, Office on Smoking and Health, 1986.

Streissguth, A. P., H. M. Barr, P. D. Sampson, et al. "IQ at Age 4 in Relation to Maternal Alcohol Use and Smoking During Pregnancy." *Developmental Psychology* 25 (1989): 3–11.

Wachsman, L., S. Schuetz, L. S. Chan, et al. "What Happens to Babies Exposed to Phencyclidine (PCP) in Utero?" *American Journal of Drug and Alcohol Abuse* 15 (1989): 31–39.

Zuckerman, B., D. A. Frank, R. Hingson, et al. "Effects of Maternal Marijuana and Cocaine Use on Fetal Growth." *New England Journal of Medicine* 320 (1989): 762–68.

19. Drugs and Sports

Alfano, P., and M. Janofsky. "A 'Guru' Who Spreads the Gospel of Steroids." *The New York Times*, November 18, 1988, 1.

———. "On the Black Market, Drugs Are in Easy Reach of Public." *The New York Times*, November 18, 1988, A1.

Altman, L. K. "New Olympic Drug Test Foiled Sprinter (Ben Johnson)." *The New York Times*, October 4, 1988, 1.

Atkin, C., J. Hocking, and M. Block. "Teenage Drinking: Does Advertising Make a Difference?" *Journal of Communication* 34 (1984): 157–67.

Bracciale, D., and E. G. Remmers. "Athletes and Steroids: A Losing Proposition." *ACSH News & Views* 8 (1987): 5, 11.

Buckley, W. E., C. E. Yesalis III, K. E. Friedl, et al. "Estimated Prevalence of Anabolic Steroid Use Among Male High School Seniors." *Journal of the American Medical Association* 260 (1988): 3441–45.

Cowart, V. S. "Issues of Drugs and Sports Gain Attention as Olympic Games Open in South Korea." *Journal of the American Medical Association* 260 (1988): 1517–18.

Cowart, V. S. "Blunting 'Steroid Epidemic' Requires Alternatives, Innovative Education." *Journal of the American Medical Association* 264 (1990): 1641.

———. "Erythropoietin: A Dangerous New Form of Blood Doping." *The Physician and Sports Medicine* 17 (1989): 115–18.

———. "National Institute on Drug Abuse May Join in Anabolic Steroid Research." *Journal of the American Medical Association* 261 (1989): 1855–56.

Hallagan, J. B., L. F. Hallagan, and M. B. Snyder. "Anabolic-Androgenic Steroid Use by Athletes." *New England Journal of Medicine* 321 (1989): 1042–45.

Haupt, H. A., and G. D. Rovere. "Anabolic Steroids: A Review of the Literature." *American Journal of Sports Medicine* 12 (1984): 469–84.

Janofsky, M. "U.S., Soviets Agree on Drug-Test Plan for Their Athletes." *The New York Times,* November 22, 1988, A1.

Johnson, W. O. "Sports and Suds: The Beer Business and the Sports World Have Brewed Up a Potent Partnership." *Sports Illustrated* 69 (1988): 68–82.

Kashkin, K. B., and H. D. Kleber. "Hooked on Hormones? An Anabolic Steroid Addiction Hypothesis." *Journal of the American Medical Association* 262 (1989): 3166–70.

Lamb, D. R. "Anabolic Steroids in Athletics: How Well Do They Work and How Dangerous Are They?" *American Journal of Sports Medicine* 12 (1984): 31–38.

Ledwith, F. "Does Tobacco Sports Sponsorship on Television Act as Advertising to Children?" *Health Education Journal* 43 (1984): 85–88.

Marshall, E. "The Drug of Champions." *Science* 242 (1988): 183–84.

Penn, S. "Muscling In; As Ever More People Try Anabolic Steroids, Traffickers Take Over; Dope Dealers Smuggle Drugs from Mexico for Athletes and for the Merely Vain; Sideline Business at the Gym." *The Wall Street Journal,* October 4, 1988, A1.

Scott, W. C. "The Abuse of Erythropoietin to Enhance Athletic Performance." *Journal of the American Medical Association* 264 (1990): 1660.

Somerville, J. "Sports, Medical Groups Crack Down on Steroids." *American Medical News,* November 4, 1988, 4.

"Steroid Use Found Off Season." *American Medical News,* September 19, 1988, 16.

Taylor, W. N. "Growth Hormone: Preventing Its Abuse in Sports." *Technological Review,* October 1985, 14.

20. Why Has the War Against Drugs Failed?

"Afghan Opium Yield Up as Pakistan Curbs Crop." *The New York Times,* April 14, 1988, A16.

Ayers, B. D., Jr. "Washington Finds Drug War Is Hardest at Home." *The New York Times,* December 9, 1988, A13.

Barrett, P. M. "A Year After Drug War Was Declared, Bennett Renews Efforts to Rally Troops." *The Wall Street Journal,* September 5, 1990, A16.

Goldstein, A., and H. Kalant. "Drug Policy: Striking the Right Balance." *Science* 249 (1990): 1513–21.

Health Objectives for the Nation. *Morbidity and Mortality Weekly Report* 39 (1990): 256–58.

Kerr, P. "Cocaine Glut Pulls New York Market into Drug Rings' Tug-of-War." *The New York Times,* August 24, 1988, B1.

Kondracke, M. "Don't Legalize Drugs: The Costs Are Still Too High." *The New Republic,* June 27, 1988, 16–19.

Labaton, S. "Canada Seen As Major Haven for Laundering Drug Money." *The New York Times,* September 28, 1989, A1.

———. "The Cost of Drug Abuse: $60 Billion a Year." *The New York Times,* December 5, 1990, D1.

———. "Plan on Drug Cache Not Being Pursued." *The New York Times,* December 16, 1990, A37.

Marshall, E. "Flying Blind in the War on Drugs." *Science* 240 (1988): 1605–07.

McBride, D. C., C. Burgman-Habermehl, J. Alpert, et al. "Drugs and Homicide." *Bulletin of the New York Academy of Medicine* 62 (1986): 497–508.

Morgenthau, R. M. "We Are Losing the War on Drugs." *The New York Times,* February 16, 1988, A21.

Nadelmann, E. A. "Drug Prohibition in the United States: Costs, Consequences, and Alternatives." *Science* 245 (1989): 939–47.

Nurco, D. N., J. W. Shaffer, J. C. Ball, et al. "Trends in the Commission of Crime Among Narcotic Addicts Over Successive Periods of Addiction and Nonaddiction." *American Journal of Drug and Alcohol Abuse* 10 (1984): 481–89.

Polich, J. M., P. L. Ellickson, P. Reuter, et al. *Strategies for Controlling Adolescent Drug Use.* Santa Monica: Rand Corporation, 1984.

Reuter, P., G. Crawford, and J. Cave. *Sealing the Borders: The Effects of Increased Military Participation in Drug Interdiction.* Santa Monica: Rand Corporation, 1988.

Saavedra, S. H. "Dire Economics Drive Coca Production." *The Drug Policy Letter* 2(3) (May–June 1990): 2–6.

Savage, L. J., and D. D. Simpson. "Drug Use and Crime During a

Four-Year Posttreatment Follow-Up." *American Journal of Drug and Alcohol Abuse* 8 (1981): 1–16.

Shenon, P. "The Score on Drugs: It Depends on How You See the Figures." *The New York Times,* April 22, 1990, 6.

Trebach, A. S. *The Great Drug War, and Radical Proposals That Could Make America Safe Again.* New York: Macmillan, 1987.

Weissman, J. "Understanding the Drugs and Crime Connection: A Systematic Examination of Drugs and Crime Relationships." *Journal of Psychedelic Drugs* 10 (1978): 171–92.

Appendix A. Drug Use Reporting Sources

Berke, R. L. "Poll Finds Many in U.S. Back Bush Strategy on Drugs." *The New York Times,* September 12, 1989, A14.

Community Epidemiology Work Group. *Epidemiologic Trends in Drug Abuse Proceedings.* Rockville, Md.: National Institute on Drug Abuse, 1989.

Johnston, L. P., M. O'Malley, and J. G. Bachman. *Drug Use, Drinking and Smoking: National Survey Results from High School, College and Young Adult Population, 1975–1988.* Rockville, Md.: National Institute on Drug Abuse. Alcohol, Drug Abuse, and Mental Health Administration, 1989.

Overview of the 1988 National Household Survey on Drug Abuse. NIDA Capsules. Rockville, Md.: National Institute on Drug Abuse, 1989.

Washton, A. M., and M. S. Gold. "Recent Trends in Cocaine Abuse: A View from the National Hotline, '800-COCAINE.' " *Advances in Alcohol & Substance Abuse* 6(2) (1986): 31–47.

Appendix B. Drug-Testing Technology

Hansen, H. J., S. P. Caudill, and D. J. Boone. "Crisis in Drug Testing: Results of CDC Blind Study." *Journal of the American Medical Association* 253 (1985): 2382–87.

Hawks, R. L., and C. N. Chiang, eds. "Urine Testing for Drugs of Abuse." NIDA Research Service Monograph 73. USPHS ADAMHA. Rockville, Md.: National Institute on Drug Abuse, 1986.

Marshall, E. "Testing Urine for Drugs." *Science* 241 (1988): 150–52.

O'Keefe, A. M. "The Case Against Drug Testing." *Psychology Today* 21 (1987): 34–38.

Schmeck, H. M., Jr. "Drug-Testing Technology Speeds Up." *The New York Times,* November 20, 1988, E7.

Index

DATE DUE			
SEP 30			
NOV 12			
NOV 17			
MAR 31			
APR 22			
MAR 03			
4/1/03